New Mechanisms of Action of Natural Antioxidants in Health and Disease

New Mechanisms of Action of Natural Antioxidants in Health and Disease

Special Issue Editors

Silvana Hrelia
Cristina Angeloni

MDPI • Basel • Beijing • Wuhan • Barcelona • Belgrade

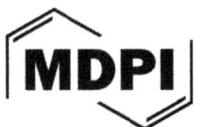

Special Issue Editors
Silvana Hrelia
University of Bologna
Italy

Cristina Angeloni
University of Camerino
Italy

Editorial Office
MDPI
St. Alban-Anlage 66
4052 Basel, Switzerland

This is a reprint of articles from the Special Issue published online in the open access journal *Antioxidants* (ISSN 2076-3921) from 2019 to 2020 (available at: https://www.mdpi.com/journal/antioxidants/special_issues/natural_antioxidants).

For citation purposes, cite each article independently as indicated on the article page online and as indicated below:

LastName, A.A.; LastName, B.B.; LastName, C.C. Article Title. *Journal Name* **Year**, *Article Number*, Page Range.

ISBN 978-3-03936-268-4 (Pbk)
ISBN 978-3-03936-269-1 (PDF)

© 2020 by the authors. Articles in this book are Open Access and distributed under the Creative Commons Attribution (CC BY) license, which allows users to download, copy and build upon published articles, as long as the author and publisher are properly credited, which ensures maximum dissemination and a wider impact of our publications.

The book as a whole is distributed by MDPI under the terms and conditions of the Creative Commons license CC BY-NC-ND.

Contents

About the Special Issue Editors vii

Preface to "New Mechanisms of Action of Natural Antioxidants in Health and Disease" . . . ix

Silvana Hrelia and Cristina Angeloni
New Mechanisms of Action of Natural Antioxidants in Health and Disease
Reprinted from: *Antioxidants* **2020**, *9*, 344, doi:10.3390/antiox9040344 1

Paola Antonia Corsetto, Gigliola Montorfano, Stefania Zava, Irma Colombo, Bergros Ingadottir, Rosa Jonsdottir, Kolbrun Sveinsdottir and Angela Maria Rizzo
Characterization of Antioxidant Potential of Seaweed Extracts for Enrichment of Convenience Food
Reprinted from: *Antioxidants* **2020**, *9*, 249, doi:10.3390/antiox9030249 6

Mariantonia Logozzi, Rossella Di Raimo, Davide Mizzoni, Mauro Andreotti, Massimo Spada, Daniele Macchia and Stefano Fais
Beneficial Effects of Fermented Papaya Preparation (FPP®) Supplementation on Redox Balance and Aging in a Mouse Model
Reprinted from: *Antioxidants* **2020**, *9*, 144, doi:10.3390/antiox9020144 21

Federica Tonolo, Federico Fiorese, Laura Moretto, Alessandra Folda, Valeria Scalcon, Alessandro Grinzato, Stefania Ferro, Giorgio Arrigoni, Alberto Bindoli, Emiliano Feller, Marco Bellamio, Oriano Marin and Maria Pia Rigobello
Identification of New Peptides from Fermented Milk Showing Antioxidant Properties: Mechanism of Action
Reprinted from: *Antioxidants* **2020**, *9*, 117, doi:10.3390/antiox9020117 38

Cheng-Chung Chou, Chi-Ping Wang, Jing-Hsien Chen and Hui-Hsuan Lin
Anti-Atherosclerotic Effect of *Hibiscus* Leaf Polyphenols against Tumor Necrosis Factor-alpha-Induced Abnormal Vascular Smooth Muscle Cell Migration and Proliferation
Reprinted from: *Antioxidants* **2019**, *8*, 620, doi:10.3390/antiox8120620 62

Luminita Capatina, Razvan Stefan Boiangiu, Gabriela Dumitru, Edoardo Marco Napoli, Giuseppe Ruberto, Lucian Hritcu and Elena Todirascu-Ciornea
Rosmarinus officinalis Essential Oil Improves Scopolamine-Induced Neurobehavioral Changes via Restoration of Cholinergic Function and Brain Antioxidant Status in Zebrafish (*Danio rerio*)
Reprinted from: *Antioxidants* **2020**, *9*, 62, doi:10.3390/antiox9010062 83

Jijun Tan, Yanli Li, De-Xing Hou and Shusong Wu
The Effects and Mechanisms of Cyanidin-3-Glucoside and Its Phenolic Metabolites in Maintaining Intestinal Integrity
Reprinted from: *Antioxidants* **2019**, *8*, 479, doi:10.3390/antiox8100479 97

Pasquale Marrazzo, Cristina Angeloni and Silvana Hrelia
Combined Treatment with Three Natural Antioxidants Enhances Neuroprotection in a SH-SY5Y 3D Culture Model
Reprinted from: *Antioxidants* **2019**, *8*, 420, doi:10.3390/antiox8100420 113

Rafael Franco, Gemma Navarro and Eva Martínez-Pinilla
Hormetic and Mitochondria-Related Mechanisms of Antioxidant Action of Phytochemicals
Reprinted from: *Antioxidants* **2019**, *8*, 373, doi:10.3390/antiox8090373 129

You-Cheng Hseu, Xuan-Zao Chen, Yugandhar Vudhya Gowrisankar, Hung-Rong Yen, Jing-Yuan Chuang and Hsin-Ling Yang
The Skin-Whitening Effects of Ectoine via the Suppression of α-MSH-Stimulated Melanogenesis and the Activation of Antioxidant Nrf2 Pathways in UVA-Irradiated Keratinocytes
Reprinted from: *Antioxidants* **2020**, *9*, 63, doi:10.3390/antiox9010063 . . . . **141**

About the Special Issue Editors

Silvana Hrelia graduated with a degree in Chemistry and completed her Ph.D. in Biochemistry at the University of Bologna, where she is now a full-time professor of Biochemistry. Her research interest covers the field of cellular and nutritional biochemistry. Her studies are focused on the protective/preventive role of nutraceutical bioactive components in the diet, and the prevention/ counteraction of chronic degenerative diseases, such as cardiovascular and neurodegenerative diseases. Prof. Hrelia is the author of more than 160 peer review papers in international journals, and has participated in national and international (EU FP VII and Horizon 2020) projects. She was the Coordinator of the Nutritional and Environmental Biochemistry Group of the Italian Society of Biochemistry and Molecular Biology, and she is now a member of the Board of the Society.

Cristina Angeloni is a professor of Biochemistry at the School of Pharmacy, at the University of Camerino, Italy. She received her MS degree in Computer Science in 1992, her MS degree in Food Science and Technology in 2000, and completed her Ph.D. degree in Biochemistry and Physiopathology of Aging in 2005. She also has a Master's degree in Bioinformatics, which she completed in 2005. She completed all of these qualifications at the University of Bologna, Italy. Prof. Angeloni is the author of four book chapters and more than seventy peer reviewed articles. The main focus of her research is the study of the mechanisms of action of dietetic natural compounds in counteracting neurodegeneration and delaying the aging process. In particular, she studies radical scavenging activity, the induction of phase II enzymes, the inhibition of apoptosis, and the modulation of signal transduction pathways by natural compounds, in in vitro and in vivo models.

Preface to "New Mechanisms of Action of Natural Antioxidants in Health and Disease"

The current understanding of the complex role of ROS in the organism, and pathological sequelae of oxidative stress, points to the necessity of comprehensive studies of antioxidant reactivities and interactions with cellular constituents. Many of the protective actions of natural antioxidants in health and diseases have been ascribed to their antioxidant properties, but in recent years, many studies have suggested that their classic hydrogen-donating antioxidant activity is unlikely to be the sole explanation for their effects. First of all, natural antioxidants are broadly metabolized in vivo, resulting in significant modifications. Moreover, the concentrations of natural antioxidants and their metabolites in vivo are lower than those usually utilized in vitro. Consequently, natural antioxidants do not exert their biological action in vivo via simply reacting with ROS. Accumulating evidence suggests that the cellular effects of natural antioxidants may be mediated by their interactions with specific proteins that are central to intracellular signaling cascades, modulating the expression and activity of key proteins, influencing epigenetic mechanisms, or modulating gut microbiota. This Special Issue includes 10 peer-reviewed papers, including eight original research papers and two reviews. Together, they represent the most recent advances in the state-of-the-art of new mechanisms of action of natural antioxidants, in both health and disease. The reviews include overviews on the function and mechanisms of cyanidin-3-glucoside and its phenolic metabolites in maintaining intestinal integrity, and on hormetic and mitochondria-related mechanisms of the antioxidant action of phytochemicals. The research papers present data on the antioxidant potential of seaweed extracts, fermented papaya preparation, and peptides from fermented milk. The neuroprotective activities of Rosmarinus officinalis essential oil in a zebrafish model and the neuroprotective effect of three phytochemicals (sulforaphane, epigallocatechin gallate, and plumbagin), alone or in combination, in a 3D neuroblastoma cell culture model, were reported. Moreover, the anti-atherosclerotic effect of Hibiscus leaf polyphenols in vascular smooth muscle cells was investigated. Finally, the skin whitening effect of ectoine was studied in keratinocytes, promoting antioxidant application in the cosmetic field. We would like to thank all the authors for their valuable contributions and all the reviewers for their availability to review the papers and their suggestions to improve scientific quality. Thank you also to the journal's publishing team for their help in disseminating the call for papers and in every step of the publishing process.

Silvana Hrelia, Cristina Angeloni
Special Issue Editors

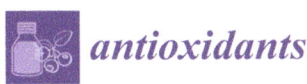

Editorial

New Mechanisms of Action of Natural Antioxidants in Health and Disease

Silvana Hrelia [1] and Cristina Angeloni [2,*]

[1] Department for Life Quality Studies, Alma Mater Studiorum, University of Bologna, Corso d'Augusto 237, 47921 Rimini (RN), Italy; silvana.hrelia@unibo.it
[2] School of Pharmacy, University of Camerino, Via Gentile III da Varano, 62032 Camerino (MC), Italy
* Correspondence: cristina.angeloni@unicam.it

Received: 20 April 2020; Accepted: 21 April 2020; Published: 23 April 2020

Natural antioxidants have been proposed to have beneficial effects on health and on different disease states, such as neurodegenerative and cardiovascular diseases, diabetes and cancer [1–4]. The use of natural plant antioxidant products to handle different diseases has very ancient roots; well before the development of modern medicine with synthetic drugs and antioxidants. A lot of the biological activities of natural antioxidants have been ascribed to their ability to scavenge reactive oxygen species (ROS) that counteract oxidative stress. In the last years, a multitude of studies have suggested that their classical hydrogen-donating antioxidant activity is unlikely to be the sole explanation for their effects [5]. First of all, natural antioxidants are subjected to an extensive metabolism in vivo that modifies their redox potentials. Moreover, the concentration of natural antioxidants and their metabolites in vivo are lower than that usually utilized in vitro. Accumulating evidence suggests that the cellular effects of natural antioxidants may also be mediated by their interactions with specific proteins central to intracellular signaling cascades [6–8], their modulation of the expression and activity of key proteins [9–11], their influencing of epigenetic mechanisms [12,13] or their modulation of the gut microbiota [14,15].

This special issue, concerning new mechanisms in the action of natural antioxidants in health and disease, contains nine contributions, seven research articles and two reviews, and details recent advances on this topic.

In recent years, increasing attention has been paid to natural dietetic antioxidants and their potential effect on human health.

Corsetto et al. [16] focused on edible brown seaweeds, a rich source of natural antioxidants, extensively investigated for their ability to prevent and/or counteract different diseases [17,18]. In particular, the authors studied the possible mechanisms of *Fucus vesiculosus*'s antioxidant action and considered its bioactivity during the production of enriched rye snacks. They used a multiple-method approach, including chemical assays and cell-based bioassays, to characterize the potential mechanisms of the antioxidant action of seaweed extracts. They demonstrated that the antioxidant action of *Fucus vesiculosus* extracts is due to their high level of polyphenols, but also to their high Fe^{2+}-chelating activity. Moreover, rye snacks enriched with *Fucus vesiculosus* showed a higher antioxidant potential, suggesting the use of these extracts to design functional foods.

Fermented foods are considered prominent constituents of the human diet because of their content in health-promoting compounds [19]. Fermentation is one the most ancient methods of food preparation, which increases the shelf life and improves the flavor of food matrices like soy, milk, meat, fruit and vegetables.

Fermented Papaya Preparation (FPP®) is a product obtained from the yeast fermentation of non-genetically modified Carica Papaya Linn, and has been shown to represent a valuable approach in obtaining systemic antioxidant effects. The study of Logozzi et al. [20] was aimed at verifying FPP®'s in vivo anti-aging effect, together with the modulation of the intracellular antioxidant system.

Mice (C57BL/6J) were treated daily with FPP® from either the 6th week or the 51st week of age. After a 10 month treatment, FPP® led to an increase in telomeres length in the bone marrow and ovary, together with an increase in the plasmatic levels of telomerase activity and antioxidant levels, and a decrease of ROS. Interestingly, the treatment started at six weeks of age was more effective, suggesting a potential preventive role of FPP® against molecular damages induced by age when started precociously.

Tonolo et al. [21] studied the antioxidant activity of different peptides extracted from fermented milk proteins. Bioactive peptides generated from milk can originate both from whey proteins and from caseins. Fermented milk was produced using Lactobacillus acidophilus NCFM®, Lactobacillus delbrueckii subs. bulgaricus and Streptococcus thermophilus. The authors identified four peptides, N-15-M, E-11-F, Q-14-R, and A-17-E, as the most effective against oxidative stress, and demonstrated that these bioactive peptides exert their antioxidant activity through the activation of the Keap1/ erythroid 2-related factor 2 (Nrf2) pathway.

Cardiovascular diseases are the leading cause of death in the world, and atherosclerosis, a chronic inflammatory process that involves a complex of pathophysiological effects, is one of the major risk factors. The development of atherosclerosis is related to the proliferation and migration of vascular smooth muscle cells (VSMCs) following stimulation with proinflammatory cytokines [22]. In recent years, phytochemicals have attracted considerable attention in the prevention and/or counteraction of atherosclerosis. The paper of Chou et al. [23] reported that a polyphenol-rich extract of *Hibiscus sabdariffa* leaves was able to inhibit matrix metalloproteinase expression and cell migration in VSMC A7r5 cells pretreated with TNF-a, by modulating protein kinase B (PKB) and inducing cell cycle G0/G1 arrest by inducing the expression of p53 and its downstream factors. The extract could also trigger a decrease in ROS production following TNF-a stimulation. In a well-established atherosclerotic New Zealand white rabbit model, the authors confirmed the in vitro data on the anti-atherosclerotic effect of *Hibiscus sabdariffa* leaf extract, suggesting that this extract could contribute to the protection against atherosclerosis and consequently against cardiovascular diseases.

Neurodegenerative disorders, like Alzheimer's disease (AD), affect millions of people in the world and cause important memory impairment. Presently, there is no drug able to treat dementia-related afflictions, so phytochemical bioactive compounds are acquiring importance as a source of anti-AD agents. Capatina et al. [24], using a zebrafish (*Danio rerio*) model treated with 100 µM scopolamine (a muscarinic acetylcholine receptor blocker known to induce amnestic effects), investigated the potential antidepressant-like and cognitive-enhancing effect of *Rosmarinus officinalis* essential oil (REO). The authors demonstrated that REO prevents the anxiogenic-like effect of scopolamine, in a dose-dependent manner, and that it exhibited an anxiolytic and memory-enhancing profile. Moreover, REO treatment significantly reduced acetylcholinesterase activity, as compared to the scopolamine treated group, and counteracted the scopolamine-induced reduction in antioxidant enzyme activities in the zebrafish brain. Therefore, REO could be considered as a promising bioactive source for fighting cognitive performance-decrease and anxiety increase.

As previously underlined, the use of natural plant antioxidant products has very ancient origins, but nowadays research has made many steps forward, and the evolution of separative techniques has made it possible to identify specific active antioxidants compounds in natural sources, and develop them as potential therapeutic agents.

In their review, Tan et al. [25] analyzed the function and mechanisms of cyanidin-3-glucoside and its phenolic metabolites in maintaining intestinal integrity. Cyanidin-3-glucoside is an anthocyanin, naturally present in black rice, black bean, purple potato and many berries. Cyanidin-3-glucoside is extensively metabolized in the gastrointestinal tract and gives rise to a series of secondary phenolic metabolites, including protocatechuic acid, phloroglucinaldehyde, vanillic acid and ferulic acid. Those metabolites have multiple effects, as they regulate the gut's microbiota and modulate Nrf2 antioxidant and inflammatory pathways. Thanks to these effects, cyanidin-3-glucoside and its metabolites play a key role in maintaining intestinal integrity and function.

In recent years, a lot of studies have underlined the synergic effect of different natural compounds when administered in combination [26]. On these bases, Marazzo et al. [27], using a three-dimensional neuronal cell culture, investigated the protective effect of three natural antioxidants (sulforaphane, epigallocatechin gallate, and plumbagin) alone or in combination, focusing on their activity against hydrogen peroxide-induced oxidative stress. Interestingly, the treatment with the combination of the three natural antioxidants was more effective than the treatments with the single compounds. In particular, the combined treatment positively modulated reduced glutathione (GSH), antioxidant enzymes (heme oxygenase 1, glutathione reductase and thioredoxin reductase) and insulin-degrading enzymes, and downregulated nicotinamide adenine dinucleotide phosphate (NADPH) oxidase 1 and 2, in respect to peroxide-treated cells.

Franco et al. [28] reviewed the indirect antioxidant mechanisms of natural antioxidants, in particular hormesis, a mechanism that triggers the upregulation of enzymes essential for the innate detox pathways and/or the modulation of vitagenes expression [29]. Moreover, they suggested that natural antioxidants present in the chloroplast and mitochondria of plant cells may reach the mitochondria of mammalian cells, and make electron transport and oxidative phosphorylation more efficient. They concluded stressing the fact that, very often, in vitro antioxidant measures do not correlate with antioxidant action at the physiological level.

Natural antioxidants have been widely studied also as effective topical natural cosmetic agents [30]. Hseu et al. [31] focused their attention on Ectoine, a natural extremolyte produced from several species of microorganisms under stressful conditions. Using UVA-irradiated human keratinocytes (HaCaT), they evaluated the effect of low Ectoine concentrations (0.5–1.5 µM) on depigmenting and anti-melanogenic parameters. They demonstrated that Ectoine treatment decreased ROS levels, α-melanocyte-stimulating hormone production, and proopiomelanocortin expression. Ectoine mediated the nuclear translocation of Nrf2 via p38, Akt and protein kinase C (PKC) pathways, and therefore the expression of antioxidant enzymes heme oxygenase-1, NAD(P)H dehydrogenase [quinone 1], and γ-glutamate-cysteine ligase catalytic subunit.

The conditioned medium, obtained from the Ectoine pre-treated and UVA-irradiated HaCaT cells, downregulated the tyrosinase, tyrosinase-related proteins and microphthalmia-associated transcription factor expressions in melanoma B16F10 cells, thus inhibiting melanin synthesis and evidencing a whitening effect. The authors concluded that Ectoine could be suggested as a potential and natural-based skin whitening agent to the cosmetic industry.

In conclusion, this special issue contributed to increasing the knowledge on the mechanisms of action of natural antioxidants, evidencing their pleiotropic role in the prevention and/or counteraction of degenerative diseases, and promoting also their application in the functional food and cosmetic field.

Conflicts of Interest: The authors declare no conflict of interest.

References

1. Pohl, F.; Lin, P.K.T. The potential use of plant natural products and plant extracts with antioxidant properties for the prevention/treatment of neurodegenerative diseases: In vitro, in vivo and clinical trials. *Molecules* **2018**, *23*, 3283. [CrossRef]
2. Kizhakekuttu, T.J.; Widlansky, M.E. Natural antioxidants and hypertension: Promise and challenges. *Cardiovasc. Ther.* **2010**, *28*. [CrossRef] [PubMed]
3. Zatalia, S.R.; Sanusi, H. The role of antioxidants in the pathophysiology, complications, and management of diabetes mellitus. *Acta Med. Indones.* **2013**, *45*, 141–147. [PubMed]
4. Mates, J.; Segura, J.; Alonso, F.; Marquez, J. Natural Antioxidants: Therapeutic Prospects for Cancer and Neurological Diseases. *Mini-Reviews Med. Chem.* **2009**, *9*, 1202–1214. [CrossRef] [PubMed]
5. Williams, R.J.; Spencer, J.P.E.; Rice-Evans, C. Flavonoids: Antioxidants or signalling molecules? *Free Radic. Biol. Med.* **2004**, *36*, 838–849. [CrossRef] [PubMed]

6. Ho, H.H.; Chang, C.S.; Ho, W.C.; Liao, S.Y.; Wu, C.H.; Wang, C.J. Anti-metastasis effects of gallic acid on gastric cancer cells involves inhibition of NF-κB activity and downregulation of PI3K/AKT/small GTPase signals. *Food Chem. Toxicol.* **2010**, *48*, 2508–2516. [CrossRef] [PubMed]
7. Al-Rasheed, N.M.; Fadda, L.M.; Ali, H.M.; Abdel Baky, N.A.; El-Orabi, N.F.; Al-Rasheed, N.M.; Yacoub, H.I. New mechanism in the modulation of carbon tetrachloride hepatotoxicity in rats using different natural antioxidants. *Toxicol. Mech. Methods* **2016**, *26*, 243–250. [CrossRef] [PubMed]
8. Angeloni, C.; Malaguti, M.; Rizzo, B.; Barbalace, M.C.; Fabbri, D.; Hrelia, S. Neuroprotective Effect of Sulforaphane against Methylglyoxal Cytotoxicity. *Chem. Res. Toxicol.* **2015**, *28*, 1234–1245. [CrossRef] [PubMed]
9. Moongkarndi, P.; Srisawat, C.; Saetun, P.; Jantaravinid, J.; Peerapittayamongkol, C.; Soi-Ampornkul, R.; Junnu, S.; Sinchaikul, S.; Chen, S.T.; Charoensilp, P.; et al. Protective effect of mangosteen extract against β-amyloid-induced cytotoxicity, oxidative stress and altered proteome in SK-N-SH cells. *J. Proteome Res.* **2010**, *9*, 2076–2086. [CrossRef]
10. Angeloni, C.; Leoncini, E.; Malaguti, M.; Angelini, S.; Hrelia, P.; Hrelia, S. Role of quercetin in modulating rat cardiomyocyte gene expression profile. *Am. J. Physiol. Hear. Circ. Physiol.* **2008**, *294*. [CrossRef]
11. Giusti, L.; Angeloni, C.; Barbalace, M.C.; Lacerenza, S.; Ciregia, F.; Ronci, M.; Urbani, A.; Manera, C.; Digiacomo, M.; Macchia, M.; et al. A proteomic approach to uncover neuroprotective mechanisms of oleocanthal against oxidative stress. *Int. J. Mol. Sci.* **2018**, *19*, 2329. [CrossRef] [PubMed]
12. Izzo, S.; Naponelli, V.; Bettuzzi, S. Flavonoids as Epigenetic Modulators for Prostate Cancer Prevention. *Nutrients* **2020**, *12*, 1010. [CrossRef] [PubMed]
13. Carrera, I.; Martínez, O.; Cacabelos, R. Neuroprotection with Natural Antioxidants and Nutraceuticals in the Context of Brain Cell Degeneration: The Epigenetic Connection. *Curr. Top. Med. Chem.* **2019**, *19*, 2999–3011. [CrossRef] [PubMed]
14. Khan, M.S.; Ikram, M.; Park, J.S.; Park, T.J.; Kim, M.O. Gut Microbiota, Its Role in Induction of Alzheimer's Disease Pathology, and Possible Therapeutic Interventions: Special Focus on Anthocyanins. *Cells* **2020**, *9*, 853. [CrossRef] [PubMed]
15. Choi, Y.; Lee, S.; Kim, S.; Lee, J.; Ha, J.; Oh, H.; Lee, Y.; Kim, Y.; Yoon, Y. Vitamin E (α-tocopherol) consumption influences gut microbiota composition. *Int. J. Food Sci. Nutr.* **2020**, *71*, 221–225. [CrossRef]
16. Corsetto, P.A.; Montorfano, G.; Zava, S.; Colombo, I.; Ingadottir, B.; Jonsdottir, R.; Sveinsdottir, K.; Rizzo, A.M. Characterization of antioxidant potential of seaweed extracts for enrichment of convenience food. *Antioxidants* **2020**, *9*, 249. [CrossRef]
17. Barbalace, M.C.; Malaguti, M.; Giusti, L.; Lucacchini, A.; Hrelia, S.; Angeloni, C. Anti-inflammatory activities of marine algae in neurodegenerative diseases. *Int. J. Mol. Sci.* **2019**, *20*, 3061. [CrossRef]
18. Hannan, M.A.; Sohag, A.A.M.; Dash, R.; Haque, M.N.; Mohibbullah, M.; Oktaviani, D.F.; Hossain, M.T.; Choi, H.J.; Moon, I.S. Phytosterols of marine algae: Insights into the potential health benefits and molecular pharmacology. *Phytomedicine* **2020**, *69*, 153201. [CrossRef]
19. Şanlier, N.; Gökcen, B.B.; Sezgin, A.C. Health benefits of fermented foods. *Crit. Rev. Food Sci. Nutr.* **2019**, *59*, 506–527. [CrossRef]
20. Logozzi, M.; Di Raimo, R.; Mizzoni, D.; Andreotti, M.; Spada, M.; Macchia, D.; Fais, S. Beneficial effects of fermented papaya preparation (FPP®) supplementation on redox balance and aging in a mouse model. *Antioxidants* **2020**, *9*, 144. [CrossRef]
21. Tonolo, F.; Fiorese, F.; Moretto, L.; Folda, A.; Scalcon, V.; Grinzato, A.; Ferro, S.; Arrigoni, G.; Bindoli, A.; Feller, E.; et al. Identification of new peptides from fermented milk showing antioxidant properties: Mechanism of action. *Antioxidants* **2020**, *9*, 117. [CrossRef]
22. Bennett, M.R.; Sinha, S.; Owens, G.K. Vascular Smooth Muscle Cells in Atherosclerosis. *Circ. Res.* **2016**, *118*, 692–702. [CrossRef]
23. Chou, C.C.; Wang, C.P.; Chen, J.H.; Lin, H.H. Anti-atherosclerotic effect of Hibiscus leaf polyphenols against tumor necrosis factor-alpha-induced abnormal vascular smooth muscle cell migration and proliferation. *Antioxidants* **2019**, *8*, 620. [CrossRef] [PubMed]
24. Capatina, L.; Boiangiu, R.S.; Dumitru, G.; Napoli, E.M.; Ruberto, G.; Hritcu, L.; Todirascu-Ciornea, E. Rosmarinus officinalis essential oil improves scopolamine-induced neurobehavioral changes via restoration of cholinergic function and brain antioxidant status in Zebrafish (Danio rerio). *Antioxidants* **2020**, *9*, 62. [CrossRef] [PubMed]

25. Tan, J.; Li, Y.; Hou, D.X.; Wu, S. The effects and mechanisms of cyanidin-3-glucoside and its phenolic metabolites in maintaining intestinal integrity. *Antioxidants* **2019**, *8*, 479. [CrossRef]
26. Angeloni, C.; Businaro, R.; Vauzour, D. The role of diet in preventing and reducing cognitive decline. *Curr. Opin. Psychiatry* **2020**, *1*. [CrossRef] [PubMed]
27. Marrazzo, P.; Angeloni, C.; Hrelia, S. Combined treatment with three natural antioxidants enhances neuroprotection in a SH-SY5Y 3D culture model. *Antioxidants* **2019**, *8*, 420. [CrossRef] [PubMed]
28. Franco, R.; Navarro, G.; Martínez-Pinilla, E. Hormetic and mitochondria-related mechanisms of antioxidant action of phytochemicals. *Antioxidants* **2019**, *8*, 373. [CrossRef]
29. Calabrese, V.; Cornelius, C.; Trovato-Salinaro, A.; Cambria, M.; Locascio, M.; Rienzo, L.; Condorelli, D.; Mancuso, C.; De Lorenzo, A.; Calabrese, E. The Hormetic Role of Dietary Antioxidants in Free Radical-Related Diseases. *Curr. Pharm. Des.* **2010**, *16*, 877–883. [CrossRef]
30. Hatem, S.; Nasr, M.; Elkheshen, S.A.; Geneidi, A.S. Recent Advances in Antioxidant Cosmeceutical Topical Delivery. *Curr. Drug Deliv.* **2018**, *15*, 953–964. [CrossRef]
31. Hseu, Y.C.; Chen, X.Z.; Gowrisankar, Y.V.; Yen, H.R.; Chuang, J.Y.; Yang, H.L. The skin-whitening effects of ectoine via the suppression of α-MSH-stimulated melanogenesis and the activation of antioxidant Nrf2 pathways in UVA-irradiated keratinocytes. *Antioxidants* **2020**, *9*, 63. [CrossRef] [PubMed]

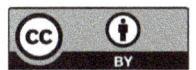

© 2020 by the authors. Licensee MDPI, Basel, Switzerland. This article is an open access article distributed under the terms and conditions of the Creative Commons Attribution (CC BY) license (http://creativecommons.org/licenses/by/4.0/).

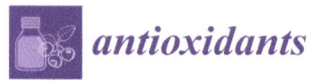

Article

Characterization of Antioxidant Potential of Seaweed Extracts for Enrichment of Convenience Food

Paola Antonia Corsetto [1,*], Gigliola Montorfano [1], Stefania Zava [1], Irma Colombo [1], Bergros Ingadottir [2], Rosa Jonsdottir [2], Kolbrun Sveinsdottir [2] and Angela Maria Rizzo [1]

1. Department of Pharmacological and Biomolecular Sciences, Università degli Studi di Milano, 20133 Milan, Italy; gigliola.montorfano@unimi.it (G.M.); stefania.zava@unimi.it (S.Z.); irma.colombo@unimi.it (I.C.); angelamaria.rizzo@unimi.it (A.M.R.)
2. Matis ohf, Vinlandsleid 12, 113 Reykjavik, Iceland; bergros@gmail.com (B.I.); rosa@matis.is (R.J.); kolbrun@matis.is (K.S.)
* Correspondence: paola.corsetto@unimi.it; Tel.: +30-025-031-5779

Received: 31 January 2020; Accepted: 15 March 2020; Published: 19 March 2020

Abstract: In recent years, there has been a growing interest in natural antioxidants as replacements of synthetic compounds because of increased safety concerns and worldwide trend toward the usage of natural additives in foods. One of the richest sources of natural antioxidants, nowadays largely studied for their potential to decrease the risk of diseases and to improve oxidative stability of food products, are edible brown seaweeds. Nevertheless, their antioxidant mechanisms are slightly evaluated and discussed. The aims of this study were to suggest possible mechanism(s) of *Fucus vesiculosus* antioxidant action and to assess its bioactivity during the production of enriched rye snacks. Chemical and cell-based assays indicate that the efficient preventive antioxidant action of *Fucus vesiculosus* extracts is likely due to not only the high polyphenol content, but also their good Fe^{2+}-chelating ability. Moreover, the data collected during the production of *Fucus vesiculosus*-enriched rye snacks show that this seaweed can increase, in appreciable measure, the antioxidant potential of enriched convenience cereals. This information can be used to design functional foods enriched in natural antioxidant ingredients in order to improve the health of targeted consumers.

Keywords: natural antioxidant; seaweed; algae; *Fucus vesiculosus*

1. Introduction

Antioxidants are attractive as supplements because of their potential preventive role in several diseases associated with oxidative stress, occurring when the balance between antioxidants and reactive oxygen species (ROS) is disrupted because of either depletion of antioxidants or accumulation of ROS [1–3]. There are many in vitro studies allowing speculation in this sense; however, clinical evidences for some of these molecules are weak. For instance, a 2007 systematic review assessed the effect of antioxidant supplements, such as β carotene, vitamins A, E and C, and selenium, on overall mortality in primary or secondary prevention randomized clinical trials. It concluded not only that β carotene and vitamins A and E do not have beneficial effects on mortality, but that they seem to increase the death risk [4]. Indeed, most trials included in this review investigated the effects of supplements administrated in higher doses than those usually found in a balanced diet, and some of the trials used doses well above the recommended daily allowances and even above the upper tolerable intake levels. Furthermore, very heterogeneous populations have been examined in this review and the impact of different types of supplements was evaluated in the general population or in patients with gastrointestinal, cardiovascular, neurological, skin, ocular, renal, endocrinological, rheumatoid, and undefined diseases in a stable phase. However, one possible effective approach for preventing or treating these ROS-mediated disorders is based on a diet rich in natural antioxidants, which is supported by many international health agencies. In this context, there is a growing interest in natural antioxidants as replacements of synthetic compounds because of increased safety concerns and a worldwide trend toward the usage of natural additives in foods [5]. In addition, natural antioxidants derived from various plants and marine algae not only have demonstrated health-promoting benefits, but have also shown a great potential for improving oxidative stability of food products [6]. Under extreme conditions, different types of edible seaweeds, including *Fucus vesiculosus (F. vesiculosus)*, develop unique metabolic systems to survive leading to the synthesis of a high number of secondary metabolites, most of which are potent antioxidant molecules [7].

Seaweeds are a rich source of nutrients and of different kinds of bioactive substances, including sulphated polysaccharides, such as fucoidans, carotenoid pigments, such as fucoxanthin, and phlorotannins, a subgroup of polyphloroglucinol polyphenols only found in brown seaweeds, with potential health benefits [8]. The antioxidant activity of phlorotannins is closed to phenol rings, which act as electron traps to scavenge ROS. Phlorotannins have been found to possess multiple physiological activities, with anti-carcinogenic, antibacterial, antiviral, anticancer, and anti-inflammatory properties [9–11].

Moreover, polysaccharides, such as fucoidans, are particularly abundant in seaweed, especially in *F. vesiculosus*; they may act as antioxidants by either directly scavenging ROS, or induction of the activity of cellular endogenous antioxidant defenses, including superoxide dismutase (SOD), catalase (CAT), glutathione transferase, and glucose-6-phosphate dehydrogenase [12].

Seaweeds are also a source of dietary fibers, prebiotics, and other functional ingredients that induce a decrease of glucose and cholesterol blood levels [13]. Indeed, seaweed consumption has been related to a lower incidence of chronic diseases, such as dyslipidemia, and coronary heart disease [14,15].

The usage and industrial applications of seaweeds are abundant in Eastern tradition, whereas in Western countries, seaweeds are particularly used for phycocolloids production [16]. Due to their excellent gel properties, the polysaccharide fibers of seaweeds, especially alginic acid, have also been used as stabilizing and water-holding agents. For this reason, seaweeds are very important industrial components in many fields, including cosmetic and pharmaceutical/medical, but also in food industry as thickeners, gels, emulsifiers, and stabilizers. However, since biological activities of seaweeds support their potential role as a natural antioxidant, seaweed extracts and purified compounds may be used as active ingredients to improve oxidative stability of functional foods and nutraceuticals [17].

On the basis of scientific and technological developments since 1997, the Regulation (EU) 2015/2283 of the European Parliament and of the Council reviews, clarifies and updates the categories of food that constitute novel foods. For this Regulation, food consisting of fungi or algae, isolated or produced from microorganisms, are defined as "novel food." Then, although scientific research highlights various bioactivity in seaweed species, marketing it as a novel or functional food with health claims requires scientific evidences, which must be provided by an application submitted to EU, an extensive and time-consuming procedure. In this contest, some *F. vesiculosus* extract or purified molecule are already recognized as Generally Recognized As Safe (GRAS) or novel foods.

Baked foods, such as snacks, cookies, and biscuits, that are consumed and stored for extended periods before consumption, need to preserve their quality to remain competitive on the economic market [18]. To ameliorate shelf life, antioxidants, antimicrobials, and anti-browning additives are mostly used by the food industry [5]. The utilization of synthetic antioxidants has been correlated to possible toxicity and side effects, such as carcinogenesis [19], and the use of synthetic antioxidants has declined due to consumer awareness and demand for natural protection. Only a few natural food antioxidants are commercially available on the market. Among these, rosemary extracts have been the most successful natural plant-based antioxidants commercialized [20].

F. vesiculosus is a brown algae species whose high antioxidant activity, in addition to other unique properties (e.g., anti-inflammatory and anti-diabetic activities), makes it particularly attractive for its use in various food systems [21]. Due to the strong market demand and very positive preliminary tests, it is believed that its extracts can be highly competitive on the market and find various uses in food.

In this paper, we describe the bioactive properties of *F. vesiculosus* extracts using different chemical and cell-based methods in order to provide evidences of possible antioxidant mechanism(s). Moreover, we present data related to the ability of extracts to increase the antioxidant potential of enriched convenience cereals. This information can be used to define a broad range of categories of convenience food to improve the health of targeted consumers.

2. Materials and Methods

2.1. Chemicals

All chemicals were of analytical grade and obtained from Sigma–Aldrich (St. Louis, MO, USA), Fluka (Buchs, Switzerland) or Sigma–Aldrich (Steinheim, Germany). All the solvents used were of HPLC grade and of analytical grade and obtained from Sigma–Aldrich (St. Louis, MO, USA and Steinheim, Germany) or Carlo Erba Reagents (Cornaredo, Milan, Italy).

2.2. Production of Fucus Vesiculosus Extracts

The brown seaweed *Fucus vesiculosus* was strategically collected in the Hvassahraun coastal area, southwestern Iceland, during peaks in bioactive content: in particular, the raw materials of batches for this study were collected in two different periods, in July 2013 and July 2014, and the batches were named B200314 and B290814, respectively. They were used as feedstocks for a pilot-scale extraction. The seaweeds were stored at −18 °C until cleaned and shredded in preparation for extract production. The preparation of seaweed extract was performed according to Wang et al. [22]. Briefly, the extracts were produced as follows: the seaweeds were soaked and rinsed in cold water to remove sand and other debris, wet-milled, mixed with water, extracted, filtered (refined), and the extracted liquid collected and frozen at −20 °C until further processing. Finally, the defrosted liquid extract was spray dried. During the process, unprocessed seaweed/water mixtures, liquid extracts, and lyophilized extracts were analyzed for microorganisms, to exclude contamination. Two aqueous seaweed extracts were produced.

2.3. Production of Extruded Rye Snacks

Development of prototypes of extruded rye snacks enriched with seaweed extracts was performed by Ruislandia, a small and medium enterprises (SME) involved in the European EnRichMar project (606023) and VTT (Finland). Several rye snack samples enriched with various amounts of seaweed extracts and three different flavorings (garlic or basil + tomato or rosemary), have been produced by an optimized extrusion and roasting processes. An overview of the parameters (time and temperature) of different production phases is reported in Table S1.

2.4. Bioactivity by Chemical Assays

Bioactivity evaluation was performed on seaweed extracts, raw materials, mixed flour, and extruded snacks, by means of different chemical assays.

2.4.1. Total Polyphenol Content

Total polyphenol content (TPC) was determined according to the method of Turkmen et al. [23] and Koivikko et al. [24] with slight modifications. For rye snacks, 100 mg was dissolved in 10 mL water to obtain a 10 mg/mL solution. Briefly, 20 µL of sample was mixed with 100 µL of 0.2N Folin-Ciocalteu phenyl reagent and allowed to stand at room temperature for 5 min. Then, 80 µL of 7.5% Na_2CO_3 was added and the solution was incubated for 10 sec at 800 W in microwave and put on a shaker for 30 min at room temperature. Absorbance was read at 720 nm with a microplate reader (POLARstar Optima BMG labtech, Offenburg, Germany). Phloroglucinol was used as a standard, and the results are expressed as gram of phloroglucinol equivalents (PGE) per 100 g of extract.

2.4.2. Oxygen Radical Absorbance Capacity

The oxygen radical absorbance capacity (ORAC) assay was performed according to Ganske and Dell [25]; the method was adapted to microplates and measurements were carried out with a microplate reader (POLARstar OPTIMA, BMG Labtech, Offenburg, Germany). The samples were incubated for 10 min at 37 °C, and after incubation, 30 µL of 120 mM 2,2′-azobis(2-amidinopropane) dihydrochloride (AAPH) solution was added rapidly using a POLARstar OPTIMA injector to trigger the oxidation reaction. The fluorescence was recorded every minute for 100 min. The filters used were 485 nm for λ excitation and 520 nm for λ emission. The ORAC values are expressed as µmol of Trolox Equivalents (TE) per gram of sample, using a standard calibration curve obtained by increasing concentrations of Trolox.

2.4.3. DPPH Radical Scavenging Activity

DPPH (2,2-DiPhenyl-1-PicrylHydrazyl, Sigma USA) radical scavenging activity was determined as recommended by Sharma and Bhat (2009). Extracts were first dissolved in 70% methanol and centrifuged at 2500× g for 5 min. Then, 150 µL of the supernatant was collected and mixed with 50 µL DPPH in methanol. The blank contained 150 µL of 70% ethanol solution instead of supernatant, while the control was prepared with 50 µL of 70% ethanol instead of DPPH solution. L-ascorbic acid was used as reference standard. Absorbance (A) was measured for 30 min at 520 nm with a microplate reader (POLARstar Optima BMG labtech, Offenburg, Germany). The scavenging effect is expressed as:

$$[(A_{blank} - A_{control}) - (A_{sample} - A_{control})]/(A_{blank} - A_{control}) \times 100$$

Increasing concentrations of extracts were used to construct a linear curve, calculated plotting extract concentrations against percentage scavenging effects, and deduce the half maximal inhibitory concentration (IC50) of the extracts: the concentration that was able to quench 50% of the DPPH radical.

2.4.4. Ferrous Ion Chelating Ability

The Fe^{2+}-chelating activity (FCA) was determined according to the method of Boyer (1988) [26] with slight modifications. Samples were dissolved in water in ratio 1/1 and centrifuged at 2500× g for 5 min; 100 µL of the supernatant were mixed with 50 µL of 2 mM ferrous chloride and 100 µL of 5 mM ferrozine for 30 min at room temperature. The absorbance was read at 560 nm using a microplate reader (POLARStar OPTIMA, BMG Labtech, Offenburg, Germany). The metal chelating activity was calculated as follows:

$$\text{Chelating activity } (\%) = \left(\frac{A_{blank} - (A_{sample} - A_{control})}{A_{blank}} \right) \times 100$$

where Ablank, Asample, and Acontrol are the absorbance of the blank, the sample, and the control at 520 nm, respectively.

2.4.5. ABTS Assay

ABTS, or 2,2′-azino-bis(3-ethylbenzothiazoline-6-sulfonic acid) diammonium salt assay, was performed following the Sigma manufacturer's instructions (Sigma-Aldrich, Missouri USA). Briefly, 0.0016 g potassium persulphate was dissolved in 25 mL of water and 0.096 g ABTS was dissolved in potassium persulfate. The solution was allowed to stabilize 12 h, stored at dark and room temperature. Then, 0.0064 g Trolox was dissolved in 25 mL methanol, stored at 5 °C during the working day. Samples were weighted, extracted with water, and solutions were centrifuged at 2500× g for 5 min. ABTS solution was added to the blank, Trolox, and samples. The calibration curve was obtained by different concentrations of Trolox. Results were referred to the Trolox standard curve and are expressed as µmol of Trolox equivalent per gram of extract.

2.5. Bioactivity by Cell-Based Assays

2.5.1. Cellular Antioxidant Activity

Cellular antioxidant assay (CAA) was performed using HepG2 cells (ATCC, USA) maintained in Minimum Essential Medium α (MEMα), supplemented with 10% (v/v) heat-inactivated fetal bovine serum, penicillin (50 units/mL), and streptomycin (50 µg/mL). Cells were incubated at 37 °C in a fully humidified environment under 5% CO_2, and HepG2 cells at passage 80–100 were used for the experiments. Cells were subcultured at 7 days intervals before reaching 90% confluence.

CAA assay was performed on spray dried extracts using HepG2 cells at a density of 6×10^4 cells/well seeded black 96-well plates (BD Falcon™) in 100 µL growth medium/well according to Wolfe and Liu (2007) [27] and Samaranayaka et al. (2010) [28] with minor modifications. Briefly, 24 hours after cell seeding, 100 µL of DCFH-DA probe (1 µM in HBSS) was added to the cells and incubated at 37 °C in the dark for 30 min. Cells were then treated with different concentrations of extract and incubated for 1 h at 37 °C. Subsequently, after removal of the antioxidant-tested compounds, 100 µL of peroxyl radical initiator AAPH (750 µM in HBSS) were added to the cultured cells. Fluorescence readings (λexcitation = 493 nm, λemission = 527 nm) were recorded using a POLARstar OPTIMA (BMG Labtech) every 10 min for 90 min after addition of AAPH. Each plate included four replicates of both blank and controls: the blank consisted of cells exposed to only the DCFH-DA probe, and the control consisted of cells with the DCFH-DA probe and the AAPH added, but in the absence of test compounds.

2.5.2. Cell Protective Effects against Induced Oxidative Stress

HepG2 cells were seeded in culture T75 flasks (16.9×10^4 cells/cm^2), and after 24 h, they were incubated with 62.5 µg/mL seaweed extract (batch B200314) for 48 h. Finally, 200 µM of tert-butyl hydroperoxide (TBUT) (Sigma-Aldrich, Missouri, USA) was added and incubated for 3 h. Experiments included untreated cells that were not exposed to seaweed and/or TBUT. Cells were harvested using trypsin/EDTA and centrifuged at $1000 \times g$ for 5 min. The supernatant was removed and the cell pellets were subjected to enzymatic assays and glutathione extraction with 10% metaphosphoric acid.

To this aim, cells were homogenized on ice in H_2O, and the supernatant was assayed for protein content according to Lowry method (1951) [29] and used to perform enzyme assays as previously described [30].

Briefly, catalase activity was assayed by measuring the consumption of H_2O_2 at 240 nm for 1 min at 30 °C according to Aebi (1984) [31]. The incubation mixture included: 50 µL H_2O_2 200 mM, 50–100 µg of proteins of sample, and Na-phosphate buffer (50 mM pH 7.0) to reach a final volume of 1 mL. One unit of catalase activity is defined as amount of enzyme required to catalyze the decomposition of 1 µmol H_2O_2 min^{-1}.

The glutathione reductase (GR) activity was assayed according to Pinto et al. (1984) [32]. Briefly, GSSG reduction and NADPH consumption were recorded at 340 nm. The incubation mixture included: 20 µL GSSG 125 mM, 11 µL NADPH 11 mM, 50–100 µg of proteins of sample, and K-phosphate buffer (100 mM pH 7.0) to 1 mL final volume.

The activity of selenium-dependent glutathione peroxidase (GPx) was assayed according to Prohaska and Ganther (1976) [33] by following the decrease in the absorbance at 340 nm for 5 min, which corresponds to the rate of GSH oxidation to GSSG in the presence of NADPH and GR. The incubation mixture included: 20 µL GSH 100 mM, 10 µL NADPH 11 mM, GR 1 Unit, 10 µL TBUT 20 mM, 50–100 µg of proteins of sample, and EDTA-K phosphate buffer to 1 mL final volume. One unit of GR or GPx activity is defined as the amount of enzyme required to catalyze the oxidation of 1 mmol NADPH min^{-1}.

Total glutathione content was assayed according to Griffith (1985) [34] with slight modifications. Briefly, the sulfhydryl group of GSH, also generated from GSSG by adding GR, reacts with DTNB (5,50-dithio-bis-2-nitrobenzoic acid) and produces a yellow-colored 5-thio-2-nitrobenzoic acid (TNB).

The rate of TNB production is directly proportional to the concentration of GSH in the sample. Measurement of the absorbance of TNB at 412 nm provides an accurate estimation of the GSH level present in the sample.

The end product of lipid peroxidation, malonyldialdehyde (MDA) was measured in cell extracts and quantified using an HPLC-UV system (Jasco, Japan) as previously described [35]. The MDA standard and sample preparation was carried out according to Karatas et al. (2002) [36]. To prepare MDA standards, 10 µL of 1,1,3,3-tetraethoxypropane (TEP) were accurately diluted to 10 mL with 0.1 M HCl in a screw-capped test tube and placed in a boiling water bath for 5 min and then rapidly cooled on ice, producing hydrolyzed acetal. A working stock solution of MDA was prepared by adding 1 mL of the hydrolyzed acetal to 99 mL of water; the working stock solution was 40 µM MDA. The stock solution was further diluted and used to construct the calibration curve. MDA was determined by HPLC (Jasco, Japan) equipped with a UV detector. A C18 column (Waters, 1.7 µm, 50 × 2.1 mm) was used at room temperature. Samples were suspended in water and $HClO_4$ 0.1 M, centrifuged at 4500× g for 5 min and supernatants were used for HPLC analysis. The mobile phase was KH_2PO_4/CH_3OH/acetonitrile (72/18/11; $v/v/v$) and the flow rate was 1.0 mL/min. Chromatograms were monitored at 254 nm and injection was 20 µl (0.5 × 10^6 cells). The retention time of MDA was 2.5–3 min.

2.6. Statistical Analysis

The data were analyzed by one way-ANOVA (Graphpad-Prism 6.0) with multiple comparisons by Fisher's Least Significant Difference (LSD) test; the level of statistical significance was set to $p < 0.05$. Data are reported as mean ± standard deviation (SD).

3. Results

3.1. Bioactive Properties of Fucus Vesiculosus Extracts

The antioxidant potential and the potential mechanism(s) of antioxidant action of seaweed extracts were characterized by a multiple-method approach, which include well-documented chemical assays and cell-based bioassays.

3.1.1. Total Polyphenol Content and Antioxidant Activity

The evaluation of total polyphenol content (TPC) is a reference assay largely used to measure polyphenols in foods. The TPC of the two batches of seaweed extracts (B200314 and B290814) was 0.26 and 0.30 g PGE/g extract, respectively (Table 1). The secondary metabolite composition of the *F. vesiculosus* was already studied in our laboratories, by HPLC-DAD-ESI-MS [21]. In accordance with the literature, we have described several phlorotannin compounds in seaweed extracts. In particular, we have detected phlorotannin tetramers, whose proposed structures were fucodiphlorethol A, and hexamer compounds at *m/z* 729, 622/621, and at *m/z* 462, whose proposed structures were trifucodiplorethol isomers. The lack of standards represents a limitation of the analytical method for these compounds.

The antioxidant capacity of the seaweed extracts was assessed by mean of ORAC, DPPH radical scavenging activity, and ferrous ion-chelating ability. The oxygen radical absorbance capacity expressed by ORAC value, a reference to compare the antioxidant value of foods, was 1545 µmol TE/g extract in B200314 and 1840 µmol TE/g extract in B290814 (Table 1). DPPH IC50 values of the extracts were 0.614 mg/mL for B200314 and 0.608 mg/mL for B290814 (Table 1). The ability of the extracts, B200314 and B290814, to chelate transition metal ions, especially Fe^{2+} and Cu^{2+}, demonstrated that their ferrous ion chelating ability (FCA) was higher (59% and 53%) at a concentration of 10 mg/mL, respectively (Table 1).

Table 1. Bioactive properties of the *Fucus vesiculosus* extracts assessed by different chemical assays.

Extract	TPC [1]	ORAC [2]	DPPH IC50 [3]	FCA 1.0 mg/mL	FCA 5.0 mg/mL	FCA 10 mg/mL
B200314	0.26 ± 0.02	1545 ± 220	0.614	15.0 ± 4.5	49.7 ± 5.3	59.2 ± 2.1
B290814	0.30 ± 0.01	1840 ± 3	0.608	21.5 ± 2.8	50.4 ± 6.7	53.0 ± 3.8

TPC, total polyphenol content; ORAC, oxygen radical absorbance capacity; DPPH. 2,2-DiPhenyl-1-PicrylHydrazyl radical scavenging activity, FCA, Fe^{2+}-chelating activity. [1] g PhloroGlucinol Equivalents/g extract; [2] µmol Trolox Equivalents/g extract; [3] mg extract/mL.

3.1.2. Cellular Antioxidant Activity of the *Fucus Vesiculosus* Extracts

To obtain a better prediction of the antioxidant activity of seaweed extracts we measured their ability to prevent the radical formation by CAA assay using HepG2 cells. The results, presented in Figure 1, indicate that both seaweed extracts were able *in vitro* to scavenge 50–60% of the AAPH-induced radicals. The extracts were active at very low concentrations (62.5 µg/mL and 31.3 µg/mL for B200314 and B290814, respectively); Trolox (50 µM = 12.5 µg/mL), used as a positive control, exhibited 98% cellular antioxidant activity.

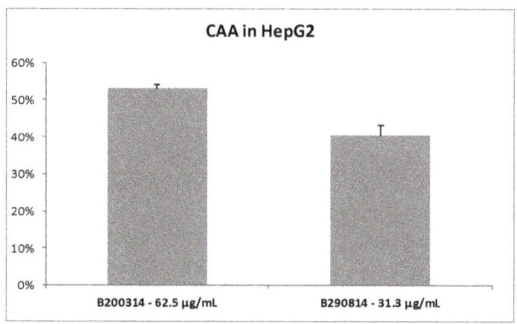

Figure 1. Cellular antioxidant activity (CAA) in HepG2 cells as a % of the control. The control consisted of cells with the DCFH-DA probe and the AAPH peroxyl radical initiator, but in the absence of samples; the blank consisted of cells exposed to only the DCFH-DA probe. The values shown are the mean ± SD of three independent experiments.

3.1.3. Cell Protective Effects of Seaweed Extract against Induced Oxidative Stress

To assess the preventive capacity of seaweed extracts to protect cells from oxidative stress we assayed the activities of the major antioxidant enzymes in HepG2 cells pre-treated with seaweed extract and then stimulated with TBUT. Cells were exposed to 62.5 µg/mL B200314, the batch that was further implemented in the rye-snacks.

The results, shown in Figure 2, demonstrate that at this concentration, the seaweed extract displayed a protective effect on hepatic cells. In fact, the pretreatment with seaweed (Sw) extract determines a significant reduction of GSH reductase activity induced by TBUT exposure (Sw + TBUT vs. TBUT $p < 0.05$). Moreover, we observed a slight decrease of catalase activity induced by TBUT stress in cells pretreated with seaweeds, although this was not statistically significant. GSH peroxidase activity and total glutathione content remained to the level of stressed cells. No effects were observed in malonyldialdehyde (MDA) levels, the typical marker of lipid peroxidation, which were slightly increased by TBUT treatment.

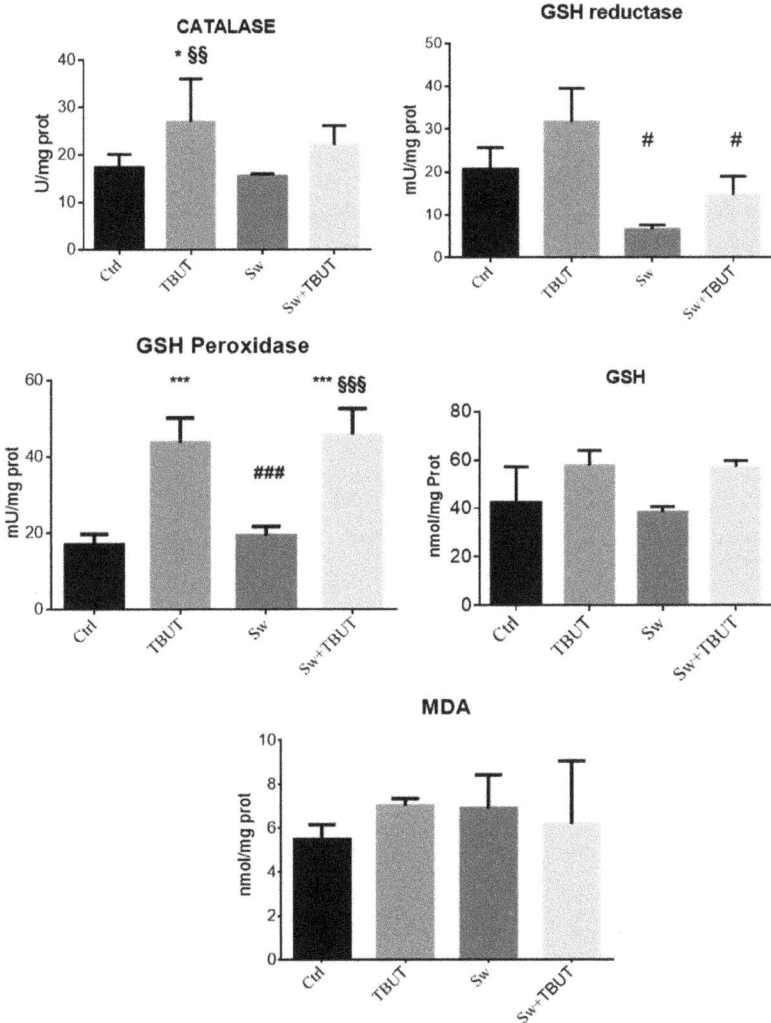

Figure 2. Protective effects of seaweed extract assessed in HepG2 cells exposed to oxidative stress (TBUT) with or without 62.5 µg/mL seaweed extract (Sw). The main antioxidant enzymes are represented together with glutathione (GSH) and malonyldialdehyde (MDA) cell content. Values are expressed as mean ± SD of three independent experiments. * vs. Ctrl (* $p < 0.05$, *** $p < 0.001$); § vs. Sw (§§: $p < 0.01$, §§§: $p < 0.001$) and # vs. TBUT (#: $p < 0.05$, ###: $p < 0.001$).

3.1.4. Development and Test of Enriched Rye Snacks

To test the ability of *F. vesiculosus* to increase snack antioxidant power, several rye snack samples enriched with various amounts of seaweed extract B200314 were produced by an optimized extrusion process (Table S1). This study included a rye snack model, as it was: (1) suitable due to uniformity of product; (2) interesting with regard to production process/heat treatment; and (3) interesting for its improved nutritional profile (iodine) and stability (potential antioxidant activity).

Several rye snack samples enriched with various amounts of seaweed extract were produced by extrusion, and the extrusion process was optimized. In spite of their health promoting impact, seaweeds cause an off-flavor to some extent in rye snacks. Thus, several experiments aiming to mask the off-flavor perceived in the snacks were also conducted.

To this aim, sensorial tests were performed and numerous snack samples were screened by a trained sensory expert panel ($n = 5$) by scoring and/or go/no go assessments. Promising samples were assessed by VTT's trained sensory panel. The test method used in sensory assessments was descriptive profiling. VTT's trained sensory panel ($n = 10$ or $n = 2 \times 10$, i.e., duplicate session of the 10-member panel) evaluated the intensities of the sensory attributes on a linear scale 0–10, which was verbally anchored from both ends (0 = the attribute not perceived, 10 = the attribute very clearly perceived). In addition, the panelists gave verbal descriptions on the samples. The Compusense software collected data.

From these analyses, suitable snack options for the study were found. The most effective flavorings were garlic (G), basil+tomato (B/T), and rosemary (R). To increase the palatability of the snacks, roasting was also utilized. The development of prototypes of extruded rye snacks enriched with seaweed powder for production by Ruislandia were performed in parallel. The list of the produced and analyzed snacks, roasted and unroasted, is reported in Tables S2 and S3.

The antioxidant activity of the prototype snacks was firstly analyzed by chemical assays, taking into account the single components (raw materials) and their mixtures (mix of flour) before and after the extrusion process.

As shown in Figure 3, an appreciable increase of antioxidant activity, correlated to the increase of seaweed concentration, is evident in both the mix of flour and extruded snacks, even if the extract displays less activity compared to the same concentration of pure seaweed extract, showed in the raw material panel.

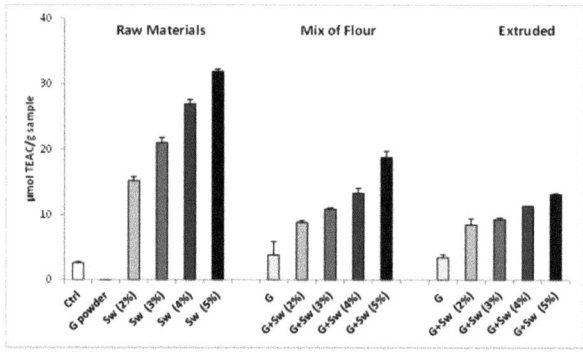

(A)

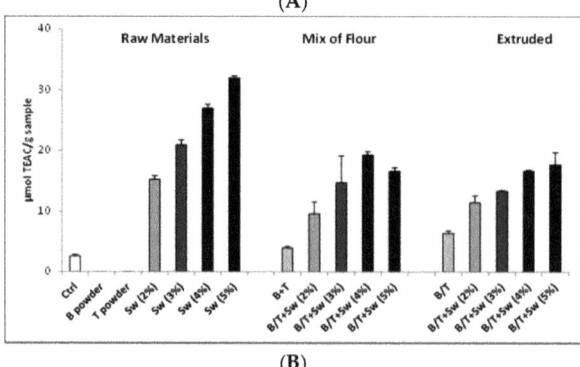

(B)

Figure 3. *Cont.*

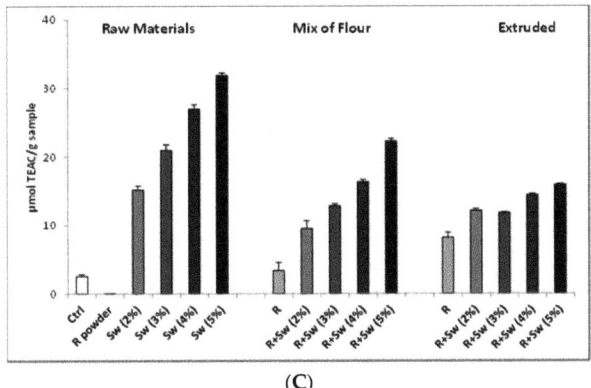

(C)

Figure 3. Trolox equivalent antioxidant capacity (TEAC) values for raw materials, mix of flour and extruded snacks with (**A**) 1% Garlic (G), (**B**) 0.5% Basil (B) + 3% Tomato (T), and (**C**) 0.5% Rosemary (R) powders and increasing concentration of seaweed extract (Sw). Ctrl consists in rye mix. Data are expressed as mean ± SD of three independent experiments.

Interestingly, the different flavorings, when added to mix of flour, showed an increment of TEAC value also in the absence of seaweed. Additionally, flavored extruded samples, without seaweed, showed an antioxidant potential in particular for rosemary and basil + tomatoes. Moreover, in a mix of flour and extruded snacks with different concentrations of seaweed, the antioxidant activity was similar, suggesting that the extrusion process did not modified the biological activity.

As regard to the palatability of the snacks, the 2% seaweed-enriched snack was considered the more interesting product, with a TEAC above 10 µmol/g sample.

In the final development of the products, extruded rye snacks were produced with 2.1% seaweed extract, corresponding to a theoretical 2500 ORAC value per portion (60 g), and flavored with garlic, basil+tomato, and rosemary, in roasted and unroasted conditions.

On these prototypes (Supplemental Table S3), we have evaluated the total polyphenol content and the oxygen radical absorbance capacity (Figure 4). The control snacks contained only 0.8% Himalayan salt as all other prototypes.

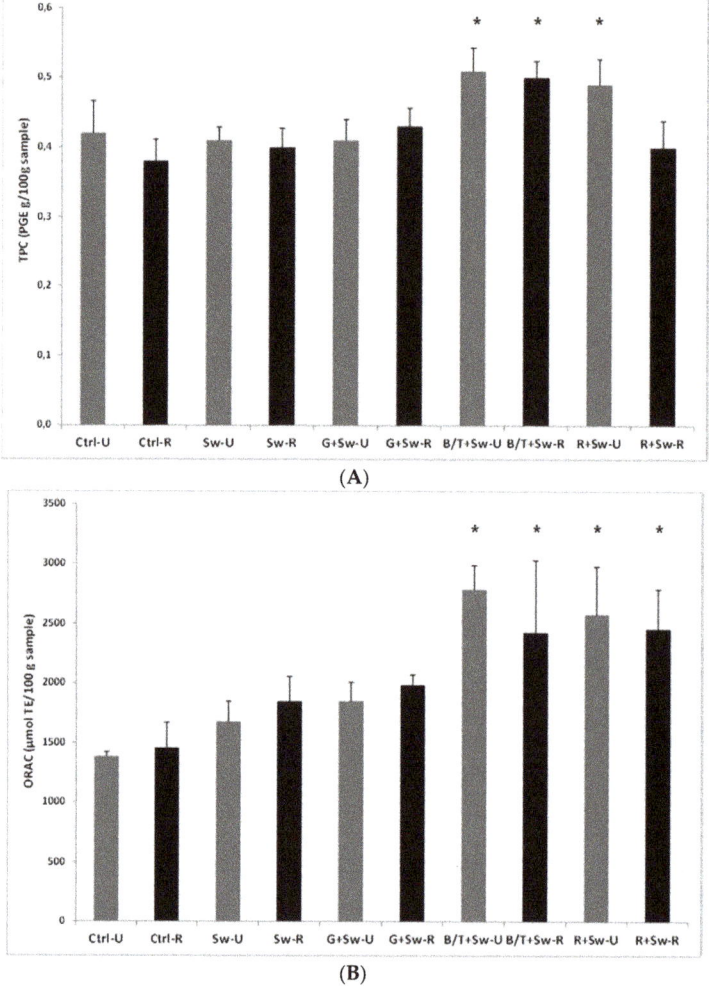

Figure 4. (**A**) TPC and (**B**) ORAC values (μmol TE in 100 g sample) of roasted (R) and unroasted (U) rye snacks containing different flavorings, i.e., 1% garlic (G), 0.5% basil (B) + 3% tomato (T) or 0.5% rosemary (R) powder. All groups contained rye mix, 0.8% Himalayan salt and 2.1% seaweed extract (Sw, batch B200314), except the control group, which only contained rye mix and 0.8% Himalayan salt (Ctrl). Data are expressed as mean ± SD of four independent experiments. * $p < 0.05$ vs. Sw-U and Sw-R groups.

The addition of basil (0.5%) + tomato powder (3%) (B/T) or rosemary (0.5%) (R) to the seaweed enriched rye snack resulted in significantly ($p < 0.05$) higher TPC compared to other groups (Figure 4A). Similar trend was evident in the ORAC measures (Figure 4B) with significantly higher values in rye snacks containing the same flavorings. No changes were observed for different roasting processes.

4. Discussion

Seaweeds are a rich source of nutrients, but they are also an important source of different kinds of bioactive substances, including sulphated polysaccharides, carotenoid pigments, and phlorotannins, with potential health benefits. In particular, phlorotannins, derived primarily from brown algae, have been recently found to possess multiple physiological activities, such as antioxidant, antibacterial, and anti-inflammatory [37].

Moreover, seaweeds provide health benefits due to biological effects attributed to some poly- and/or oligosaccharides. These include prebiotic effects, immunomodulation, affecting the ability of white blood cells to attack tumor cells, reduction of the symptoms of respiratory tract infections, and protection against infectious diseases [30].

The link between the tissue oxidative damage caused by the increase of intracellular content of ROS and several pathophysiological conditions, such as aging, obesity, non-alcoholic fatty liver disease (NAFLD), type 2 diabetes mellitus, and cognitive decline, is highlighted by many preclinical and clinical studies [38–40]. However, an intracellular basal content of ROS, physiologically generated from both normal mitochondria and peroxisomes metabolism and different cytosolic enzyme systems, is important for some physiological processes. Therefore, the maintenance of intracellular redox homeostasis is fundamental. It depends on efficient antioxidant systems that provide a decrease of ROS production and scavenging free radicals. This antioxidant system includes antioxidants and antioxidant enzymes, such as vitamin E, vitamin C, glutathione, superoxide dismutase, glutathione peroxidase, and catalase [41].

Moreover, oxidative stress is also associated with lipid accumulation and peroxidation. High ROS levels induce the production of lipid peroxyl radicals, which can generate other extremely reactive products as malonyldialdehyde (MDA), 4-hydroxy-2-nonenal (4-HNE), and 4-hydroxy-2-hexenal (4-HHE), typically used as markers of lipid oxidation [42]. Since the Western diet notably involves increased fat intake, thereby resulting in oxidative stress and impaired inflammation status, antioxidant compounds are frequently added into food.

In the last decades, the food industry has been focused in replacing synthetic antioxidants with natural compounds; of current interest are those related to bioactive compounds extracted from the edible seaweeds. Among these marine algae, *F. vesiculosus* is the most well-known species from the *Fucus* genus [25], representing an abundant and widely distributed kind of brown, perennial and edible seaweed. It is present in the cold-temperate waters of the northern hemisphere and can counteract oxidative stress. In fact, several studies have shown that it may act as an antioxidant either by direct scavenging ROS or stimulating the activity of endogenous antioxidant enzyme system [43]. Moreover, some of these studies confirmed the antioxidant effects of seaweed extracts, related to their significant polyphenol content.

The phlorotannins represent the major polyphenolics present in brown seaweed. These compounds are a subgroup of tannins, which are formed by the polymerization of phloroglucinol units. *F. vesiculosus* contains low molecular weight (LMW) phlorotannins between 4 and 8 phloroglucinol units, but also phlorotannins highly polymerized of up to 16 phloroglucinol units. In fact, Iceland colleagues have isolated in *F. vesiculosus* extracts both oligomeric and polymeric phlorotannins that have more antioxidant activity than monomeric compounds.

In our study, biochemical assays have confirmed that *F. vesiculosus* extracts, produced for healthy snack supplementation, have efficient antioxidant properties and a high content of polyphenols.

Moreover, both seaweed extracts, B200314 and B290814, prevent ROS formation in cell-based assays. Indeed, catalase and GSH reductase activities, measured in HepG2 cells, pre-incubated with seaweed extract B200314, do not increase in stress condition induced by TBUT exposure.

Other antioxidant mechanisms are rarely evaluated and discussed. In our study, we have observed the seaweed extracts capability to chelate Fe^{2+} ions, and only one report from the literature [44] until now has suggested that seaweeds are metal-chelating agents, removing the metals and reducing their redox potential.

Essential heavy metals are cofactors in several biological processes: Cu, Zn, Fe, and Co are involved in oxygen utilization, cell growth, enzymatic reactions, biomolecular metabolism, and immunity system. Essential heavy metals homeostasis is wisely regulated through protein transporters responsible for their uptake, distribution, storage, and excretion. Metal accumulation in the human body leads to damage to many organs, especially the nervous, respiratory, and reproductive systems [45]. In fact, metal accumulation induces ROS production, which results in membrane lipid peroxidation. Moreover, Fe and Cu ions catalyze hydroxyl radical's formation via Fenton-like reactions and react with DNA and proteins, resulting in their functional impairment. Finally, radicals can impact on mitochondria electron transport and metal excess in the cytoplasm can modify intracellular redox equilibrium, changing pH and protein conformation, which can lead to cellular dysfunction and apoptosis/necrosis.

Seaweeds, with their multiple polyphenols and oligo/polysaccharides enriched in a hydroxyl group and carbonyl group on ring C, have several sites for metal complexation able to chelate metal ions. Thus, *F. vesiculosus* may be considered a good chelating agent because it forms chemically inert and non-toxic complexes with metal ions.

This study was part of the VII PQ European project, EnRichMar, aimed not only at screening of the bioactivity of seaweed extracts, but also at increasing the value of convenience foods by adding functional ingredients, produced from underutilized marine based raw materials and by-products (waste) from fish processing, with confirmed bioavailability. The focus has been placed on ingredients such as powder of fish oil and seaweed extracts, which may enhance positive health effects and stability, enhance flavor, and, consequently, contribute to salt reduction of the products to meet market demand.

Our results indicate that seaweed extract can be used in convenience food to increase their stability and antioxidant potential. Data also show the ability of flavorings to enhance with their polyphenol composition the effects of *F. vesiculosus* extracts [23]. The functional properties of the enriched products have been studied also via dietary intervention.

The results collected in the EnRichMar project, and partially illustrated in this study, also suggest that rye snacks containing seaweed extracts show a higher polyphenol content and maintain antioxidant activity despite roasting process.

In conclusion, our preliminary approach suggest that seaweed-based ingredients are potential natural antioxidants that could be used as active ingredients in functional food products as well as improving oxidative stability of healthy food products for targeted consumers.

Supplementary Materials: The following are available online at http://www.mdpi.com/2076-3921/9/3/249/s1, Table S1. Overview of time and temperature during the production of the rye snack: Mixing, extrusion, drying, cooling, packaging, Table S2. List of raw materials, mix of flour, and extruded rye snacks utilized to study the antioxidant action of different flavorings and different amounts of seaweed extracts, Table S3. List of snack prototypes produced to study the effect of different flavorings and roasting on antioxidant properties of rye snacks enriched with *Fucus vesiculosus* extracts.

Author Contributions: The authors' responsibilities were as follows: R.J., K.S. and A.M.R., coordinated the analyses. G.M., S.Z., B.I. and P.A.C., conducted the experiments. A.M.R. and P.A.C. performed statistical analysis and interpreted the data. P.A.C., I.C. and A.M.R., wrote the manuscript. P.A.C., I.C., K.S., R.J. and A.M.R. revised the manuscript. All authors have read and agreed to the published version of the manuscript.

Funding: This research was funded by the European Community VII PQ SME-2013 Increased value of convenience foods by enrichment with marine based raw materials "ENRICHMAR" contract n. 606023.

Acknowledgments: The authors would like to acknowledge all the participant to the Enrichmar Consortium, in particular: the SMEs: BioActive Foods AS, Finnsnack/Ruislandia, Grímur kokkur ehf, Marinox ehf, Den Eelder; the RTD participants: Nederlandse Organisatie Voor Toegepast Natuurwetenschappelijk Onderzoek TNO, Teknologian Tutkimuskeskus VTT.

Conflicts of Interest: The authors declare no conflict of interest.

References

1. Bakir, S.; Catalkaya, G.; Ceylan, F.D.; Khan, H.; Guldiken, B.; Capanoglu, E.; Kamal, M.A. Role of dietary antioxidants in neurodegenerative diseases: Where are we standing? *Curr. Pharm. Des.* **2020**. [CrossRef] [PubMed]
2. Bungau, S.; Abdel-Daim, M.M.; Tit, D.M.; Ghanem, E.; Sato, S.; Maruyama-Inoue, M.; Yamane, S.; Kadonosono, K. Health Benefits of Polyphenols and Carotenoids in Age-Related Eye Diseases. *Oxid. Med. Cell. Longev.* **2019**, *2019*, 9783429. [CrossRef] [PubMed]

3. Sunkara, A.; Raizner, A. Supplemental Vitamins and Minerals for Cardiovascular Disease Prevention and Treatment. *Methodist Debakey Cardiovasc. J.* **2019**, *15*, 179–184. [PubMed]
4. Bjelakovic, G.; Nikolova, D.; Gluud, L.L.; Simonetti, R.G.; Gluud, C. Mortality in randomized trials of antioxidant supplements for primary and secondary prevention: Systematic review and meta-analysis. *JAMA* **2007**, *297*, 842–857. [CrossRef]
5. Caleja, C.; Barros, L.; Antonio, A.L.; Oliveira, M.B.; Ferreira, I.C. A comparative study between natural and synthetic antioxidants: Evaluation of their performance after incorporation into biscuits. *Food Chem.* **2017**, *216*, 342–346. [CrossRef]
6. Gupta, S.; Abu-Ghannam, N. Bioactive potential and possible health effects of edible brown seaweeds. *Trends Food Sci. Technol.* **2011**, *22*, 315–326. [CrossRef]
7. Rickert, E.; Wahl, M.; Heike, L.; Hannes, R.; Pohnert, G. Seasonal Variations in Surface Metabolite Composition of Fucus Vesiculosus and Fucus Serratus From the Baltic Sea. *PLoS ONE* **2016**, *11*, e0168196. [CrossRef]
8. Rengasamy, K.R.; Mahomoodally, M.F.; Aumeeruddy, M.Z.; Zengin, G.; Xiao, J.; Kim, D.H. Bioactive compounds in seaweeds: An overview of their biological properties and safety. *Food Chem. Toxicol.* **2020**, *135*, 111013. [CrossRef]
9. Brown, E.M.; Allsopp, P.J.; Magee, P.-J.; Gill, C.I.R.; Nitecki, S.; Strain, C.R.; McSrley, E.M. Seaweed and human Health. *Nutr. Rev.* **2014**, *72*, 205–216. [CrossRef]
10. Trinchero, J.; Ponce, N.M.; Cordoba, O.L.; Flores, M.L.; Pampuro, S.; Stortz, C.A.; Salomón, H.; Turk, G. Antiretroviral activity of fucoidans extracted from the brown seaweed *Adenocystis utricularis*. *Phytother. Res.* **2009**, *23*, 707–712. [CrossRef]
11. Gutiérrez-Rodríguez, A.G.; Juárez-Portilla, C.; Olivares-Bañuelos, T.; Zepeda, R.C. Anticancer activity of seaweeds. *Drug Discov. Today* **2018**, *23*, 434–447. [CrossRef]
12. Rocha de Souza, M.C.; Marques, C.T.; Guerra Dore, C.M.; Ferreira da Silva, F.R.; Oliveira Rocha, H.A.; Leite, E.L. Antioxidant activities of sulfated polysaccharides from brown and red seaweeds. *J. Appl. Phycol.* **2007**, *19*, 153–160. [CrossRef] [PubMed]
13. Sardari, R.R.R.; Nordberg Karlsson, E. Marine Poly- and Oligosaccharides as Prebiotics. *J. Agric. Food Chem.* **2018**, *66*, 11544–11549. [CrossRef] [PubMed]
14. Iso, H. Lifestyle and cardiovascular disease in Japan. *J. Atheroscler. Thromb.* **2011**, *18*, 83–88. [CrossRef] [PubMed]
15. Kim, J.; Shin, A.; Lee, J.S.; Youn, S.; Yoo, K.Y. Dietary factors and breast cancer in Korea: An ecological study. *Breast J.* **2009**, *15*, 683–686. [CrossRef]
16. Kılınç, B.; Cirik, S.; Turan, G. Seaweeds for Food and Industrial Applications. In *Food Industry*; IntechOpen: London, UK, 2013; pp. 735–748.
17. Pereira, L.; Ribeiro-Claro, P.J.A. Analysis by vibrational spectroscopy of seaweed with potential use in food, pharmaceutical and cosmetic industries. In *Marine Algae: Biodiversity, Taxonomy, Environmental Assessment, and Biotechnology*; Pereira, L., Neto, J.M., Eds.; CRC Press: Boca Raton, FL, USA, 2014; pp. 228–250.
18. Reddy, V.; Urooj, A.; Kumar, A. Evaluation of antioxidant activity of some plant extracts and their application in biscuits. *Food Chem.* **2005**, *90*, 317–321. [CrossRef]
19. Dellarosa, N.; Laghi, L.; Martinsdóttir, E.; Jónsdóttir, R.; Kolbrún Sveinsdóttir, K. Enrichment of convenience seafood with omega-3 and seaweed extracts: Effect on lipid oxidation. *Food Sci. Technol.* **2015**, *62*, 746–752. [CrossRef]
20. Nieto, G.; Ros, G.; Castillo, J. Antioxidant and Antimicrobial Properties of Rosemary (*Rosmarinus officinalis*, L.): A Review. *Medicines* **2018**, *5*, 98. [CrossRef]
21. Wang, T.; Jónsdóttir, R.; Liu, H.; Gu, L.; Kristinsson, H.G.; Raghavan, S.; Olafsdóttir, G. Antioxidant capacities of phlorotannins extracted from the brown algae *Fucus vesiculosus*. *J. Agric. Food Chem.* **2012**, *60*, 5874–5883. [CrossRef]
22. Wang, T.; Jónsdóttir, R.; Ólafsdóttir, G. Total phenolic compounds, radical scavenging and metal chelation of extracts from Icelandic seaweeds. *Food Chem.* **2009**, *116*, 240–248. [CrossRef]
23. Turkmen, N.; Sari, F.; Velioglu, Y.S. The effect of cooking methods on total phenolics and antioxidant activity of selected green vegetables. *Food Chem.* **2005**, *93*, 713–718. [CrossRef]
24. Koivikko, R.; Loponen, J.; Honkanen, T.; Jormalainen, V. Contents of soluble, cell-wall-bound and exuded phlorotannins in the brown alga *Fucus vesiculosus*, with implications on their ecological functions. *J. Chem. Ecol.* **2005**, *31*, 195–212. [CrossRef] [PubMed]

25. Ganske, F.; Dell, E.J. *ORAC Assay on the Fluorstar Optima to Determine Antioxidant Capacity*; Application note of BMG Labtech; BMG Labtech: Ortenberg, Germany, 2006.
26. Boyer, R.F.; Grabill, T.W.; Petrovich, R.M. Reductive release of ferritin iron: A kinetic assay. *Anal. Biochem.* **1988**, *174*, 17–22. [CrossRef]
27. Wolfe, K.L.; Liu, R.H. Cellular antioxidant activity (CAA) assay for assessing antioxidants, foods, and dietary supplements. *J. Agric. Food Chem.* **2007**, *55*, 8896–8907. [CrossRef] [PubMed]
28. Samaranayaka, A.G.P.; Kitts, D.D.; Li-Chan, E.C.Y. Antioxidative and Angiotensin-1-Converting Enzyme Inhibitory Potential of a Pacific Hake (*Merluccius productus*) Fish Protein Hydrolysate Subjected to Simulated Gastrointestinal Digestion and Caco-2 Cell Permeation. *J. Agric. Food Chem.* **2010**, *58*, 1535–1542. [CrossRef] [PubMed]
29. Lowry, O.H.; Rosebrough, N.J.; Farr, A.L.; Randall, R.J. Protein measurement with the Folin phenol reagent. *J. Biol. Chem.* **1951**, *193*, 265–275.
30. Berselli, P.V.R.; Zava, S.; Montorfano, G.; Corsetto, P.A.; Krzyzanowska, J.; Oleszek, W.; Berra, B.; Rizzo, A.M. A mint purified extract protects human keratinocytes from short-term, chemically induced oxidative stress. *J. Agric. Food Chem.* **2010**, *58*, 11428–11434. [CrossRef]
31. Aebi, H. Catalase In Vitro. *Methods Enzymol.* **1984**, *105*, 121–126.
32. Pinto, M.C.; Mata, A.M.; Lopez-barea, J. Reversible inactivation of Saccharomyces cerevisiae glutathione reductase under reducing conditions. *Arch. Biochem. Biophys.* **1984**, *228*, 1–12. [CrossRef]
33. Prohaska, J.R.; Ganther, H.E. Selenium and glutathione peroxidase in developing rat brain. *J. Neurochem.* **1976**, *27*, 1379–1387. [CrossRef]
34. Griffith, O.W. *Glutathione and Glutathione Disulphide. Methods of Enzymatic Analysis*; Bergmeyer, H.U., Ed.; Academic Press: New York, NY, USA, 1984; pp. 521–529.
35. Aoun, M.; Corsetto, P.A.; Nugue, G.; Montorfano, G.; Ciusani, E.; Crouzier, D.; Hogarth, P.; Gregory, A.; Hayflick, S.; Zorzi, G.; et al. Changes in Red Blood Cell membrane lipid composition: A new perspective into the pathogenesis of PKAN. *Mol. Genet. Metab.* **2017**, *121*, 180–189. [CrossRef] [PubMed]
36. Karatas, F.; Karatepe, M.; Baysar, A. Determination of free malondialdehyde in human serum by high-performance liquid chromatography. *Anal. Biochem.* **2002**, *311*, 76–79. [CrossRef]
37. Holdt, S.; Kraan, S. Bioactive compounds in seaweed: Functional food applications and legislation. *J. Appl. Phycol.* **2011**, *23*, 543–597. [CrossRef]
38. Chattopadhyay, M.; Khemka, V.K.; Chatterjee, G.; Ganguly, A.; Mukhopadhyay, S.; Chakrabarti, S. Enhanced ROS production and oxidative damage in subcutaneous white adipose tissue mitochondria in obese and type 2 diabetes subjects. *Mol. Cell. Biochem.* **2015**, *399*, 95–103. [CrossRef] [PubMed]
39. Czarny, P.; Wigner, P.; Galecki, P.; Sliwinski, T. The interplay between inflammation, oxidative stress, DNA damage, DNA repair and mitochondrial dysfunction in depression. *Prog. Neuro Psychopharmacol. Biol. Psychiatry* **2018**, *80*, 309–321. [CrossRef] [PubMed]
40. Wadhwa, R.; Gupta, R.; Maurya, P.K. Oxidative stress and accelerated aging in neurodegenerative and neuropsychiatric disorder. *Curr. Pharm. Des.* **2019**, *24*, 4711–4725. [CrossRef]
41. Liguori, L.; Russo, G.; Curcio, F.; Bulli, G.; Aran, L.; Della-Morte, D.; Gargiulo, G.; Testa, G.; Cacciatore, F.; Bonaduce, D.; et al. Oxidative Stress, Aging, and Diseases. *Clin. Interv. Aging* **2018**, *13*, 757–772. [CrossRef]
42. Draper, H.H.; Csallany, A.S.; Hadley, M. Urinary aldehydes as indicators of lipid peroxidation In Vivo. *Free Radic. Biol. Med.* **2000**, *29*, 1071–1077. [CrossRef]
43. Tan, B.L.; Norhaizan, M.E.; Liew, W.P.P.; Rahman, H.S. Antioxidant and Oxidative Stress: A Mutual Interplay in Age-Related Diseases. *Front. Pharmacol.* **2018**, *9*, 1162. [CrossRef]
44. Pinto, E.; Sigaud-kutner, T.C.S.; Leitão, M.A.S.; Okamoto, O.K.; Morse, D.; Colepicolo, P. Heavy metal–induced oxidative stress in algae. *J. Phycol.* **2003**, *39*, 1008–1018. [CrossRef]
45. Kim, J.J.; Kim, Y.S.; Kumar, V. Heavy metal toxicity: An update of chelating therapeutic strategies. *J. Trace Elem. Med. Biol.* **2019**, *54*, 226–231. [CrossRef] [PubMed]

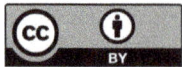

© 2020 by the authors. Licensee MDPI, Basel, Switzerland. This article is an open access article distributed under the terms and conditions of the Creative Commons Attribution (CC BY) license (http://creativecommons.org/licenses/by/4.0/).

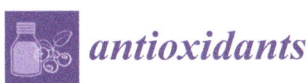

Article

Beneficial Effects of Fermented Papaya Preparation (FPP®) Supplementation on Redox Balance and Aging in a Mouse Model

Mariantonia Logozzi [1,†], Rossella Di Raimo [1,†], Davide Mizzoni [1], Mauro Andreotti [2], Massimo Spada [3], Daniele Macchia [3] and Stefano Fais [1,*]

1. Department of Oncology and Molecular Medicine, Istituto Superiore di Sanità, Viale Regina Elena 299, 00161 Rome, Italy; mariantonia.logozzi@iss.it (M.L.); rossella.diraimo@iss.it (R.D.R.); davide.mizzoni@iss.it (D.M.)
2. National Center for Global Health, Istituto Superiore di Sanità, Viale Regina Elena 299, 00161 Rome, Italy; mauro.andreotti@iss.it
3. Centro Nazionale Sperimentazione e Benessere Animale, Istituto Superiore di Sanità, Viale Regina Elena 299, 00161 Rome, Italy; massimo.spada@iss.it (M.S.); daniele.macchia@iss.it (D.M.)
* Correspondence: stefano.fais@iss.it; Tel.: +39-0649903195; Fax: +39-0649902436
† These authors contributed equally to this work.

Received: 9 January 2020; Accepted: 5 February 2020; Published: 7 February 2020

Abstract: In recent decades much attention has been paid to how dietary antioxidants may positively affect the human health, including the beneficial effects of fermented foods and beverages. Fermented Papaya Preparation (FPP®) has been shown to represent a valuable approach to obtain systemic antioxidants effect. In this study, we wanted to verify whether FPP® had a clear and scientifically supported in vivo anti-aging effect together with the induction of a systemic antioxidant reaction. To this purpose we daily treated a mouse model suitable for aging studies (C57BL/6J) with FPP®-supplemented water from either the 6th weeks (early treatment) or the 51th weeks (late treatment) of age as compared to mice receiving only tap water. After 10 months of FPP® treatment, we evaluated the telomerase activity, antioxidants and Reactive Oxygen Species ROS plasmatic levels and the telomeres length in the bone marrow and ovaries in both mice groups. The results showed that the daily FPP® assumption induced increase in telomeres length in bone marrow and ovary, together with an increase in the plasmatic levels of telomerase activity, and antioxidant levels, with a decrease of ROS. Early treatment resulted to be more effective, suggesting a potential key role of FPP® in preventing the age-related molecular damages.

Keywords: FPP®; nutraceutical supplementation; C57BL/6J; anti-aging effect; antioxidant effect; telomeres; telomerase; SOD-1; GSH

1. Introduction

Fermentation is one the most ancient methods of food preparation that exploits the growth and metabolic activities of microorganisms to preserve and transform food materials [1,2]. During this process, growth of spoilage and pathogenic organisms is inhibited by secondary metabolites produced by fermenting organisms, preserving and extending the storage of perishable foods [3,4]. Beyond conservation, fermentation gives to food a characteristic aroma and taste and enhance their organoleptic profiles and palatability, digestibility of proteins and carbohydrates, and the bioavailability of vitamins and minerals [4–7]. Since ancient times, fermented foods and beverages have been a fundamental part of human diet and their beneficial effects in reducing cholesterol levels and blood pressure, boosting immune system, protecting from toxic pathogens and in the prevention of carcinogenesis, osteoporosis, diabetes, cardiovascular and hepatic diseases have been widely characterized [8]. Moreover, fermented foods and beverages have a strong impact on human gut microbiota. It is well established that intestinal bacteria modulate the metabolic profile of the host, also influencing the immune system [9,10] and maintaining the structure and function of the intestinal tract [11,12]. The interactions between ingested fermented food and microbiota constitute a rapidly expanding field of study, focusing in particular on human health impact [12–16].

More than 100 years ago Metchnikoff, Nobel prize winner for the discovery of macrophages, already claimed that the longevity of some populations of Eastern Europe was due to the high quantity of fermented food in their diet [17] and more recently it has been shown that microbiota in the elderly is strongly influenced by diet, opening up that healthy ageing is associated with microbial diversity [18,19].

Fermented Papaya Preparation (FPP®, Immun'Âge®) is one of the fermented foods that have proven positive effects on brain health; FPP® is a product resulting from yeast fermentation of non-genetically modified *Carica Papaya* Linn, which is marketed as a natural dietary functional health supplement under the brand name of Immun'Âge® [20,21]. FPP® is a powerful antioxidant and nutraceutical adjuvant in combined therapies against various diseases [22–29], including cancer [22,25,30]. The FPP® more documented actions are as a free radical regulator [31], as immunomodulator [32–36] and as antioxidant [37,38]. In fact, FPP® has shown a powerful *in vitro* anti-oxidative activity on brain cells [39], as well on *in vivo* experimental model of epilepsy consistently reducing neural release of epileptogenic monoamine [40]. Moreover, FPP® showed a clear action in reducing the derangement of oxidant/antioxidant balance at the brain level in elderly rats and in experimental ischemia-reperfusion model [20,41,42]; FPP® modulates oxidative DNA damage, protecting brain from oxidative damage in hypertensive rats and reducing genotoxic effect of H_2O_2 [43], and protecting the body from the aging-related diseases [44–47], including neurodegenerative diseases [47–49]. However, a clear *in vivo* action of FPP® on the molecular signature of aging, such as telomerase activity and telomeres length has not been provided yet.

In this study we investigated the role of in vivo FPP® administration in the induction of an antioxidant action together with an anti-aging effect. The experimental design provided that the mice received the FPP® in water either from 6 weeks (ET-FPP® group: early treatment with FPP®), or from 51 weeks of life (LT-FPP® group: late treatment with FPP®), as compared to mice receiving FPP®-free tap water (CTR group). For both treatment groups, at the end of treatment period (10 months), we evaluated antioxidants (Total Antioxidant Capacity, SOD-1 and GSH), ROS and telomerase activity levels in blood samples, and telomeres length in single cell suspensions from the bone morrow and the ovaries of the mice. Our results showed the effect of FPP® in inducing a clear systemic antioxidant reaction (higher of SOD-1 and GSH plasma levels) along with an increased telomerase activity and longer telomeres in both the bone marrow and the ovaries of the treated mice. Lastly, FPP® was more effective when it starts at an early age as compared to late treatment.

2. Materials and Methods

2.1. Immun'Âge®-FPP® (Fermented Papaya Preparation)

The FPP® (Immun'Âge®, patent number 6401792, Osato Research Institute, Gifu, Japan), used in the present study was obtained from *Carica papaya* L. cultivated in Hawaii, followed by yeast fermentation for 10 months and batch-to-batch checking at the Osato Research Institute. FPP® was dissolved in tap water and administrated every day without interruption.

2.2. In Vivo Studies

For our analysis, we have chosen an aging female mouse model (C57BL/6J), in order to have available cells from organs with either gender-independent (i.e., the bone marrow) or gender-dependent (i.e., ovaries) functions, and divided mice into two groups: FPP® was daily administered to the first group for 10 months from 6 weeks old (6 to 51 weeks of age) (ET-FPP®: early treatment with FPP®) and to the second group for 10 months from 51 weeks old (51 to 96 weeks of age) (LT-FPP: late treatment with FPP®); in both conditions a control group was included receiving tap water only (ET-CTR and LT-CTR). Each group consisted of 10 animals for statistical significance. To compare the mice treatment groups to the human age, ET treatment corresponded to women starting FPP®at 13 years and ending FPP® at 41 years of age; while LT treatment starting at 41 years and ending at 63 years of age. (Figure 1).

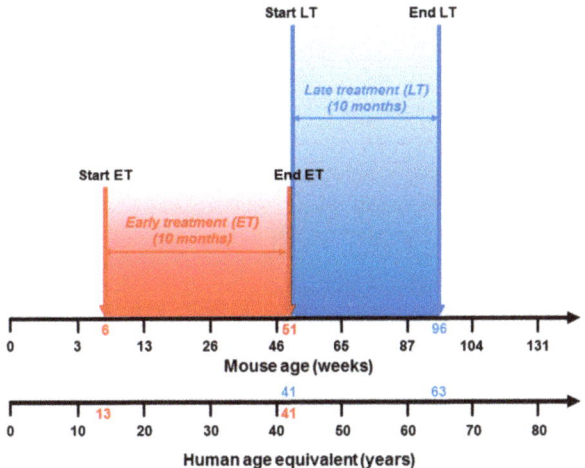

Figure 1. Equivalence between mice age and human age. Early treatment of mice from 6 weeks to 51 weeks of age corresponds to treatment in humans from 13- to 41-years old. Late treatment of mice from 51 weeks to 96 weeks of age corresponds to treatment in humans from 41- to 63-years old.

Each treated mice drank 1 mL of FPP®-supplemented water every day, corresponding to 6 mg/mouse/day of FPP®. Just before mice sacrifice, blood was withdrawn from mice eyes. Immediately after the sacrifice, bone marrow was isolated from both tibias and femurs of the mice hind legs, while ovaries were retrieval from reproductive system. Blood, bone marrow cells and ovarian germ cells were used for subsequent experimental analysis of aging parameters.

All the studies were approved by the ethical committee of the Italian National Institute of Health (Rome, Italy) and were conducted in accordance with the current Italian Law (Law 26/2014), authorization n∘792/2017-PR (prot. D9997.49 27/06/2017), that regulates experiments in laboratory animals. 40 C57BL/6J female mice between 16 and 20 g (4 weeks of age) were purchased from Charles River Laboratories Italia s.r.l., (Calco, Lecco, Italy), and housed in the animal facility of the Italian National Institute of Health. Mice had 10 and 14 h periods of light and darkness respectively, were housed in a different number of animal cages, depending on the experiment, with ad libitum mice chow (Mucedola, Settimo Milanese (MI), Italy) and water intake. Accordingly to the guidelines for a correct laboratory practice and signs of poor quality of life, a veterinarian responsible for animal welfare checked mice twice a week, to monitor signs of sufferance such as weight loss, decreased water and food consumption, poor hair coat, decreased activity levels and tumor ulcerations

2.3. Total Antioxidant Power Assay (PAO Test Kit)

Detection and quantification of Total Antioxidant Power was performed in FPP®-supplemented water using a colorimetric assay: PAO Test kit for Total Antioxidant Capacity (JaICA, Japan). The assay can detect not only hydrophilic antioxidants such as Vitamin C, glutathione, but also can detect hydrophobic antioxidants such as Vitamin E. The determination of the antioxidant power is carried out using the reduction of the cupric ion (Cu^{++} to Cu^{+}). Briefly, samples were incubated for 3 min at room temperature with Cu^{++} solution, Cu^{++} are reduced by antioxidants to form Cu^+ that reacts with chromatic solution (bathocuproine), and can be detected by absorbance at wavelength 480 to 490 nm. Antioxidant capacity can be calculated from the Cu^+ formed. Absorbance was recorded at 490 nm.

2.4. Ascorbic Acid Assay

Detection and quantification of Ascorbic Acid in FPP®-supplemented water was performed using a fluorometric Ascorbic Acid Assay Kit (Abcam, Cambridge, UK). Samples were diluted in ascorbic acid buffer in 96-well plate and subsequently to each well was added catalyst and then reaction mix. After 3 min of incubation, fluorescence was read in microplate reader at Ex/Em = 535/590 nm.

2.5. Collection and Processing of Murine Plasma from Blood Samples

Blood samples collection from each group mice was performed by retro-orbital bleeding (ROB) immediately before the sacrifice. This safe phlebotomy technique allowed to obtain high-quality samples of adequate volume (500 µL/mouse) for analysis [50]. Blood samples were collected in K3-EDTA-coated collection tubes. To obtain plasma samples, EDTA-treated whole blood from each mouse was centrifuged at 400 g for 20 min. Plasma samples (250 µL/mouse) were then collected and immediately analyzed or stored at −80 °C until analysis.

2.5.1. Total Antioxidant Power Assay (PAO Test kit)

Detection and quantification of Total Antioxidant Power was in mice plasma obtained before the sacrifice using a colorimetric assay: PAO Test kit for Total Antioxidant Capacity (JaICA). After centrifugation of blood at 400× g for 20 min, supernatant was collected and immediately analyzed. Briefly, samples were incubated for 3 minutes at room temperature with Cu^{++} solution, subsequently Stop Solution was added to each well. Absorbance was recorded at 490 nm.

2.5.2. Superoxide Dismutase (SOD) Activity Assay

The Superoxide Dismutase Activity kit (Thermo Fisher, Waltham, MA, USA), a colorimetric assay, was used for detection and quantification of superoxide dismutase activity in mice plasma preparations. Plasma samples were incubated for 20 min at room temperature after the addition of the sample and substrate and chromogenic detection reagent. The optical densities were recorded at 450 nm.

2.5.3. Reduced Glutathione (GSH) Detection and Quantification Assay

Glutathione Colorimetric Detection Kit (Thermo Fisher), a colorimetric assay, was used for detection and quantification of reduced glutathione (GSH) levels in plasma preparations. Detection reagent and reaction mixture were added to samples and after 20 min of incubation at room temperature the optical densities were recorded at 405 nm.

2.5.4. Total Reactive Oxygen Species (ROS) Assay

Total Reactive Oxygen Species (ROS) Assay Kit 520 nm (Thermo Fisher) was used to analyze the total ROS levels in mice plasma preparations. 10 µl of each plasma sample were added to 100 µL of 1× ROS Assay Stain. After for 60 min of incubation at 37 °C and 5% CO_2, signals were analyzed using a fluorescent microplate reader off the 488 nm (blue laser) in the FITC channel.

2.5.5. Detection of telomerase by ELISA Assay

Quantitative determination of mouse telomerase concentrations was performed in plasma preparations using a colorimetric sandwich-ELISA assay, Mouse TE(telomerase) ELISA Kit (Elabsciences®, Houston, TX, USA. The optical density (OD) was measured at 450 ± 2 nm.

2.6. Bone Marrow Cells Recovery from Mice

Immediately after the sacrifice of CTR, ET-FPP® and LT-FPP® mice, bone marrow was obtained from both tibias and femurs of the hind legs of mice [51–54]. Bone marrow was then placed in physiological solution (NaCl) and disrupted with the blunt end of a 5-mL syringe plunger. Bone marrow cells were isolated using a Falcon® 100 µm cell strainer (Corning, Corning, NY, USA), obtaining a uniform single-cell suspension from bone marrow. The single-cell suspensions were washed twice in PBS and immediately processed for following analysis.

2.7. Ovarian Germ Cells Recovery from Mice

Immediately after the sacrifice of CTR, ET-FPP® and LT-FPP® mice, ovaries were dissected [51–53,55], placed in physiological solution (NaCl) with 1% of trypsin and 0.1 µM of EDTA, separated from the remaining reproductive system with a cutter and disrupted with the blunt end of a 5-mL syringe plunger. Ovarian germ cells were isolated using a Falcon® 100 µm cell strainer (Corning), connective tissue and debris were allowed to settle, obtaining a uniform single-cell suspension from ovarian tissue. The single-cell suspensions were washed twice in PBS and immediately processed for following analysis.

2.8. Detection of Telomeres by PNA Kit/FITC for Flow Cytometry

Detection of telomeres was performed in bone marrow cells and in ovarian germ cells of CTR, ET-FPP® and LT-FPP® mice obtained immediately after the sacrifice. To this purpose a Telomere PNA Kit/FITC for Flow Cytometry (Dako-Agilent, Santa Clara, CA, USA) was used. The kit allows detection of telomeres in nucleated haematopoietic cells using a fluorescence in situ hybridization and a fluorescein-conjugated peptide nucleic acid (PNA) probe. Results were evaluated by flow cytometry using a light source with excitation at 488 nm.

2.9. Statistical Analysis

Results in the text are reported as means ± standard error (SE), and calculation were done using the GraphPad Prism software (San Diego, CA, USA). Unpaired t-test (Student's t-test) was applied to analyze the results. Statistical significance was set at $p < 0.05$.

3. Results

3.1. Evaluation of FPP®-Supplemented Water Effectiveness

The experimental design has been set up in order to evaluate *in vivo* the effectiveness of FPP® supplementation on redox balance and molecular signature of aging. Although the greater efficacy of FPP® was proven when taken sublingually [28], we found that this administration was very stressful for mice [30], so we decided to dissolve FPP® in the daily water.

In order to verify the real *in vivo* effectiveness of the non-orthodox FPP® administration following dissolution in water, we have first evaluated the papaya antioxidant capacity when dissolved in water by a colorimetric test. Each day a sachet of FPP® (3 g) was dissolved in 500 mL of water and administered to mice; each FPP® mouse drank about 1 mL a day, with the resulting dose of 6 mg/mouse/day FPP® taken every day. Therefore, same doses of papaya dissolved in water (500 mL for each cage) and taken by each mouse were analyzed for quantification of antioxidant power. We used a test that allowed us to estimate the total content of both hydrophilic (for example Ascorbic Acid) and hydrophobic antioxidants. As shown in Table 1, FPP® in 500 mL of water had a Total Antioxidant Power of 6.7 ± 0.6 M, and in 1 mL taken by each FPP-treated mouse 13.48 ± 0.9 mM. Ascorbic acid is one of the hydrophilic antioxidants that can be quantified and, as for the Total Antioxidant Power, we measured ascorbic acid concentrations of a FPP® sachet dissolved in 500 mL and of FPP® dose taken by the mouse daily by fluorimetric assay. The papaya sachet in 500 mL of water had an ascorbic acid content equal to 192.2 ± 3.5 ng, while the mouse daily dose was 0.4 ± 0.03 ng (Table 1).

Table 1. Total Antioxidant Power and Ascorbic Acid quantification in FPP®-supplemented water.

	FPP® in 500 mL Water (the Amount in a Bottle for Each Cage)	FPP® Drank by Mice Daily
Total Antioxidant Power	6.7 ± 0.6 M	13.48 ± 0.9 mM
Ascorbic Acid	192.2 ± 3.5 ng	0.4 ± 0.03 ng

Data are expressed as mean ± SE of three experiments.

3.2. Early Treatment with FPP®: from 6 to 51 Weeks of Age

3.2.1. Oral Administration of FFP® Increases Plasma Levels of Antioxidants

To the purpose of evaluating comparable effect in our experimental model, we first measured the Total Antioxidant Power in plasma samples of FPP® in both treated and untreated mice; this test allows to detect both hydrophilic and hydrophobic antioxidant in blood samples. The results showed that mice daily treated with FPP® (Figure 2A) had an increased antioxidant power (ET-FPP® 11.9 ± 1.4 mM, $p < 0.05$) as compared to the control group (ET-CTR 7.6 ± 0.4 mM).

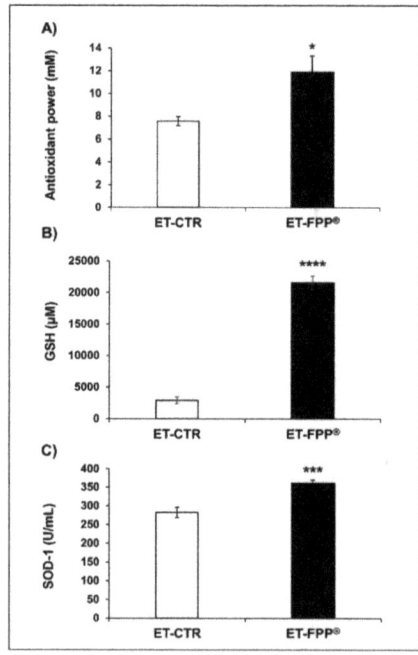

Figure 2. Antioxidant effect of FPP® in C57BL/6J female mice by measuring the plasma antioxidant levels (antioxidant power, GSH and SOD-1). Plasma samples collected from both untreated (ET-CTR group) and treated (ET-FPP®group) mice were analyzed. (**A**) Analysis of the quantification and detection of the total antioxidant power (mM). (**B**) Analysis of the quantification and detection of GSH activity (μM). (**C**) Analysis of the quantification and detection of SOD-1 activity (U/mL). Data are normalized on total plasma and expressed as means ± SE. * $p < 0.05$, *** $p < 0.001$, **** $p < 0.0001$.

Thus, we measured the enzymatic activities of superoxide dismutase-1 (SOD-1) and plasmatic levels of reduced glutathione (GSH). SOD-1 is an enzymatic antioxidant responsible for the dissociation of superoxide anion into hydrogen peroxide and dioxygen; glutathione is a non-enzymatic antioxidant as represented by the glutathione reduced form (GSH), that plays the important role of protector against oxidative stress neutralizing reactive oxygen species.

The results showed that ET-FPP® -treated mice presented a significant increase of GSH plasmatic levels ($p < 0.0001$) of about 7.5-fold higher as compared to control plasma samples (ET-FPP® 21558 ± 1100 μM, ET-CTR 2896 ± 574 μM) (Figure 2B). Comparable results were obtained with SOD-1 analysis, where SOD-1 plasmatic levels in FPP® treated mice were significantly higher (ET-FPP® 361 ± 9 U/mL, $p < 0.001$) as compared to control mice (ET-CTR 282 ± 13 U/mL) (Figure 2C). These results supported a potentially powerful in vivo antioxidant action exerted by FPP® administered to mice from 6 weeks of age (early treatment), even when administered as dissolved in the water.

3.2.2. Oral Administration of FFP® Reduces Plasma Levels of ROS

Although Reactive Oxygen Species (ROS) and ROS-induced oxidative damage are not considered as the sole cause of aging, it is believed that ROS play a key role in the molecular mechanisms regulating longevity. For this reason, we evaluated and determined the effect of FPP® supplementation on plasmatic levels of ROS in our experimental model. The results in Figure 3 showed a significant decrease ($p < 0.005$) of plasmatic ROS levels in ET-FPP® mice (7737 ± 331 a.u.) as compared to ET-CTR group (10962 ± 692 a.u.).

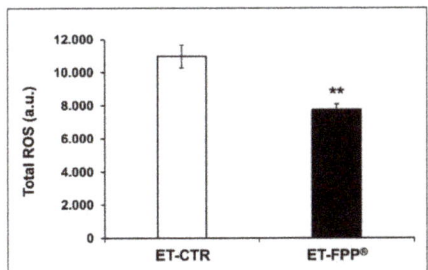

Figure 3. Effect of FPP® on total ROS blood levels in C57BL/6J female mice. Analysis of the total ROS levels (arbitrary units, a.u.) on the plasma samples collected from both ET-CTR and ET-FPP®. Data are normalized on total plasma and expressed as means ± SE. ** $p < 0.005$.

3.2.3. Oral Administration of FFP® Increases Plasmatic Telomerase Activity

Telomerase (TE) is an enzyme that adds repetitive sequences of DNA to the chromosomal ends (telomeres); at each DNA replication, the telomeres undergo shortening and the task of telomerase is to maintain their integrity. In fact, in the absence of telomerase, the telomeres progressively shorten until they reach a threshold value where cell division stops, thus inducing cell senescence. Telomerase activity and telomeres length are currently considered the molecular signature of aging. To this purpose, we first determined and quantified the telomerase activity in the plasmas of FPP®-treated mice (ET-FPP®) as compared to the control group (ET-CTR).

As shown in Figure 4, we observed an increase in telomerase concentration of mice daily treated with FPP® as compared to mice drinking tap water. More in details, ET-FPP® mice had a concentration of TE 1.6-fold higher ($p < 0.005$) as compared to ET-CTR (ET-FPP® mice: 88.5 ± 4.5 ng/mL, ET-CTR mice: 55.9 ± 6.6 ng/mL).

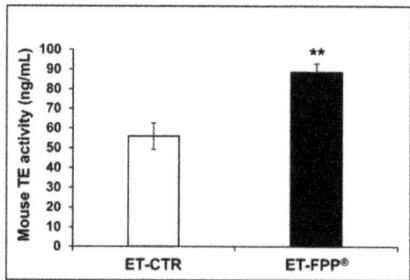

Figure 4. Effect of FPP® on telomerase (TE) activity in plasma samples from C57BL/6J female mice. Quantitative determination of mouse telomerase (TE) activity (ng/mL) was performed on plasma samples obtained from both ET-CTR and ET-FPP® groups immediately before the sacrifice. Data are normalized on total plasma and expressed as means ± SE. ** $p < 0.005$.

3.2.4. Oral Administration of FFP® Increases Telomeres Length in Bone Marrow Cells and Ovarian Germ Cells

In order to evaluate the effect of FPP® treatment on telomeres length, we analyzed single cell suspensions obtained from both bone marrow and ovaries of either FPP® treated or untreated mice. To this purpose bone marrow and ovaries were obtained from each mouse and the single cell suspensions were isolated as described in the Materials and Methods section; subsequently bone marrow and ovarian germ cells were counted by trypan blue exclusion under optical microscope. In ET-FPP® mice bone marrow and ovarian germ cells were respectively almost 4-fold and 2-fold more than the ET-CTR cells (data not shown).

Comparable numbers of cells obtained from both organs were analyzed by hybridization of a fluorescein-conjugated probe (PNA) recognizing the sequence of six nucleotides (TTAGGG) repeated in the telomeres. The results, expressed as mean intensity of fluorescence (M.I.F.), are summarized in Figure 5. TTAGGG sequence in telomeres correlated with the value of the M.I.F.

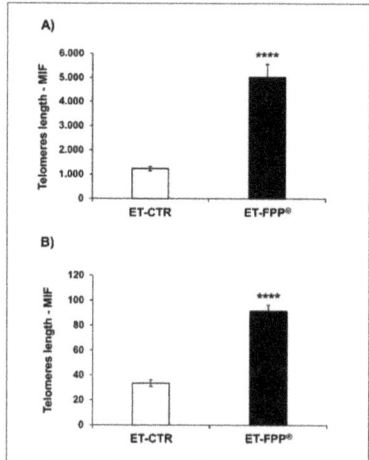

Figure 5. Effect of FPP® on telomeres length in bone marrow cells and in ovarian germ cells from C57BL/6J female mice. The analysis of telomeres length was performed on nucleated haematopoietic cells from (**A**) bone marrow and (**B**) on ovarian germ cells. Cells were retrieved from both ET-CTR and ET-FPP® groups immediately after the sacrifice. Data are expressed as mean ± SE of M.I.F. (Mean Intensity Fluorescence) normalized on total cells. **** $p < 0.0001$.

The results showed that ET-FPP® mice had an impressive increase of telomeres length than ET-CTR in both organs. In details the telomeres lenght in bone marrow cells was 4-fold higher than in control group (ET-FPP®: 5020 ± 542 M.I.F, ET-CTR: 1228 ± 88 M.I.F., $p < 0.0001$) (Figure 5A), while in ovarian germ cells the telomeres length was 2.7-fold higher as compared to controls (ET-FPP®: 91 ± 5 M.I.F., ET-CTR 33 ± 3 M.I.F., $p < 0.0001$) (Figure 5B).

3.3. Late Treatment with FPP®: from 51 to 96 Weeks of Age

This set of experiments was aimed at evaluating the FPP® anti-aging effect in a group of mice that started the treatment later in their life (10 months) (LT-FPP®). As for ET-FPP® mice, we measured antioxidants and ROS levels and telomerase in the blood and the telomeres length in single cell suspensions obtained from the bone marrow and the ovaries of the mice.

3.3.1. Oral Administration of FFP® Increases Plasma Levels of Antioxidants

The results showed that Total Antioxidant Power levels in LT-FPP® (8 ± 0.17 mM) were comparable ($p > 0.05$, not significant) to LT-CTR (7.5 ± 0.13 mM) (Figure 6A); similarly to previous results in ET-FPP® mice, GSH plasmatic levels resulted to be 279.5 ± 24.9 µM in LT-FPP® mice ($p < 0.05$) and 208.9 ± 11.2 µM in LT-CTR (Figure 6B), and SOD-1 levels 89.9 ± 1.5 U/mL in LT-FPP® mice ($p < 0.05$) and 78.3 ± 4.3 U/mL in LT-CTR group (Figure 6C). It is clear from the figures that while the significant increase in the SOD-1 and GSH plasma levels in the FPP® -treated mice, the absolute values are lower than in the group of mice that started the FPP® treatment earlier in their life (Figure 2).

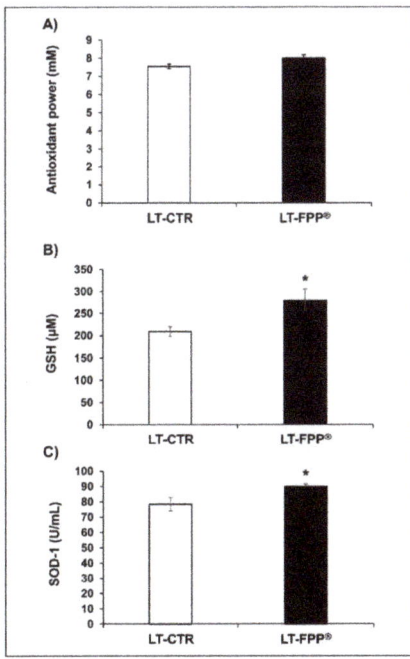

Figure 6. Antioxidant effect of FPP® in C57BL/6J female mice by measuring the plasma antioxidant levels (antioxidant power, GSH and SOD-1). Plasma samples collected from both untreated (LT-CTR group) and treated (LT-FPP® group) mice were analyzed. (**A**) Analysis of the quantification and detection of the total antioxidant power (mM). (**B**) Analysis of the quantification and detection of GSH activity (µM). (**C**) Analysis of the quantification and detection of SOD-1 activity (U/mL). Data are normalized on total plasma and expressed as means ± SE. * $p < 0.05$.

3.3.2. Oral Administration of FFP® Reduces Plasma Levels of ROS

This set of results did not show significant difference in the plasmatic ROS levels between the FPP®-treated and untreated mice ($p > 0.05$, not significant). In fact, LT-FPP® mice had ROS levels of 10727 ± 157 a.u. and LT-CTR mice 11266 ± 198 a.u. (Figure 7).

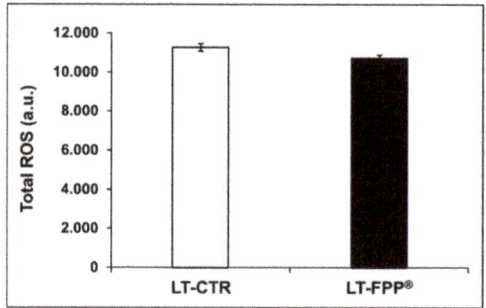

Figure 7. Effect of FFP® on total ROS blood levels in C57BL/6J female mice. Analysis of the total ROS levels (arbitrary units, a. u.) on the plasma samples collected from both LT-CTR and LT-FPP®. Data are normalized on total plasma and expressed as means ± SE. p = NS (>0.05).

3.3.3. Oral Administration of FFP® Increases Plasmatic Telomerase Activity

Analysis of telomerase activity was performed also for LT-FPP® mice LT-CTR controls. As for the early treatment, in this case the mice that received water supplemented with FPP® showed a higher telomerase concentration (LT-FPP®: 124.0 ± 9.0 ng/mL, $p < 0.05$) than the mice that drank only tap water (LT-CTR: 92.5 ± 6.5 ng/mL) (Figure 8).

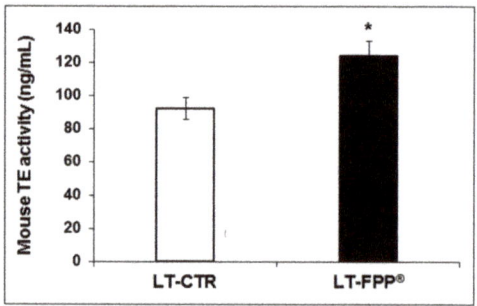

Figure 8. Effect of FFP® on telomerase (TE) activity in plasma samples from C57BL/6J female mice. Quantitative determination of mouse telomerase (TE) activity (ng/mL) was performed on plasma samples obtained from both LT-CTR and LT-FPP® groups immediately before the sacrifice. Data are normalized on total plasma and expressed as means ± SE. * $p < 0.05$.

3.3.4. Oral Administration of FFP® Increases Telomeres Length in Bone Marrow Cells and Ovarian Germ Cells

As previously described, bone marrow and ovarian germ cells were obtained from each mouse and hybridized of with a fluorescein-conjugated probe (PNA) for telomeres length analysis. As for the previous group of experiments cells were counted by trypan blue exclusion under optical microscope and the results showed that the number of bone marrow and ovarian germ cells in LT-FPP® mice was increased 1.8-fold and 2-fold, respectively, as compared to cells obtained from LT-CTR mice. The results on telomeres length showed that cells from the bone marrow of LT-FPP® treated mice had 2-fold longer telomeres (121 ± 6 M.I.F., $p < 0.0005$) as compared to LT-CTR 59 ± 9 M.I.F. (Figure 9A).

Similarly, telomeres analyzed from ovarian germ cells of LT-FPP® mice were significantly longer (8.69 ± 0.25 M.I.F., $p < 0.05$) than telomeres from untreated mice (7.29 ± 0.44 M.I.F.) (Figure 9B). Consistent with the anti-oxidant reaction the M.I.F. signals in both bone marrow and ovarian germ cells were significantly decreased in LT-FPP® as compared to ET-FPP®.

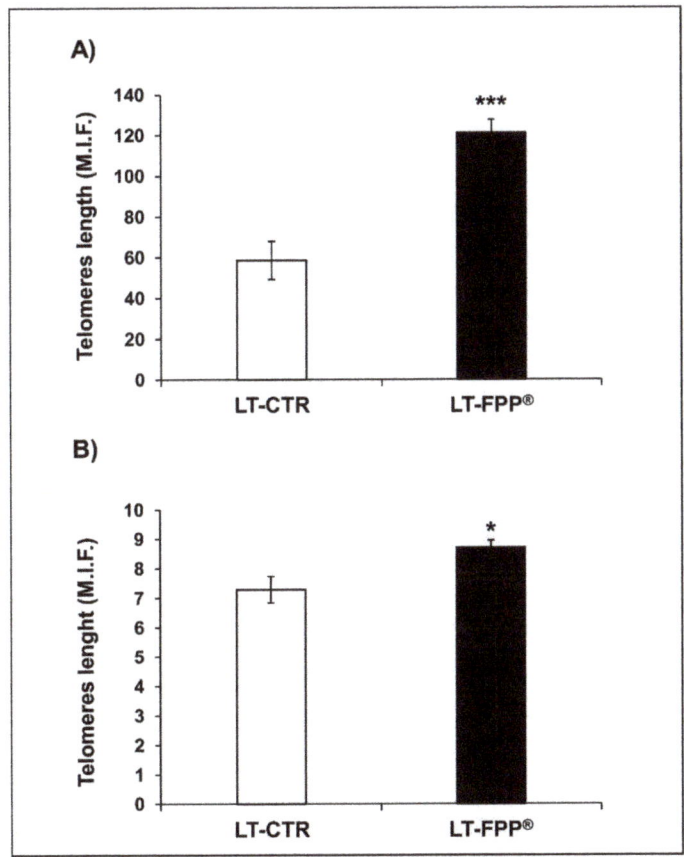

Figure 9. Effect of FPP® on telomeres length in bone marrow cells and in ovarian germ cells from C57BL/6J female mice. The analysis of telomeres length was performed on nucleated haematopoietic cells from (**A**) bone marrow and (**B**) on ovarian germ cells. Cells were retrieved from both LT-CTR and LT-FPP® groups immediately after the sacrifice. Data are expressed as mean ± SE of M.I.F. (Mean Intensity Fluorescence) normalized on total cells. * $p < 0.05$, *** $p < 0.0005$.

3.4. Comparison of FPP® Effectiveness between Early Treatment and Late Treatment Supplementation

We thus wanted to compare the early to the late FPP® treatment in terms of percentage of ratio between FPP®-treated mice and untreated controls. As shown in Table 2, the most beneficial effects are observed with the early treatment.

Comparing ET-FPP® and LT-FPP® values with their respective control, we could observe that the early treatment with FPP® was impressively more effective in increasing the plasmatic levels of the antioxidant power (increase of 56%) as compared to the late treatment (1%) that was in fact comparable to CTR.

In the case of GSH the differences between early and late treatment were straightforward: in the case of ET mice GSH plasmatic level was increased of 640% compared to control, while we observed only 34% of increase in the LT group. Also SOD-1 levels were higher in the early treated mice (30%), as compared to the late treatment (15%). Moreover, FPP® showed a greater effect in decreasing total ROS levels when administered early (30% of decrease) than in LT-FPP® group (5% of decrease).

Comparable results were obtained with telomerase levels (58% increase in ET-FPP® mice and 34% in LT-FPP®) as compared to controls, and telomeres length in bone marrow and ovarian germ cells (length increase of 300% and 174% in ET-FPP® and 101% and 19% in LT-FPP®, respectively). All in all this analysis allows to conclude that the early treatment with FPP® starting from 6 weeks of life was the most effective.

Table 2. Comparison between ET- and LT-treatment.

	ET-FPP®	LT-FPP®
Total Antioxidant Power	+56%	+1%
GSH	+640%	+34%
SOD-1	+30%	+15%
Total ROS	−30%	−5%
Telomerase	+58%	+34%
Telomeres length of bone marrow cells	+300%	+101%
Telomeres length of ovarian germ cells	+174%	+19%

Results are expressed as percentage ratio between value of FPP® mice and respective control.

4. Discussion

The improved living conditions, reduced rate of child mortality and advances in the medical field have led to an increased life expectancy compared to past decades. Despite this, aging and in particular age-related diseases are still major causes of mortality worldwide. Aging is characterized by a loss of fitness over time, with a series of molecular and macromolecular damages over the course of a lifetime. Faulty regulation of cellular processes could damage physiological integrity of cells and let to accumulation of damaged bioproducts. Among the various phenomena associated with aging, there is oxidative stress, characterized by the loss of balance of antioxidants/reactive oxygen species, with an accumulation of ROS at the cellular level. At the molecular level, there is a progressive shortening of the telomeres that, reached a threshold level, lead to cellular senescence and/or apoptosis. Crucial is the role of telomerase, a polymerase that can elongate telomeres by de novo addition of TTAGGG sequence repeated in telomeres.

In this study, we evaluated the effect of FPP® on redox balance (antioxidant and ROS levels) together with an anti-aging effect on telomerase concentration and telomeres length in a mice model of aging treated with FPP®-supplemented water from 6 weeks of age (early treatment) and from 51 weeks of age (late treatment). Interestingly, we showed that FPP® dissolved in water had a higher Total Antioxidant Power and it contains measurable amount of Ascorbic Acid and we were able to measure the daily dose of ascorbic acid taken by the FPP®-treated mice. The dual action of ascorbic acid as scavenging antioxidant and pro-antioxidant and the direct correlation between ascorbic acid dietary intake and the increased amount of antioxidants levels (i.e. glutathione) have been previously demonstrated [56–60].

Our data are consistent with previous works, where the correlation between dietary antioxidants from fruits and vegetables and the effects on the increase of antioxidant levels in the treated subjects has been extensively studied [9,10]. Our results showed that the daily intake of FPP® significantly increased the levels of antioxidants in the blood (Total Antioxidant Power, GSH and SOD-1) and decreased the levels of total ROS, together with a clear anti-aging effect as shown by the length of telomeres and telomerase quantification in FPP® treated mice. These results are consistent with previous studies where the crucial role of FPP® in reducing oxidative stress and inducing the antioxidant defense response have been extensively investigated [22–29,37,38,61]. Previous reports have shown that FPP® is able to modulate characteristic phenomena of elderly people, such as the pro-inflammatory profile [31] and the oxidative damage [44,45]. Moreover, FPP® supplementation induced several beneficial effects in patients with neurodegenerative diseases and Electromagnetic Field Intolerance Syndrome [21,43,47,48]. Supporting these reports we have shown that plasmatic telomerase concentration and the telomeres length in bone marrow and ovarian germ cells, are significantly increased by the daily FPP® administration. In our experiment, we have shown that although papaya has an effect even in beginning treatment later in life, the early treatment is far more effective. This is conceivably due to the fact that the anti-aging action of FPP® in maintaining telomeres length and mitigating progressive age-related shortening, is reduced when at a later age the telomeres have reached a shorter length. These results are consistent with previous reports on the attenuation of telomere length by antioxidants during aging [62,63] and on FPP® action in modulating aging mechanisms [44–47,49].

Similarly considering the redox balance, in ET-FPP® mice we have much higher antioxidants levels and a greater reduction of ROS than in LT-FPP® mice. The plasma levels of antioxidants, in particular GSH and SOD-1, usually decrease with increasing age [64–67], therefore in the case of LT-FPP® mice, FPP® induces an increase in GSH and SOD-1, but starting from lower basal levels, thus failing to trigger a minimally comparable anti-aging action.

5. Conclusions

Our results showed the beneficial effect of FPP® on the redox balance and anti-aging effect in mice drinking daily FPP® dissolved in water. Furthermore, our data showed that early treatment induced greater effects than late treatment. Lastly, while administered in a non-orthodox way (i.e., dissolved in water, rather than sublingually) the daily FPP® intake has shown to be highly effective in increasing the body anti-oxidant reaction and in improving the molecular signatures of aging.

Author Contributions: Conceptualization, M.L. and S.F.; Data curation, M.L., R.D.R., D.M. (Davide Mizzoni), M.A., M.S. and D.M. (Daniele Macchia); Formal analysis, M.L., R.D.R., D.M. (Davide Mizzoni)., M.A., M.S. and D.M. (Daniele Macchia); Funding acquisition, S.F.; Methodology, M.L., R.D.R., D.M. (Davide Mizzoni)., M.A., M.S. and D.M. (Daniele Macchia); Project administration, S.F.; Supervision, M.L. and S.F.; Validation, R.D.R. and D.M. (Davide Mizzoni); Visualization, R.D.R. and D.M. (Davide Mizzoni); Writing—original draft, M.L., R.D.R., D.M. (Davide Mizzoni) and S.F.; Writing—review & editing, M.L., R.D.R. and S.F. All authors have read and agreed to the published version of the manuscript.

Funding: This work was supported by OLIMED LIMITED: "The effects of fermented papaya fermentation on prevention and control of aggressive melanoma in an immunocompetent mouse model", (National Institute of Health internal classification: Fasc K66).

Conflicts of Interest: The authors declare no conflict of interest.

References

1. Nuraida, L. A review: Health Promoting Lactic Acid Bacteria in Traditional Indonesian Fermented Foods. *Food Sci. Hum. Wellness* **2015**, *4*, 47–55. [CrossRef]
2. Frias, J.; Martinez-Villaluenga, C.; Peñas, E. *Fermented Foods in Health and Disease Prevention*; Elsevier: Amsterdam, The Netherlands, 2017.
3. Dimidi, E.; Cox, S.R.; Rossi, M.; Whelan, K. Fermented Foods: Definitions and Characteristics, Impact on the Gut Microbiota and Effects on Gastrointestinal Health and Disease. *Nutrients* **2019**, *11*, 1806. [CrossRef] [PubMed]
4. Terefe, N.S. Food Fermentation. In *Reference Module in Food Science*; Elsevier: Amsterdam, The Netherlands, 2016; p. 978008100596503420.
5. Altay, F.; Karbancıoğlu-Güler, F.; Daskaya-Dikmen, C.; Heperkan, D. A Review on Traditional Turkish Fermented Non-Alcoholic Beverages: Microbiota, Fermentation Process and Quality Characteristics. *Int. J. Food Microbiol.* **2013**, *167*, 44–56. [CrossRef] [PubMed]
6. Hwang, J.; Kim, J.-C.; Moon, H.; Yang, J.-Y.; Kim, M. Determination of Sodium Contents in Traditional Fermented Foods in Korea. *J. Food Compos. Anal.* **2017**, *56*, 110–114. [CrossRef]

7. Şanlier, N.; Gökcen, B.B.; Sezgin, A.C. Health Benefits of Fermented Foods. Crit. *Rev. Food Sci. Nutr.* **2019**, *59*, 506–527. [CrossRef]
8. Tamang, J.P. *Fermented Foods and Beverages of the World*; CRC Press: Boca Raton, FL, USA, 2010; ISBN 978-1-4200-9495-4.
9. Rubio, C.A.; Schmidt, P.T. Severe Defects in the Macrophage Barrier to Gut Microflora in Inflammatory Bowel Disease and Colon Cancer. *Anticancer Res.* **2018**, *38*, 3811–3815. [CrossRef]
10. Gao, J.; Xu, K.; Liu, H.; Liu, G.; Bai, M.; Peng, C.; Li, T.; Yin, Y. Impact of the Gut Microbiota on Intestinal Immunity Mediated by Tryptophan Metabolism. *Front. Microbiol.* **2018**, *8*, 13. [CrossRef]
11. Jandhyala, S.M.; Talukdar, R.; Subramanyam, C.; Vuyyuru, H.; Sasikala, M.; Reddy, D.N. Role of the Normal Gut Microbiota. *World J. Gastroenterol.* **2015**, *21*, 8787–8803. [CrossRef]
12. Sánchez, B.; Delgado, S.; Blanco-Míguez, A.; Lourenço, A.; Gueimonde, M.; Margolles, A. Probiotics, Gut Microbiota, and Their Influence on Host Health and Disease. *Mol. Nutr. Food Res.* **2017**, *61*, 1600240. [CrossRef]
13. Singh, R.K.; Chang, H.-W.; Yan, D.; Lee, K.M.; Ucmak, D.; Wong, K.; Abrouk, M.; Farahnik, B.; Nakamura, M.; Zhu, T.H.; et al. Influence of Diet on the Gut Microbiome and Implications for Human Health. *J. Transl. Med.* **2017**, *15*, 73. [CrossRef]
14. Howarth, G.S.; Wang, H. Role of Endogenous Microbiota, Probiotics and Their Biological Products in Human Health. *Nutrients* **2013**, *5*, 58–81. [CrossRef] [PubMed]
15. Gonzalez-Sarrias, A.; Romo-Vaquero, M.; García-Villalba, R.; Cortés-Martín, A.; Selma, M.V.; Espín, J.C. The Endotoxemia Marker Lipopolysaccharide-Binding Protein is Reduced in Overweight-Obese Subjects Consuming Pomegranate Extract by Modulating the Gut Microbiota: A Randomized Clinical Trial. *Mol. Nutr. Food Res.* **2018**, *62*, 1800160. [CrossRef] [PubMed]
16. Bell, V.; Ferrão, J.; Pimentel, L.; Pintado, M.; Fernandes, T. One Health, Fermented Foods and Gut Microbiota. *Foods* **2018**, *7*, 195. [CrossRef] [PubMed]
17. Mackowiak, P.A. Recycling Metchnikoff: Probiotics, the Intestinal Microbiome and the Quest for Long Life. *Front. Public Health* **2013**, *1*, 52. [CrossRef] [PubMed]
18. Biagi, E.; Nylund, L.; Candela, M.; Ostan, R.; Bucci, L.; Pini, E.; Nikkïla, J.; Monti, D.; Satokari, R.; Franceschi, C.; et al. Through Ageing, and Beyond: Gut Microbiota and Inflammatory Status in Seniors and Centenarians. *PLoS ONE* **2010**, *5*, e10667. [CrossRef]
19. Lynch, D.B.; Jeffery, I.B.; Cusack, S.; O'Connor, E.M.; O'Toole, P.W. Diet-Microbiota-Health Interactions in Older Subjects: Implications for Healthy Aging. *Interdiscip. Top Gerontol.* **2015**, *40*, 141–154.
20. Aruoma, O.I.; Hayashi, Y.; Marotta, F.; Mantello, P.; Rachmilewitz, E.; Montagnier, L. Applications and Bioefficacy of the Functional Food Supplement Fermented Papaya Preparation. *Toxicology* **2010**, *278*, 6–16. [CrossRef]
21. Irigaray, P.; Catherine, G.; Carine, H.; Pierre, M.; Dominique, B. Beneficial Effects of a Fermented Papaya Preparation for the Treatment of Electrohypersensitivity Self-Reporting Patients: Results of a Phase I-II Clinical Trial with Special Reference to Cerebral Pulsation Measurement and Oxidative Stress Analysis. *Funct. Foods Health Dis.* **2018**, *8*, 122–144. [CrossRef]
22. Aruoma, O.I.; Somanah, J.; Bourdon, E.; Rondeau, P.; Bahorun, T. Diabetes as a Risk Factor to Cancer: Functional Role of Fermented Papaya Preparation as Phytonutraceutical Adjunct in the Treatment of Diabetes and Cancer. *Mutat. Res. Mol. Mech. Mutagen.* **2014**, *768*, 60–68. [CrossRef]
23. Dickerson, R.; Banerjee, J.; Rauckhorst, A.; Pfeiffer, D.R.; Gordillo, G.M.; Khanna, S.; Osei, K.; Roy, S. Does Oral Supplementation of a Fermented Papaya Preparation Correct Respiratory Burst Function of Innate Immune Cells in Type 2 Diabetes Mellitus Patients? *Antioxid. Redox Signal.* **2015**, *22*, 339–345. [CrossRef]
24. Marotta, F.; Koike, K.; Lorenzetti, A.; Jain, S.; Signorelli, P.; Metugriachuk, Y.; Mantello, P.; Locorotondo, N. Regulating Redox Balance Gene Expression in Healthy Individuals by Nutraceuticals: A Pilot Study. *Rejuvenation Res.* **2010**, *13*, 175–178. [CrossRef] [PubMed]
25. Otsuki, N.; Dang, N.H.; Kumagai, E.; Kondo, A.; Iwata, S.; Morimoto, C. Aqueous Extract of Carica Papaya Leaves Exhibits Anti-Tumor Activity and Immunomodulatory Effects. *J. Ethnopharmacol.* **2010**, *127*, 760–767. [CrossRef] [PubMed]
26. Fibach, E.; Rachmilewitz, E.A. The Effect of Fermented Papaya Preparation on Radioactive Exposure. *Radiat. Res.* **2015**, *184*, 304–313. [CrossRef] [PubMed]

27. Somanah, J.; Bourdon, E.; Rondeau, P.; Bahorun, T.; Aruoma, O.I. Relationship between Fermented Papaya Preparation Supplementation, Erythrocyte Integrity and Antioxidant Status in Pre-Diabetics. *Food Chem. Toxicol.* **2014**, *65*, 12–17. [CrossRef]
28. Marotta, F.; Chui, D.H.; Jain, S.; Polimeni, A.; Koike, K.; Zhou, L.; Lorenzetti, A.; Shimizu, H.; Yang, H. Effect of a Fermented Nutraceutical on Thioredoxin Level and TNF-alpha Signalling in Cirrhotic Patients. *J. Biol. Regul. Homeost. Agents* **2011**, *25*, 37–45.
29. Tomella, C.; Catanzaro, R.; Illuzzi, N.; Cabeca, A.; Zerbinati, N.; Celep, G.; Milazzo, M.; Sapienza, C.; Italia, A.; Lorenzetti, A.; et al. The Hidden Phenomenon of Oxidative Stress during Treatment of Subclinical-Mild Hypothyroidism: A Protective Nutraceutical Intervention. *Rejuvenation Res.* **2014**, *17*, 180–183. [CrossRef]
30. Logozzi, M.; Mizzoni, D.; Di Raimo, R.; Macchia, D.; Spada, M.; Fais, S. Oral Administration of Fermented Papaya (FPP®) Controls the Growth of a Murine Melanoma through the in Vivo Induction of a Natural Antioxidant Response. *Cancers* **2019**, *11*, 118. [CrossRef]
31. Marotta, F.; Koike, K.; Lorenzetti, A.; Naito, Y.; Fayet, F.; Shimizu, H.; Marandola, P. Nutraceutical Strategy in Aging: Targeting Heat Shock Protein and Inflammatory Profile through Understanding Interleukin-6 Polymorphism. *Ann. N. Y. Acad. Sci.* **2007**, *1119*, 196–202. [CrossRef]
32. Collard, E.; Roy, S. Improved Function of Diabetic Wound-Site Macrophages and Accelerated Wound Closure in Response to Oral Supplementation of a Fermented Papaya Preparation. *Antioxid. Redox Signal.* **2010**, *13*, 599–606. [CrossRef]
33. Das, A.; Dickerson, R.; Das Ghatak, P.; Gordillo, G.M.; Chaffee, S.; Saha, A.; Khanna, S.; Roy, S. May Dietary Supplementation Augment Respiratory Burst in Wound-Site Inflammatory Cells? *Antioxid. Redox Signal.* **2018**, *28*, 401–405. [CrossRef]
34. Dickerson, R.; Deshpande, B.; Gnyawali, U.; Lynch, D.; Gordillo, G.M.; Schuster, D.; Osei, K.; Roy, S. Correction of Aberrant NADPH Oxidase Activity in Blood-Derived Mononuclear Cells from Type II Diabetes Mellitus Patients by a Naturally Fermented Papaya Preparation. *Antioxid. Redox Signal.* **2012**, *17*, 485–491. [CrossRef] [PubMed]
35. Marotta, F.; Catanzaro, R.; Yadav, H.; Jain, S.; Tomella, C.; Polimeni, A.; Mantello, P. Functional foods in genomic medicine: a review of fermented papaya preparation research progress. *Acta Biomed.* **2012**, *83*, 21–29. [PubMed]
36. Rimbach, G.; Guo, Q.; Akiyama, T.; Matsugo, S.; Moini, H.; Virgili, F.; Packer, L. Ferric Nitrilotriacetate Induced DNA and Protein Damage: Inhibitory Effect of a Fermented Papaya Preparation. *Anticancer Res.* **2000**, *20*, 2907–2914. [PubMed]
37. Prus, E.; Fibach, E. The Antioxidant Effect of Fermented Papaya Preparation Involves Iron Chelation. *J. Boil. Regul. Homeost. Agents* **2012**, *26*, 203–210.
38. Rimbach, G.; Park, Y.C.; Guo, Q.; Moini, H.; Qureshi, N.; Saliou, C.; Takayama, K.; Virgili, F.; Packer, L. Nitric Oxide Synthesis and TNF-alpha Secretion in RAW 264.7 Macrophages: Mode of Action of a Fermented Papaya Preparation. *Life Sci.* **2000**, *67*, 679–694. [CrossRef]
39. Marotta, F.; Celep, G.S.; Cabeca, A.; Polimeni, A. Novel Concepts on Functional Foods and Nutrigenomics in Healthy Aging and Chronic Diseases: A Review of Fermented Papaya Preparation Research Progress. *Funct. Foods Health Dis.* **2012**, *2*, 120. [CrossRef]
40. Santiago, L.A.; Osato, J.A.; Hiramatsu, M.; Mori, A. Fermented Papaya Preparation Quenched Free Radicals and Inhibited Lipids Peroxidation in Iron- Induced Epileptic Focus in Rats. *Oxyg. Rad.* **1992**, *4*, 405–408.
41. Santiago, L.A.; Osato, J.A.; Ogawa, N.; Mori, A. Antioxidant Protection of Bio-Normalizer in Cerebral Ischaemia-Reperfusion Injury in the Gerbil. *NeuroReport* **1993**, *4*, 1031–1034. [CrossRef]
42. Zhang, J.; Mori, A.; Chen, Q.; Zhao, B. Fermented Papaya Preparation Attenuates Beta-Amyloid Precursor Protein: Beta-Amyloid-Mediated Copper Neurotoxicity in Beta-Amyloid Precursor Protein and Beta-Amyloid Precursor Protein Swedish Mutation Overexpressing SH-SY5Y Cells. *Neuroscience* **2006**, *143*, 63–72. [CrossRef]
43. Aruoma, O.I.; Colognato, R.; Fontana, I.; Gartlon, J.; Migliore, L.; Koike, K.; Coecke, S.; Lamy, E.; Mersch-Sundermann, V.; Laurenza, I.; et al. Molecular Effects of Fermented Papaya Preparation on Oxidative Damage, MAP Kinase Activation and Modulation of the Benzo[a]Pyrene Mediated Genotoxicity. *BioFactors* **2006**, *26*, 147–159. [CrossRef]

44. Marotta, F.; Weksler, M.; Marandola, P.; Naito, Y.; Yoshida, C.; Yoshioka, M. Nutraceutical Supplementation: Effect of a Fermented Papaya Preparation on Redox Status and DNA Damage in Healthy Elderly Individuals and Relationship with GSTM1 Genotype: A Randomized, Placebo-Controlled, Cross-Over Study. *Ann. N. Y. Acad. Sci.* **2006**, *1067*, 400–407. [CrossRef] [PubMed]
45. Marotta, F.; Pavasuthipaisit, K.; Yoshida, C.; Albergati, F.; Marandola, P. Relationship Between Aging and Susceptibility of Erythrocytes to Oxidative Damage: In View of Nutraceutical Interventions. *Rejuvenation Res.* **2006**, *9*, 227–230. [CrossRef] [PubMed]
46. Bertuccelli, G.; Zerbinati, N.; Marcellino, M.; Kumar, N.S.N.; He, F.; Tsepakolenko, V.; Cervi, J.; Lorenzetti, A.; Marotta, F. Effect of a Quality-Controlled Fermented Nutraceutical on Skin Aging Markers: An Antioxidant-Control, Double-Blind Study. *Exp. Ther. Med.* **2016**, *11*, 909–916. [CrossRef] [PubMed]
47. Marotta, F.; Marcellino, M.; Solimene, U.; Cuffari, B.; Yadav, H.; Khokhlov, A.N.; Lorenzetti, A.; Mantello, A.; Cervi, J.; Catanzaro, R. A 2-year Double-Blind RCT Follow-up Study with Fermented Papaya Preparation (FPP) Modulating Key Markers in Middle-Age Subjects with Clustered Neurodegenerative Disease-Risk Factors. *Clin. Pharmacol. Biopharm.* **2017**, *6*, 1–9. [CrossRef]
48. Barbagallo, M.; Marotta, F.; Dominguez, L.J. Oxidative Stress in Patients with Alzheimer's Disease: Effect of Extracts of Fermented Papaya Powder. *Mediat. Inflamm.* **2015**, *2015*. [CrossRef]
49. Bolner, A.; Micciolo, R.; Bosello, O.; Nordera, G. Effect of Papaya Supplementation on Oxidative Stress Markers in Parkinsons Disease. *Oxid. Antioxid. Med. Sci.* **2016**, *5*, 49. [CrossRef]
50. Sharma, A.; Fish, B.L.; Moulder, J.E.; Medhora, M.; Baker, J.E.; Mader, M.; Cohen, E.P. Safety and Blood 546 Sample Volume and Quality of a Refined Retro-Orbital Bleeding Technique in Rats Using a Lateral Approach. *Lab Anim.* **2014**, *43*, 63–66. [CrossRef]
51. Rizza, P.; Santini, S.M.; A Logozzi, M.; Lapenta, C.; Sestili, P.; Gherardi, G.; Lande, R.; Spada, M.; Parlato, S.; Belardelli, F.; et al. T-cell Dysfunctions in hu-PBL-SCID Mice Infected with Human Immunodeficiency Virus (HIV) Shortly after Reconstitution: In Vivo Effects of HIV on Highly Activated Human Immune Cells. *J. Virol.* **1996**, *70*, 7958–7964. [CrossRef]
52. Santini, S.M.; Spada, M.; Parlato, S.; Logozzi, M.; Lapenta, C.; Proietti, E.; Belardelli, F.; Fais, S. Treatment of Severe Combined Immunodeficiency Mice with Anti-Murine Granulocyte Monoclonal Antibody Improves Human Leukocyte Xenotransplantation. *Transplanttion* **1998**, *65*, 416–420. [CrossRef]
53. Fais, S.; Lapenta, C.; Santini, S.M.; Spada, M.; Parlato, S.; Logozzi, M.; Rizza, P.; Belardelli, F. Human Immunodeficiency Virus Type 1 Strains R5 and X4 Induce Different Pathogenic Effects in hu-PBL-SCID Mice, Depending on the State of Activation/Differentiation of Human Target Cells at the Time of Primary Infection. *J. Virol.* **1999**, *73*, 6453–6459. [CrossRef]
54. Amend, S.R.; Valkenburg, K.C.; Pienta, K.J. Murine Hind Limb Long Bone Dissection and Bone Marrow Isolation. *J. Vis. Exp.* **2016**, e53936. [CrossRef] [PubMed]
55. Duselis, A.R.; Vrana, P.B. Retrieval of Mouse Oocytes. *J. Vis. Exp.* **2007**, 185. [CrossRef] [PubMed]
56. Meister, A. Glutathione-Ascorbic Acid Antioxidant System in Animals. *J. Biol. Chem.* **1994**, *269*, 9397–9400.
57. Lenton, K.J.; Therriault, H.; Cantin, A.M.; Fülöp, T.; Payette, H.; Wagner, J.R. Direct Correlation of Glutathione and Ascorbate and Their Dependence on Age and Season in Human Lymphocytes. *Am. J. Clin. Nutr.* **2000**, *71*, 1194–1200. [CrossRef]
58. Gebicki, J.M.; Nauser, T.; Domazou, A.; Steinmann, D.; Bounds, P.L.; Koppenol, W.H. Reduction of Protein Radicals by GSH and Ascorbate: Potential Biological Significance. *Amino Acids* **2010**, *39*, 1131–1137. [CrossRef]
59. Domazou, A.S.; Koppenol, W.H.; Gebicki, J.M. Efficient Repair of Protein Radicals by Ascorbate. *Free Radic. Biol. Med.* **2009**, *46*, 1049–1057. [CrossRef]
60. Smirnoff, N. Ascorbic Acid Metabolism and Functions: A Comparison of Plants and Mammals. *Free Radic. Biol. Med.* **2018**, *122*, 116–129. [CrossRef]
61. Marotta, F.; Yoshida, C.; Barreto, R.; Naito, Y.; Packer, L. Oxidative-Inflammatory Damage in Cirrhosis: Effect of Vitamin E and a Fermented Papaya Preparation: Oxidative Damage in Stable Liver Cirrhosis. *J. Gastroenterol. Hepatol.* **2007**, *22*, 697–703. [CrossRef]
62. Yabuta, S.; Masaki, M.; Shidoji, Y. Associations of Buccal Cell Telomere Length with Daily Intake of β-Carotene or α-Tocopherol Are Dependent on Carotenoid Metabolism-related Gene Polymorphisms in Healthy Japanese Adults. *J. Nutr. Health Aging* **2016**, *20*, 267–274. [CrossRef]

63. Prasad, K.N.; Wu, M.; Bondy, S.C. Telomere Shortening during Aging: Attenuation by Antioxidants and Anti-Inflammatory Agents. *Mech. Ageing Dev.* **2017**, *164*, 61–66. [CrossRef]
64. Jeon, J.S.; Oh, J.-J.; Kwak, H.C.; Yun, H.; Kim, H.C.; Kim, Y.-M.; Oh, S.J.; Kim, S.K. Age-Related Changes in Sulfur Amino Acid Metabolism in Male C57BL/6 Mice. *Biomol. Ther. (Seoul)* **2018**, *26*, 167–174. [CrossRef] [PubMed]
65. Zhang, Y.; Unnikrishnan, A.; Deepa, S.S.; Liu, Y.; Li, Y.; Ikeno, Y.; Sosnowska, D.; Van Remmen, H.; Richardson, A. A New Role for Oxidative Stress in Aging: The Accelerated Aging Phenotype in Sod1-/- Mice Is Correlated to Increased Cellular Senescence. *Redox Biol.* **2017**, *11*, 30–37. [CrossRef] [PubMed]
66. Ali, S.S.; Xiong, C.; Lucero, J.; Behrens, M.M.; Dugan, L.L.; Quick, K.L. Gender Differences in Free Radical Homeostasis during Aging: Shorter-Lived Female C57BL6 Mice Have Increased Oxidative Stress. *Aging Cell* **2006**, *5*, 565–574. [CrossRef] [PubMed]
67. Aliahmat, N.S.; Noor, M.R.M.; Yusof, W.J.W.; Makpol, S.; Ngah, W.Z.W.; Yusof, Y.A.M. Antioxidant Enzyme Activity and Malondialdehyde Levels Can Be Modulated by Piper Betle, Tocotrienol Rich Fraction and Chlorella Vulgaris in Aging C57BL/6 Mice. *Clinics* **2012**, *67*, 1447–1454. [CrossRef]

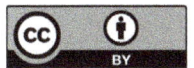

© 2020 by the authors. Licensee MDPI, Basel, Switzerland. This article is an open access article distributed under the terms and conditions of the Creative Commons Attribution (CC BY) license (http://creativecommons.org/licenses/by/4.0/).

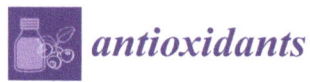

Article

Identification of New Peptides from Fermented Milk Showing Antioxidant Properties: Mechanism of Action

Federica Tonolo [1,†], Federico Fiorese [1,†], Laura Moretto [1], Alessandra Folda [1], Valeria Scalcon [1], Alessandro Grinzato [1], Stefania Ferro [1], Giorgio Arrigoni [1], Alberto Bindoli [2], Emiliano Feller [3], Marco Bellamio [3], Oriano Marin [1,*] and Maria Pia Rigobello [1,*]

[1] Department of Biomedical Sciences, University of Padova, 35131 Padova, Italy; federica.tonolo@phd.unipd.it (F.T.); federico.fiorese.1@gmail.com (F.F.); laura.moretto@unipd.it (L.M.); alessandra.folda.1@unipd.it (A.F.); valeria.scalcon@unipd.it (V.S.); alessandro.grinzato@phd.unipd.it (A.G.); stefania.ferro.1@unipd.it (S.F.); giorgio.arrigoni@unipd.it (G.A.)
[2] Institute of Neuroscience, CNR, 35131 Padova, Italy; alberto.bindoli@bio.unipd.it
[3] Centrale del Latte di Vicenza S.p.A., 36100 Vicenza, Italy; feller@centralelatte.vicenza.it (E.F.); bellamio@centralelatte.vicenza.it (M.B.)
* Correspondence: oriano.marin@unipd.it (O.M.); mariapia.rigobello@unipd.it (M.P.R.)
† These authors contributed equally to the work.

Received: 27 December 2019; Accepted: 27 January 2020; Published: 29 January 2020

Abstract: Due to their beneficial properties, fermented foods are considered important constituents of the human diet. They also contain bioactive peptides, health-promoting compounds studied for a wide range of effects. In this work, several antioxidant peptides extracted from fermented milk proteins were investigated. First, enriched peptide fractions were purified and analysed for their antioxidant capacity in vitro and in a cellular model. Subsequently, from the most active fractions, 23 peptides were identified by mass spectrometry MS/MS), synthesized and tested. Peptides **N-15-M**, **E-11-F**, **Q-14-R** and **A-17-E** were selected for their antioxidant effects on Caco-2 cells both in the protection against oxidative stress and inhibition of ROS production. To define their action mechanism, the activation of the Kelch-like ECH-associated protein 1/nuclear factor erythroid 2-related factor 2(Keap1/Nrf2) pathway was studied evaluating the translocation of Nrf2 from cytosol to nucleus. In cells treated with **N-15-M**, **Q-14-R** and **A-17-E**, a higher amount of Nrf2 was found in the nucleus with respect to the control. In addition, the three active peptides, through the activation of Keap1/Nrf2 pathway, led to overexpression and increased activity of antioxidant enzymes. Molecular docking analysis confirmed the potential ability of **N-15-M**, **Q-14-R** and **A-17-E** to bind Keap1, showing their destabilizing effect on Keap1/Nrf2 interaction.

Keywords: bioactive peptides; Keap1/Nrf2 pathway; natural antioxidants; oxidative stress

1. Introduction

In order to increase the shelf life and improve the flavour, fermentation is a process used for many years in a wide variety of food matrices such as soy, milk, meat and vegetables. Due to the presence of health-promoting compounds, fermented foods are considered important components of the human diet [1]. In fact, this type of food processing not only improves the organoleptic properties of the food matrix, but it can also increase the availability of various constituents, which can exert positive effects after consumption [2]. Among these compounds, bioactive peptides are inactive in the primary structure of proteins and can be released from them by fermenting bacteria-mediated proteolysis [3]. Many microorganisms are utilized in this process and it is well known that different fermenting strains can generate various patterns of bioactive peptides [4–6]. In particular, for dairy products, *Streptococcus thermophilus*, *Lactobacillus delbrueckii* subsp. *bulgaricus* and *Bifidobacterium* spp are usually employed [2,7]. Bioactive peptides generated from milk can originate both from whey proteins (β-lactoglobulin, α-lactalbumin, serum albumin, immunoglobulins, lactoferrin and protease-peptone fractions) and from caseins (α-, β- and κ-casein) [8–10]. Bioactive peptides are studied for their various beneficial activities, for example anti-hypertensive, anti-microbial, opioid and antioxidant [4,11–14]. The antioxidant activity of bioactive peptides can depend on their amino acid composition and position in the sequence [15]. Moreover, these compounds can exert their antioxidant activity in cell environment through activation of specific pathways [16,17]. Oxidants and electrophiles are well known molecules recognized to determine the disruption of Keap1/Nrf2 interaction [16,18,19]. However, new series of other compounds are now emerging, such as the bioactive peptides, that with specific protein-protein interactions are able to activate nuclear factor erythroid 2-related factor 2 (Nrf2). The latter, after dissociation from Kelch-like ECH-associated protein 1 (Keap1), migrates to the nucleus where interacts with the antioxidant response element (ARE), activating a large number of genes expressing antioxidant enzymes. Nrf2 translocation is one of the key events required for the regulation of Keap1/Nrf2 pathway and it is considered an evidence of the activation of the system. [20,21]

As reported in the present paper, peptide fractions from fermented milk were isolated and tested for their antioxidant properties. From the most active fractions, sequences of the most abundant peptides were identified and then synthesized. Finally, these compounds were analyzed for their antioxidant activity in vitro and in a cellular model.

This work aimed to understand the mechanism of action of fermented milk-derived peptides in the protection from oxidative stress. In particular, the interaction of these peptides with Keap1/Nrf2 pathway, the main molecular pathway involved in the protection of cells from oxidative stress conditions, was taken into account.

2. Materials and Methods

2.1. Materials

DMEM + Glutamax, trypsin + EDTA (0.25%) and fetal calf serum (FBS) were purchased from Gibco (Thermo Fisher Scientific, Waltham, MA, USA). For peptide synthesis, all *N*-α-fluorenylmethyloxycarbonyl (Fmoc) L-amino acids, *p*-benzyloxybenzyl alcohol resins (Wang resin) were obtained from Merck (Darmstadt, Germany). Coupling reagent *O*-(7-azabenzotriazole-1-yl)-*N,N,N′,N′*-tetramethyluronium hexafluorophosphate (HATU) was purchased from ChemPep (Wellington, FL, USA). Formic acid was purchased from Fluka (Ammerbuch, Germany). Chemical reagents were purchased from Sigma-Aldrich (St Louis, MO, USA) and Iris Biotech (Marktredwitz, Germany). Acetonitrile, trifluoroacetic acid (TFA), 2,2′-azinobis(3-ethylbenzo-thiazoline 6-sulfonate) (ABTS), 1,1-diphenyl-2-picrylhydrazyl (DPPH), 3-(4,5-dimethylthiazolyl-2)-2,5-diphenyltetrazolium bromide (MTT), potassium persulfate, *tert*-butyl hydroperoxide (TbOOH), PBS, isopropanol, dimethyl sulfoxide (DMSO), Trolox C and Corning Incorporated Transwell® 12 well plates were all obtained from Sigma-Aldrich (St Louis, MO, USA).

2.2. Preparation of Fermented Milk

The samples of fermented milk were collected on the day of their manufacturing. Pasteurized milk was ultrafiltered, sterilized at 120 °C for 30 s and subjected to homogenization (APV, SPX Flow Technology, Crawley, UK). At this point, milk was inoculated with 0.6 mg/L *Lactobacillus acidophilus* NCFM® and 0.2 mg/L *Lactobacillus delbrueckii* subs. *bulgaricus* and *Streptococcus thermophilus* (DUPONT DANISCO, Bologna, Italy) and the product was incubated in a maturation tank at 38 °C for 10 h. At the end, fermented milk (pH 4.5) was vigorously mixed breaking the clot, and brought to 20 °C to block the fermentation process.

2.3. Aqueous Extract of Samples

150 mL of fermented milk were mixed with 150 mL of distilled water in an orbital shaker at room temperature (RT) for 5 min. Then the solution was centrifuged at 16,800× g for 25 min at 15 °C. The supernatants were filtered through Whatman Chr 1 (GE Healthcare, Chicago, IL, USA) and the obtained aqueous extracts were stored at −20 °C until use [22].

2.4. Solid Phase Extraction of Bioactive Fractions from Aqueous Preparations

For the extraction of peptide fractions, a solid phase STRATA C18 E column (Phenomenex, Torrance, CA, USA) was employed. The column was initially conditioned with 50 mL of 100% acetonitrile (ACN) and rinsed with 125 mL of 0.1% trifluoroacetic acid (TFA) aqueous solution. Aliquots of 50 mL of aqueous extract, obtained as described above, were loaded onto the column. After washing with 125 mL of 0.1% TFA, a discontinuous gradient step of ACN was applied in order to obtain peptide enriched fractions [22]. Briefly, the column was eluted with 50 mL of 5%, 30% and 50% ACN solutions and the fractions 5–30% ACN and 30–50% ACN were collected, frozen at −80 °C and lyophilized (Freeze Drier, Edwards, Burgess Hill, west Sussex, UK), then stored at −20 °C until further analysis.

2.5. Purification of Peptide Fractions

In order to increase the resolution in peptide separation, the peptide enriched fractions obtained with solid phase extraction were further purified. 5–30% ACN fraction (35 mg) was dissolved in 2 mL of 0.1% TFA and further purified using preparative Reversed Phase-High Performance Liquid Chromatography (RP-HPLC) with a PrepNova-Pak® HR C18 column (6 µm 60 Å 25 × 10 mm; Waters, Milford, MA, UK) with a linear gradient from 5% to 40% ACN with a flow rate of 12 mL/min. Briefly, after an isocratic step at 5% ACN for 5 min, ACN was linearly increased from 5% to 40% for 24 min and then to 100% within the following 5 min. The column effluent was monitored by UV detection (λ = 220 nm). Fractions were collected every 2 min and then lyophilized.

2.6. Liquid Chromatography-Tandem Mass Spectrometry (LC-MS/MS) Analysis

The fraction of interest was dissolved in H_2O/0.1% formic acid (FA) and an amount of sample corresponding to 1 µg (2.5 µL) was subjected to LC-MS/MS analysis. For the MS analyses a LTQ-Orbitrap XL mass spectrometer (Thermo Fisher Scientific, Waltham, MA, USA) coupled online with a nano-HPLC Ultimate 3000 (Dionex-ThermoFisher Scientific, Waltham, MA, USA) was employed. A homemade 10 cm chromatographic column packed into a pico-frit (75 µm internal diameter (I.D.), 15 µm tip, New Objective, Woburn, MA, USA) with C18 material (Aeris Peptide 3.6 µm XB-C18, Phenomenex Torrance, CA, USA) was utilized for sample loading. A linear gradient from 3% to 40% of ACN, 0.1% FA in 20 min at a flow rate of 250 nL/min was chosen for peptide elution from the original sample. Data of the LC-MS/MS analysis were obtained performing on the Orbitrap a full scan at high resolution (60,000). The MS-MS fragmentation scans were conducted on the ten most intense ions acquired with collision-induced dissociation (CID) fragmentation in the linear trap (data-dependent acquisition—DDA). Furthermore, the following parameters were set for this analysis: capillary voltage 1.2 kV; source temperature 200 °C.

2.7. Database Search and Peptide Identification

In order to permit peptide identification two proteomic tools, Proteome Discoverer software (version 1.4, Thermo Fisher Scientific, Waltham, MA, USA) and the Mascot Search engine server (version 2.2.4, MatrixScience, London, UK) were utilized for processing raw LC-MS/MS data files given by Xcalibur software (version 2.2 SP1, Thermo Fisher Scientific, Waltham, MA, USA). Protein identification against the SwissProt database (version 20180703; 597363 sequences; SIB Swiss Institute of Bioinformatics, Lausanne, Switzerland) was performed using the following parameters: no enzyme, precursor tolerance 10 ppm and fragment tolerance 0.6 Da. Oxidation of methionine was set as variable modification. The Percolator algorithm was used to assess the false-discovery rate and filter the results (FDR < 0.01). Proteins were grouped in protein families according to the principle of maximum parsimony.

2.8. Peptide Synthesis

All the peptides derived from alignments with proteins of bovine milk proteome were subjected to synthesis, employing a solid-phase technique performed on a fully automated peptide synthesizer (Syro II, MultiSynTech GmbH, Witten, Germany). Wang resins preloaded with the first N-α-Fmoc-protected amino acid were utilized for stepwise assembly of the entire peptide chain. This assembly was done according to the Fmoc standard strategy and was based on the use of HATU as the coupling reagent [23,24]. The side-chain protected amino acid building blocks utilized in these peptide syntheses were Fmoc-Glu(OtBu)-OH, Fmoc-Gln(Trt)-OH, Fmoc-Asn(Trt)-OH, Fmoc-His(Trt)-OH, Fmoc-Ser(tBu)-OH, Fmoc-Lys(Boc)-OH, Fmoc-Tyr(tBu)-OH, Fmoc-Arg(Pbf)-OH, Fmoc-Asp(OtBu)-OH, Fmoc-Trp(Boc)-OH, Fmoc-Cys(Trt)-OH and Fmoc-Thr(tBU)-OH. A step of deprotection of the final peptides was conducted, followed by cleavage from the resin with a mixture of 88% (*v/v*) trifluoroacetic acid (TFA) with 5% phenol (*w/v*), 5% H_2O (*v/v*) and 2% (*v/v*) of triisopropylsylane via shaking at RT for 2.5 h. A step of vacuum filtration allowed to remove the resin from the assembled peptide chains. Then, the peptides were precipitated with cold diethyl ether and transformed into pellet by a centrifugation procedure. Two washes with cold diethyl ether were performed on the precipitated peptides. At the end, purification of the crude peptides was done through flash chromatography (SP1, Biotage, Uppsala, Sweden) on a Biotage SNAP Ultra C18 12 g cartridge packed with Biotage HP-Sphere C18 25 μm spherical silica. A final step of molecular mass confirmation was performed by mass spectroscopy on a MALDI-TOF/TOF mass spectrometer (ABI 4800, AB Sciex, Framingham, MA, USA). The mechanism of action analysis was conducted on four selected peptides, **N-15-M**, **E-11-F**, **Q-14-R** and **A-17-E**.

2.9. ABTS and DPPH Scavenging

Samples were analysed for antioxidant capacity through ABTS and DPPH tests [25]. For the first assay, 7 mM ABTS solution and 2.46 mM potassium persulfate were prepared and maintained for 18 h in the dark to obtain the radical molecule ABTS•+. The other test utilized a stable radical (1,1-diphenyl-2-picrylhydrazyl (DPPH)) dissolved in ethanol. Briefly, 0.1 mL of peptide solution (4 mg/mL) was added to 0.1 mL of 0.160 mM DPPH or 0.08 mM ABTS•+ solution. The change of absorbance was estimated at 517 nm and 415 nm for DPPH and ABTS assay, respectively, with a plate reader (Infinite® M200 PRO, Tecan, Männedorf, Switzerland). For ABTS test a calibration curve was set up using Trolox C as standard and results were expressed as Trolox Equivalent Antioxidant Capacity (TEAC). In the other assay, the results were indicated as percentage of antioxidant capacity inhibition (% DPPH scavenging).

2.10. Caco-2 Cell Culture

Caco-2 cells were obtained from DISCOG (University of Padova, Padova, Italy). The cells cultured in DMEM (high glucose) supplemented with 10% FBS, were used between 35 and 60 passages. In order to perform transepithelial transport, 8×10^4 cells were seeded on Transwell© cell culture inserts (0.4 μm pore sizes, 12 mm diameter, 1.12 cm^2 grown surface; Corning Life Sciences, Tewksbury, MA, USA). Cells were grown, differentiated for 21 days and the monolayer integrity was estimated by transepithelial electrical resistance (TEER) (Millicell® ERS-2 volt-ohmmeter, EDM Millipore, Darmstadt, Germany) showing values higher than 1100 $\Omega \times cm^2$.

2.11. Transepithelial Transport of Fractions or Peptides Through Caco-2 Cell Monolayers

The intestinal barrier crossing capacity of the fractions or synthetic peptides through Caco-2 cells monolayer was evaluated using Transwell® insert model according to Tonolo et al. [26]. Briefly, after 21 days of culturing, Caco-2 cells differentiated forming a monolayer that delimited an upper part (apical compartment) and lower part (basolateral compartment). The monolayer was rinsed three times with Hank's balanced salt solution (HBSS) and 10 mM D-glucose and equilibrated for 30 min at 37 °C. After, cells were incubated in the presence of 0.75 mL HBSS containing 150 µg fraction or 75 µg peptide in the apical chamber at 37 °C for 120 min. Samples collected from both compartments (apical and basolateral) at different times were centrifuged at 11,600× g, filtered with 0.45 µm filter, frozen and lyophilized. Subsequently, the obtained samples were dissolved in 100 µL of 0.1% TFA aqueous solution and evaluated by RP-HPLC and Matrix assisted laser desorption/ionization- time of flight/time of flight mass spectrometry (MALDI-TOF/TOF MS).

RP-HPLC and MS Analyses

The apical and basolateral compartments were evaluated in RP-HPLC using a column Onyx Monolithic C18 100 mm × 4.6 mm, LC column (Phenomenex, Torrance, CA, USA) with a Waters 2695 Separation Module (Milfold, MA, USA) with a Waters 996 Photodiode Array Detector. Separations were performed with a linear gradient from 0–60% ACN in the presence of 0.1% TFA over 20 min at a constant flow rate of 2 mL/min monitoring the peaks by UV detection (λ = 220 nm).

Subsequently, the obtained fractions were analysed with a MALDI-TOF/TOF 4800 mass spectrometer (AB Sciex, Framingham, MA, USA). After an initial full MS scan, enlargements on the MS signals of interest were acquired. For the basolateral fractions, the samples, after lyophilisation, were dissolved in 50 µL of 25% ACN and 0.1% TFA. The analysis was then performed on 2 µL of these solutions mixed with 2 µL of peptide MALDI matrix α-cyano-4-hydroxycynnamic acid (10 mg/mL aqueous 70% acetonitrile/0.1% TFA). The following analytical conditions were set for MALDI-TOF spectra acquisition: positive ion reflector mode, initial mass range 500–3500 Da (the mass range was then adapted for each enlargement), variable laser intensity (3000–3800), shots/sub-spectrum 50, total shots/spectrum 1500 and accelerating voltage of 20 kV. Final data analysis and fragments identification were done on Data Explorer software (AB Sciex, Framingham, MA, USA), utilizing external mass calibration performed with mass peptide standards (Sigma-Aldrich, St Louis, MO, USA).

2.12. Cell Viability

The analysed peptide fractions and synthetic peptides were tested with MTT assay. Caco-2 cells (1×10^4) were seeded in 96 well plates and incubated with peptide fractions (0.125 mg/mL) or synthetic peptides (0.05 mg/mL). After 24 h, medium was removed and MTT solution (0.5 mg/mL, 100 µL) in PBS (1×) was added for 3 h in the dark at 37 °C. Removed MTT solution, the reaction was stopped with 100 µL of isopropanol/DMSO (9:1). The absorbance was followed ($Abs_{595-690}$) using a plate reader (Tecan Infinite® M200 PRO, Männedorf, Switzerland).

2.13. ROS Production Estimation

ROS production in Caco-2 cell line was measured by using 5-(and 6)-chloromethyl-20,70-dichlorohydrofluorescein diacetate (CM-H_2DCFDA, Molecular Probes, Thermo Fisher Scientific, Waltham, MA, USA). Briefly, cells (1×10^4) were grown in a 96-wells plate for 48 h, and then treated with synthetic peptides (0.05 mg/mL) for 24 h. Cells washed in PBS 1×/10 mM glucose were loaded with 10 µM CM-H_2DCFDA for 20 min in the dark at 37 °C. Subsequently, the fluorescent probe was removed and cells were rinsed with PBS 1×/10 mM glucose and subjected to oxidative stress in the presence of 250 µM TbOOH. Fluorescence increase was followed at 485 nm (λ excitation) and 527 nm (λ emission) for 90 min using a plate reader (Tecan Infinite® M200 PRO, Männedorf, Switzerland).

2.14. Nrf2 Translocation to the Nucleus

In order to investigate the Keap1/Nrf2 activation, the translocation of Nrf2 to the nucleus was followed. For this purpose, nuclear and cytosolic fractions were divided according to the method described by Yao et al. (2014), with some modifications [27,28]. Briefly, Caco-2 cells (1×10^6) were grown in T25 flasks for 48 h and then treated with 0.05 mg/mL **N-15-M**, **E-11-F**, **Q-14-R** and **A-17-E**.

After 24 h, cells were rinsed with 1 mL of PBS 1× and lysed for 15 min on ice with 100 μL of buffer containing 10 mM Hepes/Tris pH 7.9, 0.1 mM EGTA, 0.1 mM EDTA, 0.1 mM PMSF, 10 mM KCl, 1 mM NaF and a protease inhibitor cocktail (Complete, Roche®, Basel, Switzerland). The samples were rapidly added of IGEPAL (5% final concentration), mixed for 15 s and centrifuged at 1000× g for 10 min at 4 °C. The pellet (nuclear fraction) was dissolved in 20 mM Hepes/Tris (pH 7.9), 1 mM EGTA, 1 mM EDTA, 0.4 M NaCl in the presence of 0.1 mM PMSF, 1 mM NaF and protease inhibitors (Complete, Roche®, Basel, Switzerland). Samples were mixed every 2 min for 10–15 s and centrifuged at 20,000× g for 10 min at 4 °C to discard the debris. Nuclear proteins (30 μg evaluated according to Lowry et al. [29]) were subjected to SDS-PAGE (10%) and subsequently to western blot analysis to define the expression level of Nrf2. Densitometric analysis of WB was carried out using NineAlliance software (Mini 9 17.01 version, Uvitec Alliance, Cambridge, UK). PCNA was used as loading reference.

2.15. Cell Lysates

Cells (5×10^5 per well) were seeded in six well plates and, after 48 h, treated with 0.05 mg/mL **N-15-M**, **E-11-F**, **Q-14-R** and **A-17-E**. After 24 h, cells were collected, rinsed with 1 mL of PBS 1× and then lysed with modified RIPA buffer in the presence of protease inhibitor cocktail (Complete, Roche®, Basel, Switzerland) [19]. Protein content was estimated with the Lowry method [29].

2.15.1. Antioxidant Enzymes Detection

Superoxide dismutase (SOD1), thioredoxin reductase 1 (TrxR1), glutathione reductase (GR) and NAD(P)H quinone dehydrogenase 1 (NQO1) were evaluated by Western blot analysis, using 30 μg of cell protein lysates subjected to SDS-PAGE (12%). The WB detection was assessed using ECL system with UVITEC (Alliance Q9 Advanced, Cambridge, UK) equipment. Densitometric quantification of antioxidant enzymes WB was performed using NineAlliance software (Mini 9 17.01 version, Uvitec Alliance, Cambridge, UK). GAPDH was used as loading reference.

2.15.2. TrxR1 and GR Activities

TrxR1 and GR activities were measured spectrophotometrically using 50 μg of cell lysates proteins and following absorbance at 412 and 340 nm, respectively as described by Tonolo F. 2018 [26].

2.16. Gene Expression Analysis

The levels of gene expression of antioxidant enzymes (TrxR1, GR, NQO1 and SOD1) were evaluated with Real-Time PCR and β-actin was used as reference. Firstly, Caco-2 cells (5×10^5) were cultured into six well plates for 48 h in a complete medium and then treated with **N-15-M**, **E-11-F**, **Q-14-R** and **A-17-E** (0.05 mg/mL) for 24 h. Cells were rinsed with 1 mL PBS 1×, lysed with 1 mL of TRIzol reagent (Invitrogen, Thermo Fisher Scientific, Waltham, MA, USA) and transferred into a new test tube. At this point, 0.2 mL of chloroform were added and vigorously mixed for 15 s. Then samples were placed at RT for 15 min and subsequently centrifuged at 12,000× g for 15 min at 4 °C. In this way, three phases were obtained and the upper one, that contain mRNA, was transferred in a new test tube. Samples were added of 0.5 mL of isopropanol, mixed and maintained at RT for 10 min and subsequently centrifuged at 12,000× g for 10 min at 4 °C. The pellets were rinsed with 1 mL of 75% ethanol and mixed vigorously for 1 min. Samples were centrifuged at 7500× g for 10 min at 4 °C and the pellets were air-dried. The extracted mRNA was diluted in 0.01 mL of RNase free water and its concentration was estimated using NanoDrop system (Thermo Fisher Scientific). mRNA (1 μg) was subjected to reverse transcription using Euroscript M-MLV Reverse Transcriptase in the presence of 25 μg/mL oligo(dT), 10 mM DNTp mix, 10 mM DTT and RNase inhibitors (Euroclone, Milan, Italy) in a final volume of 0.02 mL. Before adding the reverse transcriptase, the mRNA was denatured at 65 °C for 5 min, then the mix were placed at 42 °C for 50 min and at 70 °C for 15 min. The resulting cDNA (1.5 ng/μL) was used for the Real-Time PCR analysis using Hot FIREpol Eva Green qPCR Supermix (Solis BioDyne, Tartu, Estonia). The target cDNA was amplified as follow: an initial step for polymerase activation at 95 °C for 12 min and then 40 cycles of denaturation for 15 s at 95 °C, annealing at 65 °C for 1 min and elongation at 72 °C for 1 min. All the primers were purchased from Sigma-Aldrich (St Louis, MO, USA). GR: Fw: 5′-TCA CGC AGT TAC CAA AAG GAA A-3′, Rv: 5′-CAC ACC CAA GTC CCC TGC ATA T-3′; TrxR1: Fw: 5′-GCC CTG CAA GAC TCT CGA AAT TA-3′, Rv: 5′-GCC CAT AAG CAT TCT CAT AGA CGA-3′; NQO1: Fw: 5′-GGA GAC AGC CTC TTA CTT GCC AAG, Rv: 5′-CCA GCC GTC AGC TAT TGT GGA TAC; β-actin: Fw: 5′-ACC TGA CTG ACT ACC TCA TGA AGA-3′, Rv: 5′-GCG ACG TAG CAC AGC TTC TC-3′; SOD 1: Fw: 5′-TCA GGA GAC CAT TGC ATC ATT-3′, Rv: 5′-CGC TTT CCT GTC TTT GTA CTT TCT TC-3′.

2.17. Molecular Docking Analysis

The interaction of peptides **N-15-M**, **E-11-F**, **Q-14-R** and **A-17-E** with the Kelch domain of Keap1 was investigated trough docking simulation. The protein-peptide model was initially predicted using CASB-Dock [30], providing the peptide sequence and the chain X of the Crystal structure of Kelch domain of Keap1 bound to Neh2 domain of Nrf2 (2FLU), and refined with HADDOCK [31,32]. After 50 ns of relaxation with gromacs 2016.1 [33], the interactions between peptides and their target were evaluated using PISA [34] and UCSF Chimera [35].

2.18. Statistical Analysis

All the reported results are indicated as the mean values ± SD of at least three independent experiments. The analysis of variance was estimated by multiple comparison test employing Tukey-Kramer test and the differences with $p < 0.05$ were considered significant. The software InStat 3 (GraphPad Software, San Diego, CA, USA) was used.

3. Results

Aqueous extracts from fermented milk, obtained with three different microbial strains *Lactobacillus acidophilus*, *Lactobacillus delbrueckii subs. bulgaricus* and *Streptococcus thermophilus*, were used. Then, the samples underwent two different types of purification. To obtain peptide enriched fractions, the first one was a discontinuous step gradient of ACN (5–30% and 30–50%). The major amount of peptides was found in the 5–30% ACN step, while in the 30–50% fraction only a small amount of peptides was present. Subsequently, to provide a higher resolution in peptide separation, the fractions were further purified with RP-HPLC using a continuous gradient. The collected samples were tested for their antioxidant properties in vitro and in Caco-2 cells. The peptides present in the most active fraction were identified.

3.1. Analysis of 5–30% ACN Fraction in Caco-2 Cells: Evaluation of Cell Viability

To estimate the effects of 5–30% and 30–50% ACN fractions on Caco-2 cells, the MTT test was performed. Caco-2 cells (1×10^4) were treated with the peptide fractions (0.125 mg/mL) and, as shown in Table 1, both fractions were not cytotoxic. Moreover, when cells (1×10^4) were subjected to oxidative stress induced by 200 µM TbOOH we observed a decrease of viability. However, when cells were pretreated with the 5–30% ACN fraction a significant protective effect from oxidative stress was observed. Therefore, the further analysis was conducted only on this fraction.

Table 1. Percentage of viability (MTT test) in Caco-2 cells in the presence of the isolated 5–30% and 30–50% acetonitrile (ACN) fractions. Means of at least three experiments (eight replicates for each experiment) were compared with the treated control. (* $p < 0.05$).

Fraction	Percentage of Cell Viability	
	None	TbOOH
Control	100	73.11 ± 8.22
5–30% ACN	103.59 ± 5.20	83.60 ± 2.06 *
30–50% ACN	108.67 ± 10.15	77.80 ± 3.27

3.2. HPLC Analysis, Antioxidant Properties In Vitro and In a Cellular Model of the Purified Fractions Obtained From the 5–30% ACN Pool

Fraction 5–30% ACN, containing a large amount of peptides, was further purified, in order to isolate and identify the most active peptides. To this purpose, 35 µg of the 5–30% ACN fraction was subjected to RP-HPLC (PrepNova-Pak® HR C18) employing a linear gradient from 5% to 40% ACN with a flow rate of 12 mL/min. Collecting the eluted solution every two minutes, fifteen fractions were obtained as described in Figure 1A. In particular, fractions from 0 to 5 and from 11 to 15 were discarded, because the amount of obtained peptides was negligible and insufficient to perform further experiments, indicating a low peptide content at the beginning and at the end of the gradient. On the other hand, each fraction from 6 to 10 was analyzed for its antioxidant properties in vitro. As reported in Figure 1B, all the fractions showed an antioxidant capacity in vitro, as they exhibited moderate TEAC and DPPH scavenging values. Moreover, the effects on Caco-2 cells of the purified fractions were analyzed and the peptides did not show cytotoxicity (Figure 1C). In addition, all the fractions were evaluated for their protection from oxidative stress in cells pretreated with them and subsequently incubated with 200 µM TbOOH. As shown in Figure 1C, some fractions, in particular 6, rescued the viability of Caco-2 cells treated with the oxidative agent. For this reason, this fraction was selected for the further analysis. In order to identify the peptides, present in the most active fraction (6) and able to cross the intestinal barrier, the Transwell® insert model was used. Caco-2 cells were grown on the Transwell® insert for 21 days to reach the differentiated epithelium formation and peptide fractions were added in the apical compartment. After 10 and 120 min, apical and basolateral solutions were collected and analyzed by HPLC and mass spectrometry. As shown in Figure S1, some peptides present in the fraction 6 can cross Caco-2 monolayer.

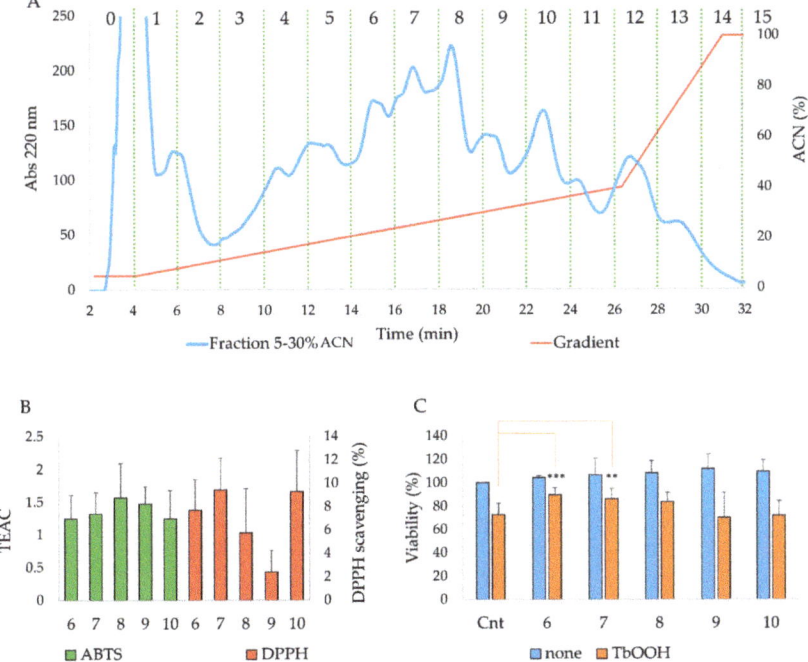

Figure 1. (**A**) Purification of the 5–30% ACN fraction with RP-HPLC. Fractions were collected every 2 min. (**B**) Analysis of antioxidant capacity of the purified fractions in vitro with 2,2'-azinobis(3-ethylbenzo-thiazoline 6-sulfonate) (ABTS) (green) and 1,1-diphenyl-2-picrylhydrazyl (DPPH) (red)

scavenging tests. (**C**) Effects of the purified fractions on cell viability in the presence and absence of TbOOH. Caco-2 cells were treated with the indicated fractions for 24 h and oxidative stress was induced by 200 µM TbOOH. Means of at least three experiments (eight replicates for each experiment) were compared with the treated control. (*** $p < 0.001$, ** $p < 0.01$).

3.3. Identification of the Peptides with Mass Spectrometry Analysis

Then, peptides included in fraction **6** were analyzed with mass spectrometry in order to identify their sequence. The investigation with the Proteome Discoverer and Mascot gave a list of peptides reported in the Table S1. The list of peptides for each protein given by the proteomic identification was aligned with the sequences of the reference proteins (Figure S2) and the candidates for the solid-phase peptide synthesis were chosen in order to obtain the maximum protein sequences coverage. Some criteria were considered as fundamental for the choice of candidate peptides, such as the maximum protein sequences coverage, the best match score between the peptides given by the Proteome Discoverer Software and the reference proteins expressed by Peptide Spectral Match (#PSM), and the peptide length. When more than one peptide covered a region, only the peptide that has the best match score, expressed by the highest value of #PSM was chosen. Of note, the same analysis were performed for fraction 7, but the identified peptides were mostly the same as those identified in fraction 6. Due to the more significant activity in cellular model of fraction 6, the further experimentation was performed with the latter. The sequences and properties of the synthesized peptides were reported in Table 2.

Table 2. Sequences and characteristics of the synthesized peptides.

Native Protein	Peptide Sequence	Name	Number of Residues	Peptide Fragment	Monoisotopic MW (Da)	Presence on BIOPEP Database [36]
κ-casein	QYVLSRYPSYGIN	Q-13-N	13	50–62	1558.76	NO
	KYIPIQYVLS	K-10-S	10	45–54	1222.68	NO
	INNQFLPYPYYAKPA	I-15-A	15	72–86	1797.89	NO
	DKTEIPTINTIASGEPT	D-17-T	17	136–152	1785.88	YES (ID 8194—Kappacin; activity: Antibacterial)
	AVRSPAQILQWQ	A-12-Q	12	87–98	1395.75	NO
	VIESPPEINTVQ	V-12-Q	12	173–184	1324.67	YES (ID 8194—Kappacin; activity: Antibacterial)
	NTVPAKSCQAQPTTm *	N-15-M	15	102–116	1591.72	NO
β-casein	NVPGEIVESL	N-10-L	10	22–31	1055.53	YES (ID: 8173—peptide derived from bovine β-casein (1–28); activity: Immunomodulating)
	VYPFPGPIPN	V-10-N	10	74–83	1099.55	YES (ID: 7564 e 9240; ACE inhibitor; activity: ACE inhibitor)
	HKEMPFPKYPVEPFTESQ	H-18-Q	18	121–138	2190.03	NO
	SQSKVLPVPQKAVPYPQ	S-17-Q	17	181–197	1865.03	NO
	SWMHQPHQPLPPT	S-13-T	13	157–169	1554.72	NO
	VVPPFLQPE	V-9-E	9	98–106	1024.54	NO
	EDELQDKIHPF	E-11-F	11	57–67	1369.64	NO
	FPKYPVEPF	F-9-F	9	126–134	1122.56	NO
αS1-casein	APSFSDIPNPIGSENSE	A-17-E	17	191–207	1759.77	NO
	KHQGLPQEVLNENLL	K-15-L	15	22–36	1730.92	YES (ID: 8171—Isracidin-peptide derived from αS1-casein (1–23); activity: Immunomodulating)
	PFPEVFGKE	P-9-E	9	42–50	1048.51	NO

Table 2. *Cont.*

Native Protein	Peptide Sequence	Name	Number of Residues	Peptide Fragment	Monoisotopic MW (Da)	Presence on BIOPEP Database [36]
αS2-casein	QGPIVLNPWDQVKR	Q-14-R	14	116–129	1648.89	NO
	ALPQYLKTVYQHQK	A-14-K	14	190–203	1715.92	YES (ID: 8257, 8258, 8259; fragments of bovine αS2-casein; activity: Antibacterial)
	IQPKTKVIPYVRYL	I-14-L	14	209–222	1717.01	YES (ID: 8255; 8256; 8257; 8258; 8259; fragments of bovine αS2-casein; activity: Antibacterial)
	FLKKISQRYQKF	F-12-F	12	163–174	1584.90	YES (ID: Casocidin-I f(150–188); activity: antibacterial)
NaPi2B **	EKDDTGTPITKIELVPSH	E-18-H	18	36–53	1979.01	NO

*: peptide N-15-M was identified by Proteome Discoverer Software as NTVPAKSCQAQPTTm, with an oxidized Methionine at position 15, but it was synthesized with not oxidized Methionine; **: Sodium-dependent phosphate transport protein 2B.

3.4. New Identified Peptides

From the reported analysis, 23 peptides were chosen and synthetized. Of them, 15 were not retrieved on the BIOPEP database, indicating that they were completely new in the scientific investigation. The remaining 8 were already registered in the sequence database, although with activities different from the antioxidant one. These peptides were tested for their antioxidant properties in vitro and in the Caco-2 cells model. In particular, 4 of them were selected for their antioxidant effects exerted on the cells and further analyzed to understand their mechanism of action.

3.4.1. Antioxidant Properties In Vitro and In Caco-2 Cells

The 23 peptides were evaluated for their antioxidant capacity using ABTS and DPPH scavenging tests. As reported in Table 3, many peptides displayed a great antioxidant capacity with different extent, while some of them were ineffective. All the synthetic peptides were also tested in the cellular model for their potential cytotoxicity. In addition, they were also checked for their capability to protect against oxidative stress induced by 200 µM TbOOH. As reported in Table 3, column c, all peptides were not cytotoxic. Moreover, most of the synthesized peptides protected the viability of the cells once treated with the oxidative agent, in particular **V-12-Q**, **N-15-M**, **E-11-F**, **K-15-L** and **I-14-L**. These peptides showed a recovery of viability of about 10% (Table 3, column d).

Table 3. Evaluation of antioxidant properties of the identified peptides in vitro using 2,2′-azinobis(3-ethylbenzo-thiazoline 6-sulfonate) (ABTS) and 1,1-diphenyl-2-picrylhydrazyl (DPPH) scavenging tests and in Caco-2 cells pretreated with the 23 peptides. Oxidative stress was induced by 200 µM TbOOH.

Samples	In Vitro Antioxidant Tests		Percentage of Cell Viability	
	DPPH (%) Scavenging (a)	ABTS TEAC (b)	None (c)	TbOOH (d)
Cnt	n.d.	n.d.	100	73.11 ± 8.22
Q-13 N	24.44 ± 7.07	6.09 ± 1.08	104.10 ± 6.64	64.03 ± 10.15
K-10-S	19.09 ± 3.35	4.14 ± 0.82	97.27 ± 6.69	55.32 ± 10.01
I-15-A	19.40 ± 3.64	5.71 ± 1.09	104.37 ± 5.12	76.19 ± 13.27
N-10-L	13.19 ± 5.50	n. d.	119.52 ± 15.74	77.26 ± 12.44
V-10-N	12.24 ± 5.94	0.97 ± 0.48	110.89 ± 9.93	65.40 ± 17.60
F-9-F	12.69 ± 7.02	2.45 ± 0.54	109.47 ± 12.69	69.30 ± 12.78
H-18-Q	19.93 ± 5.13	1.30 ± 0.69	91.92 ± 8.99	52.61 ± 16.83
S-13-T	4.93 ± 3.45	2.96 ± 0.59	107.33 ± 12.39	71.60 ± 6.90
S-17-Q	3.74 ± 0.55	0.83 ± 0.36	101.47 ± 7.46	74.12 ± 11.76
Q-14-R	12.22 ± 4.72	1.28 ± 0.1	114.52 ± 15.55	81.47 ± 11.28
A-17-E	1.02 ± 0.15	0.64 ± 0.13	108.13 ± 13.19	78.33 ± 15.44
D-17-T	5.75 ± 0.38	0.84 ± 0.14	104.19 ± 5.62	73.36 ± 12.10
E-18-H	n. d.[a]	n. d.	103.64 ± 5.01	74.70 ± 10.52
A-12-Q	8.6± 5.98	1.39 ± 0.11	101.85 ± 4.69	78.89 ± 8.75
V-12-Q	n. d.	n. d.	112.70 ± 3.52	93.74 ± 10.68
N-15-M	16.93 ± 3.42	15.18 ± 0.04	107.99 ± 5.96	83.40 ± 5.51
V-9-E	n. d.	n. d.	106.59 ± 8.02	80.55 ± 6.62
E-11-F	n. d.	n. d.	111.51 ± 13.50	87.77 ± 4.50

Table 3. *Cont.*

Samples	In Vitro Antioxidant Tests		Percentage of Cell Viability	
	DPPH (%) Scavenging (a)	ABTS TEAC (b)	None (c)	TbOOH (d)
K-15-L	4.14 ± 2.65	n. d.	104.70 ± 14.49	83.76 ± 6.30
P-9-E	n. d.	n. d.	100.97 ± 14.49	72.56 ± 3.68
F-12-F	15.29 ± 3.33	6.38 ± 0.29	97.73 ± 19.21	75.91 ± 4.80
A-14-K	2.16 ± 0.83	7.19 ± 0.23	84.39 ± 9.69	71.51 ± 5.22
I-14-L	22.9 ± 1.21	8.56 ± 0.43	92.98 ± 13.61	84.48 ± 8.64

[a] n. d.: not detected with the used assay.

3.4.2. Inhibition of ROS Production by Bioactive Peptides

The identified peptides were further examined for their capacity to inhibit ROS production in Caco-2 cells. To this purpose, Caco-2 cells were treated with the peptides for 24 h and subsequently incubated with CM-DCFDA as described in the Material and methods. ROS production in Caco-2 cells pretreated with the peptides was similar to the untreated control, while, when the oxidative stress was induced by 250 μM TbOOH we observed a marked decrease in fluorescence after pretreatment with **N-15-M, E-11-F, Q-14-R, E-18-H, H-18-Q, A-17-E, D-17-T, S-17-Q, V-9-E, P-9-E** and **F-12-F** (Figure 2).

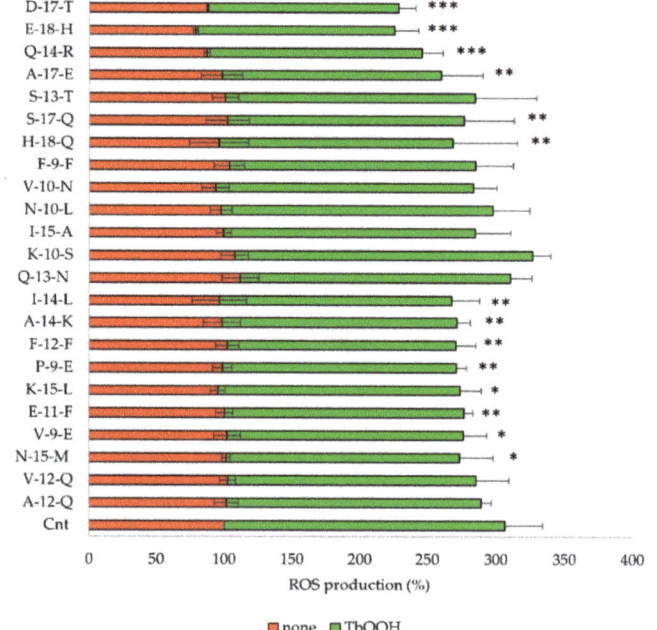

Figure 2. Estimation of reactive oxygen species (ROS) production in Caco-2 cells treated with the indicated peptides (0.05 mg/mL) in the absence (red) or presence (green) of 250 μM TbOOH. The values at 5000 s were reported and the means of at least three experiments (four replicates for each experiment) were compared with the treated control. (*** $p < 0.001$, ** $p < 0.01$, * $p < 0.05$).

3.5. Analysis of the Mechanism of Action of the Antioxidant Peptides

Considering both the protection of the viability and the inhibition of ROS production in Caco-2 cells, **N-15-M**, **E-11-F**, **Q-14-R** and **A-17-E** were selected for their powerful antioxidant effects. Therefore, these four peptides were further analyzed to define their mechanism of action.

3.5.1. Nrf2 Translocation to the Nucleus

An antioxidant action inside the cell could be due to activation of the Keap1/Nrf2 pathway. For this reason, the translocation of Nrf2 from the cytosol to the nucleus in Caco-2 cells treated with the four peptides **N-15-M**, **E-11-F**, **Q-14-R** and **A-17-E** (0.05 mg/mL) was evaluated. Cells (1×10^6) were treated for 24 h with the peptides and then processed to obtain the nuclear fraction, as described in Materials and methods. Nrf2 present in the nuclear fraction was detected by Western blot analysis. Peptides **N-15-M**, **Q-14-R** and **A-17-E** increased significantly the levels of Nrf2 in the nucleus as reported in Figure 3, while **E-11-F** was completely ineffective.

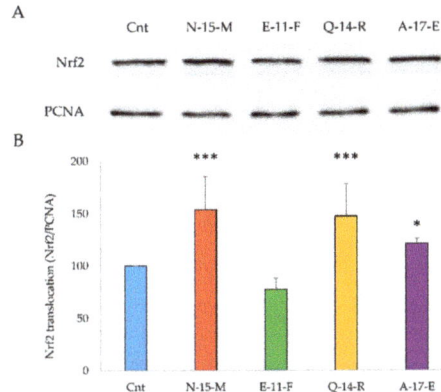

Figure 3. Nrf2 translocation from cytosol to nucleus in Caco-2 cells in the presence of **N-15-M**, **E-11-F**, **Q-14-R** and **A-17-E**. (**A**) Cells were treated with 0.05 mg/mL of each peptide for 24 h. Nuclear fractions were isolated and proteins were subjected to WB detection as indicated in paragraph 2.15. (**B**) Densitometric analysis of four experiments compared with the control were reported, using PCNA as loading control. (*** $p < 0.001$, * $p < 0.05$).

3.5.2. Antioxidant Enzymes Gene Expression Analysis

After the observation that **N-15-M**, **Q-14-R** and **A-17-E** showed a large increase of Nrf2 in the nucleus, the levels of gene expression of antioxidant enzymes were analyzed by RT-PCR. Cells (5×10^5) were treated for 24 h with the four peptides and processed as described in Section 2.16. The transcription of these enzymes is regulated by the translocation of Nrf2 to the nucleus where it can bind ARE.

As shown in Figure 4, the peptides **N-15-M**, **Q-14-R** and **A-17-E** were able to induce an increase of the *GSR*, *TXNRD1*, *NQO1* and *SOD1* mRNA levels. On the other hand, **E-11-F**, that did not show any effect on the translocation of Nrf2 to the nucleus, also in this case did not exert any effect on the antioxidant enzymes gene expression.

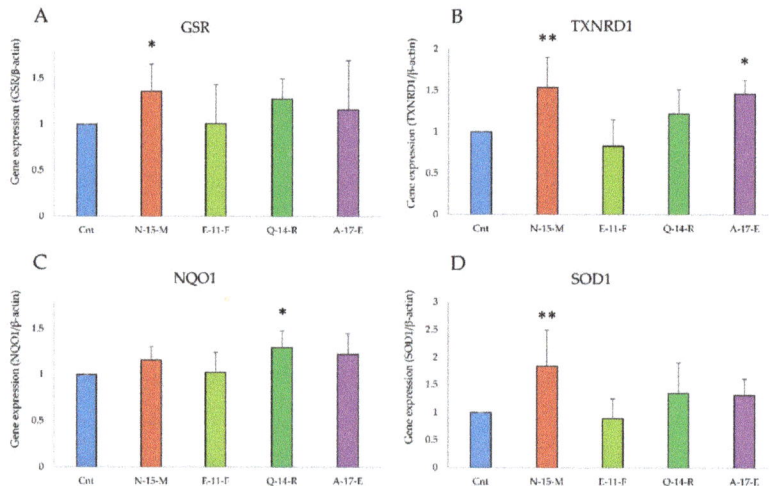

Figure 4. Antioxidant enzymes gene expression analysis. The gene expression of glutathione reductase (GRS, **A**), thioredoxin reductase (TXNRD1, **B**), NADPH quinone oxidoreductase (NQO1, **C**) and superoxide dismutase (SOD1, **D**) was evaluated in cDNA obtained from Caco-2 cells treated with **N-15-M**, **E-11-F**, **Q-14-R** and **A-17-E** (0.05 mg/mL) for 24 h. β-actin was used as reference. Means of at least four experiments were compared with the control. (** $p < 0.01$, * $p < 0.05$).

3.5.3. Antioxidant Enzymes Detection in the Presence of the Four Peptides

In order to confirm the observation regarding the increase of gene expression induced by **N-15-M**, **Q-14-R** and **A-17-E**, western blot analysis of lysates of cells treated with the four peptides was performed. Cells (5×10^5) were incubated in the presence of the four peptides (0.05 mg/mL) for 24 h. Aliquots of the samples (30 µg) were subjected to WB to detect glutathione reductase (GR), NADPH quinone oxidoreductase (NQO1), superoxide dismutase (SOD1) and thioredoxin reductase 1 (TrxR1). As shown in Figure 5, the most active peptides enhanced also the protein levels of these enzymes. In particular, cells treated with **Q-14-R** and **A-17-E** showed a large increase of GR, TrxR1 and NQO1 protein levels (Figure 5).

3.5.4. TrxR1 and GR Activities in Cell Lysates

The activities of TrxR1 and GR in cells treated with **N-15-M**, **E-11-F**, **Q-14-R** and **A-17-E** were also analyzed. Cells were incubated with the indicated peptides in the same conditions as described above and 50 µg of protein cell lysates were used to determine TrxR1 activity by following DTNB reduction at 412 nm and NADPH oxidation at 340 nm for GR. As showed in Figure 6, a slight increase of the activities of the two antioxidant enzymes was observed in cells treated with **N-15-M** and **Q-14-R.**

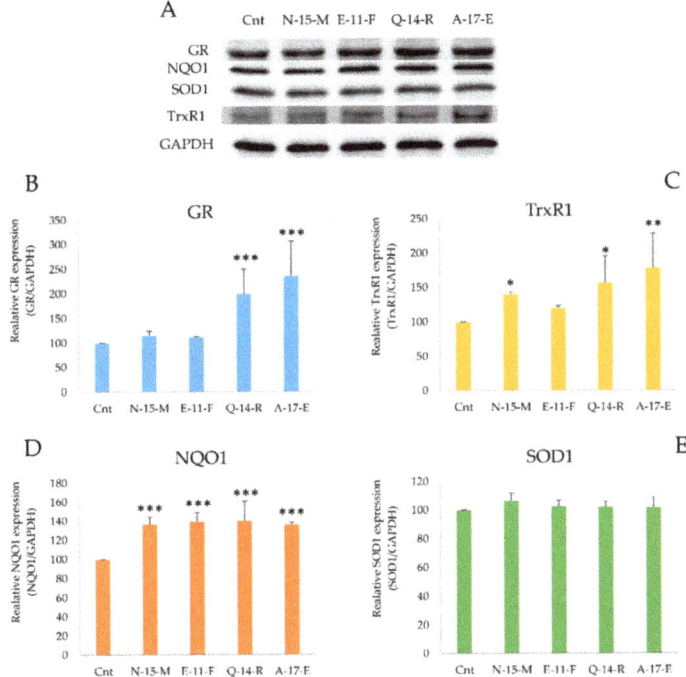

Figure 5. Antioxidant enzymes detection by WB analysis. (**A**) Protein levels of glutathione reductase (GR), thioredoxin reductase (TrxR1), NADPH quinone oxidoreductase (NQO1) and superoxide dismutase (SOD1) in Caco-2 cell lysates treated with the four peptides (0.05 mg/mL) for 24 h. (**B–E**) Densitometric analysis of four experiments were compared with the control and normalized using GAPDH as loading control. (*** $p < 0.001$, ** $p < 0.01$, * $p < 0.05$).

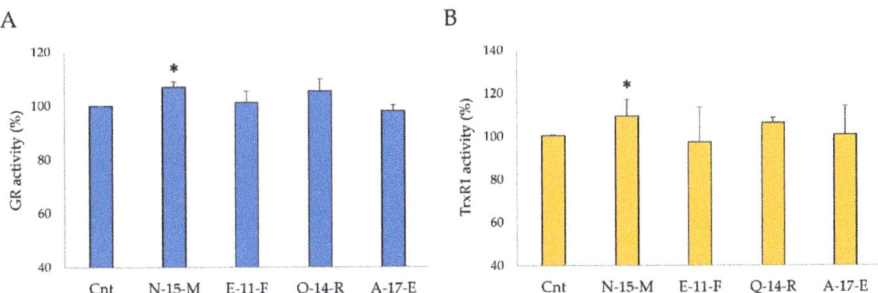

Figure 6. GR (**A**) and TrxR1 (**B**) activities in Caco-2 cells treated with **N-15-M**, **E-11-F**, **Q-14-R** and **A-17-E** (0.05 mg/mL). The activity of the two antioxidant enzymes was analyzed in Caco-2 cells treated with the four peptides for 24 h. Means of at least four experiments were compared with the control. (* $p < 0.05$).

3.5.5. Molecular Docking Analysis

In order to get a prediction of the interaction of the Kelch domain of Keap1 with **N-15-M**, **E-11-F**, **Q-14-R** and **A-17-E**, docking simulation was performed (Figure 7). The free energy of dissociation of the assemblies calculated after a simulation of 50 ns showed that peptide **E-11-F** has no binding affinity with the target protein. On the contrary, peptides **A-17-E**, **Q-14-R** and **N-15-M** formed stable assemblies with the Kelch domain of Keap1. More in details, the first Serine (Ser 3) of **A-17-E** formed hydrogen bonds with a serine (Ser 363) and an arginine (Arg 415), the first **A-17-E** asparagine (Asn 9) formed a hydrogen bond with a tyrosine (Tyr 572) and the inner glutamic acid (Glu 14) formed hydrogen bonds with another arginine (Arg 336) (Figure 7A'). The **Q-14-R** peptide formed hydrogen bonds between its backbone and asparagine (Asn 382), arginine (Arg 380), glutamine (Gln 530), threonine (Thr 576) and histidine (His 575) of the Keap1 pocket; there were also hydrogen bonds between the asparagine (Asn 7) of the peptide and asparagine (Asn 387), arginine (Arg 380) and histidine (His 432) of Kelch domain, the aspartic acid (Asp 10) formed a hydrogen bond with a tyrosine (Tyr 525) and the inner glutamine of the peptide (Gln 11) formed hydrogen bonds with an arginine (Arg 415) and a serine (Ser 508) (Figure 7B'). The backbone of the **N-15-M** formed hydrogen bonds with an asparagine (Asn 382) a glycine (Gly 509), a tyrosine (Tyr 572) and three arginines (Arg 336, Arg 380, Arg 415); the first threonine of the peptide (Thr 2) formed a hydrogen bond with a Serine (Ser 602), the lysine (Lys 6) of the peptide form hydrogen bonds with a glycine (Gly 433) and an isoleucine (Ile 435), the glutamine of the peptide (Gln 11) formed a hydrogen bond with a threonine (Thr 576) (Figure 7C'). It is crucial to notice that there is a certain recurrence among the residues of the Kelch domain involved in the interaction with the peptides. Moreover, these residues are also implicated in the interaction between Kelch domain and Nrf2 [37] (Table 4).

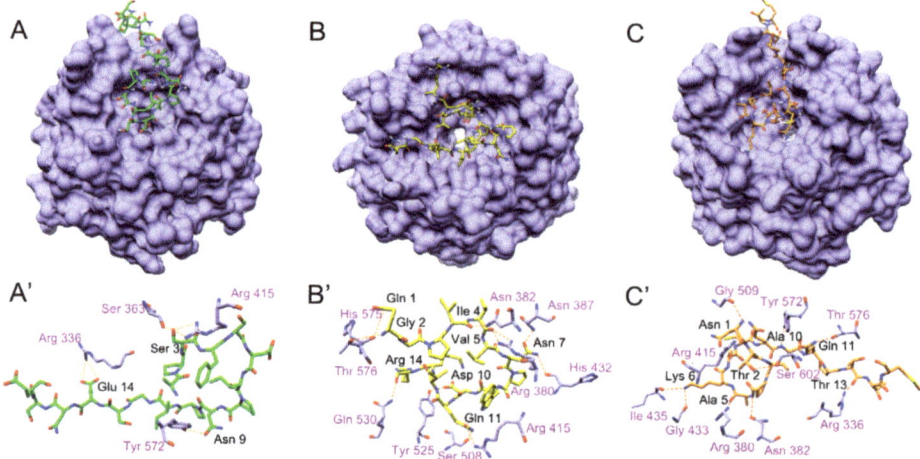

Figure 7. Molecular docking analysis of the interaction between peptides and Keap1 Kelch domain. (**A–C**) Binding geometry of **A-17-E**, **Q-14-R** and **N-15-M** in the pocket of Keap1. (**A'–C'**) Magnification of the interaction of Keap1 Kelch domain with **A-17-E** (**A'**), **Q-14-R** (**B'**) and **N-15-M** (**C'**). Amino acids involved in the hydrogen bond formation were connected with orange dashed lines and highlighted in Table 4.

Table 4. Residues involved in the binding of Keap1 with Nrf2 or the analyzed peptides.

KEAP1	NRF2	A-17-E	Q-14-R	N-15-M
ARG 336		Glu 14		Thr 13
SER 363	Glu 82	Ser 3		
ARG 380	Glu 82		Val 5, Asn 7	Ala 5
ASN 382	Glu 82, Phe 83		Ile 4	Ala 5
ASN 387			Asn 7	
ARG 415	Glu 79, Thr 80	Ser 3	Gln 11	Asn 1
HIS 432			Asn 7	
GLY 433				Lys 6
ILE 435				Lys 6
SER 508	Glu 79		Gln 11	
GLY 509				Asn 1
TYR 525	Glu 79		Asp 10	
GLN 530	Glu 78		Arg 14	
TYR 572	Leu 76, Gly 81	Asn 9		Ala 10
HIS 575			Gly 2	
THR 576			Gln 1	Gln 11
SER 602	Thr 80			Thr 2

3.5.6. Peptide Absorption Analysis

In order to evaluate the intestinal crossing capacity of the four peptides, Transwell® insert model peptide absorption, was performed. For this purpose **N-15-M**, **E-11-F**, **Q-14-R** and **A-17-E** (75 µg) were added to the differentiated Caco-2 cells grown (21 days) on the Transwell® insert. After 10 min and 120 min, apical and basolateral compartments were collected and analyzed by RP-HPLC and mass spectrometry. As shown in Figure 8, all peptides, although with different extent and fragmentation pattern, can cross the intestinal barrier model.

In the apical compartment (AP), the measured amount of **N-15-M**, **E-11-F**, **Q-14-R** and **A-17-E** after 120 min was 60.74%, 88.28%, 87.59% and 68.4%, respectively of the total amount of peptide added (Table 5). These values were due both to the absorption and to a slight fragmentation depending on the action of the brush border peptidases present in the AP. In particular, **N-15-M** gave rise to **V-13-M** and **A-11-M** and **Q-14-R** originated **N-8-R**, **V-10-R**, **I-11-R** and **G-13-R**, and, finally, **A-16-S**, **S-15-S** and **F-14-E** were produced from **A-17-E**. The peptide **E-11-F** gave rise to one fragment, **D-10-F** detectable only by mass spectrometry analysis. The increasing amount of **V-13-M** and **A-11-M** (**N-15-M**) and **A-16-S**, **S-15-E** and **F-14-E** (**A-17-E**) was visible at 120 min (Figure 8A,D, respectively). On the other hand, after 120 min a great amount of the four peptides was found in the basolateral compartment both with HPLC and with mass spectrometry analysis (Figure 8). In particular, **N-15-M**, **E-11-F**, **Q-14-R** and **A-17-E** were estimated to be 0.13%, 0.21%, 0.02% and 0.05% of the initial amount of the peptides, added in the apical compartment (Table 5). All the details about peptides and their fragments absorption analysis were reported in Table 5.

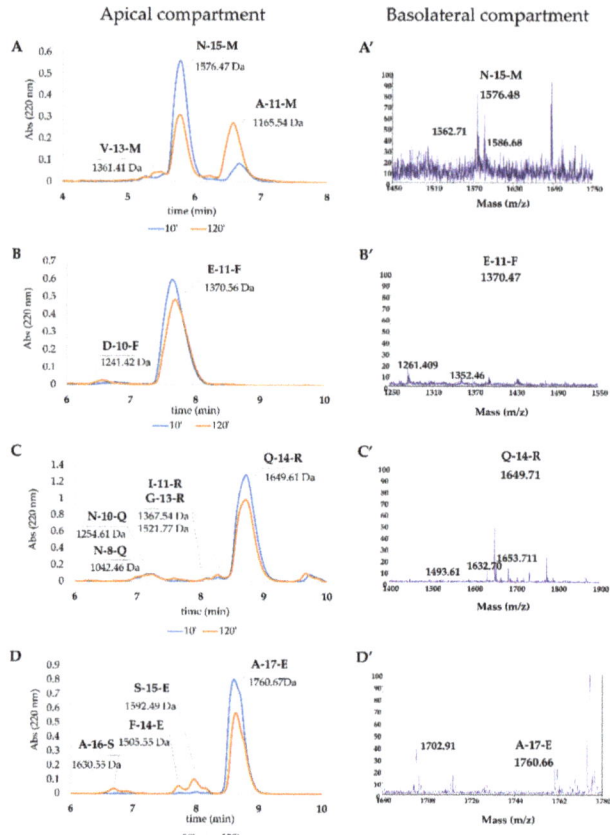

Figure 8. Uptake of the peptides by Caco-2 cells monolayer and their detection in AP and BL compartments. Each peptide (75 µg) was administered to the monolayer cells and samples of AP and BL were collected at the indicated time. (**A–D**) RP-HPLC chromatograms of the four peptides in the apical compartment at 10 and 120 min. (**A′–D′**) MS analysis of the peptides present in the basolateral side after 120 min.

Table 5. Features of the studied peptides (bold) and their produced fragments, using RP-HPLC and MS analysis.

Peptide	Sequence	Retention Time (min)	Theoretical Mass	Measured MW	RP-HPLC Estimation AP (%)	RP-HPLC Estimation BL (%)
N-15-M	NTVPAKSCQAQPTTM	5.77	1575.73	1576.46	60.76 ± 8.83	0.13 ± 0.04
V-13-M	VPAKSCQAQPTTM	5.22	1360.63	1361.41	2.21 ± 0.53	n. d. [a]
A-11-M	AKSCQAQPTTM	6.47	1164.51	1165.53	44.96 ± 9.09	0.16 ± 0.02
S-9-M	SCQAQPTTM	7.18	965.38	965.43	n. d.	0.12 ± 0.03
E-11-F	EDELQDKIHPF	7.63	1369.64	1370.56	88.28 ± 5.89	0.21 ± 0.01
D-10-F	DELQDKIHPF	6.75	1240.598	1241.42	4.17 ± 0.27	n. d.
Q-14-R	QGPIVLNPWDQVKR	8.73	1648.90	1649.60	87.59 ± 12.18	0.02 ± 0.01
G-13-R	GPIVLNPWDQVKR	8.29	1520.83	1521.76	3.19 ± 0.27	n. d.
Q-13-K	QGPIVLNPWDQVK	5.03	1492.79	1493.56	n. d.	0.07 ± 0.05
I-11-R	IVLNPWDQVKR	8.11	1366.76	1367.54	1.47 ± 0.19	n. d.
Q-11-Q	QGPIVLNPWDQ	7.19	1265.63	1266.94	n. d.	0.11 ± 0.01
N-10-Q	VLNPWDQVKR	7.28	1253.68	1254.60	7.44 ± 0.85	n. d.
N-8-R	NPWDQVKR	6.37	1041.52	1042.46	0.55 ± 0.15	n. d.
A-17-E	APSFSDIPNPIGSENSE	8.60	1759.80	1760.66	68.4 ± 4.6	0.05 ± 0.03
A-16-S	APSFSDIPNPIGSENS	6.73	1630.73	1630.45	3.22 ± 0.00	n. d.
S-15-E	SFSDIPNPIGSENSE	8.00	1591.69	1592.48	8.97 ± 0.53	0.30 ± 0.07
F-14-E	FSDIPNPIGSENSE	7.75	1504.65	1505.54	3.07 ± 0.60	n. d.

[a] n. d.: not detected with RP-HPLC analysis.

4. Discussion

In order to identify new bioactive peptides from fermented milk, antioxidant peptide enriched fractions were extracted and further purified with the aim of identify the sequence of the included peptides. More in detail, the fraction 5–30% ACN was selected for the high presence of peptides able to prevent oxidative stress. In fact, when Caco-2 cells were pretreated for 24 h with enriched peptide fractions, a protective effect on the viability was apparent when oxidative stress was induced by TbOOH (Table 1). Therefore, 5–30% ACN fraction was further purified by RP-HPLC obtaining five major fractions, selected on the basis of the highest peptide relative abundance (Figure 1). These collected fractions, called **6, 7, 8, 9** and **10**, were studied for their antioxidant properties in vitro and in Caco-2 cells (Figure 1). In particular, fraction **6** showed a powerful activity in protecting cells from oxidative stress and thus this fraction was selected for the following studies. The sequences of the peptides included in fraction **6** were identified by using LC-MS/MS analysis and the appropriate software. From these data, 23 peptides were chosen according to the peptide coverage for a specific sequence of the reference proteins (see Supplementary Materials). The novelty of the peptides was demonstrated by their absence in the BIOPEP database. When present, their function was not related to an antioxidant effect. Three criteria have been considered for peptide selection: firstly, the maximum protein sequences coverage, in order to map each protein sequence as much as possible from N-terminus to C-terminus; secondly, the best match score, indicated by #PSM, between the peptides given by the Proteome Discoverer Software and the reference proteins; thirdly, the length of peptides, as peptides with less than 20 residues were preferred instead of longer ones. Peptide sequences derived from alignments with other proteins, such as short isoform of polymeric immunoglobulin receptor, glycosylation-dependent cell adhesion molecule, histatherin and 3-phosphoshikimate 1-carboxyvinyltransferase were not taken into account, as they were considered less important. Subsequently, the selected peptides were synthesised, characterized and tested for their antioxidant properties. Two in vitro antioxidant tests, ABTS and DPPH, were performed and, as apparent in Table 3, peptides **Q-13-N, K-10-S, I-15-A, N-10-L, F-9-F,**

Q-14-R, **N-15-M**, **F-12-F** and **I-14-L** were the most active in the scavenging tests (in vitro). However, when all the 23 peptides were screened in a cellular model for their action against oxidative stress induced by TbOOH testing cell viability (Table 3), only peptides **V-10-N**, **Q-14-R**, **A-17-E**, **A-12-Q**, **V-12-Q**, **N-15-M**, **V-9-E**, **E-11-F** and **K-15-L** were effective. Subsequently, in order to confirm the antioxidant power of the peptides, ROS production was evaluated in cells pre-treated for 24 h with the peptides and then subjected to an oxidative stimulus induced by TbOOH. As shown in Figure 2, the most active peptides against ROS production were **N-15-M**, **E-11-F**, **Q-14-R**, **E-18-H**, **H-18-Q**, **A-17-E**, **D-17-T**, **S-17-Q**, **V-9-E**, **P-9-E** and **F-12-F**. From the analysis of all the obtained results (in vitro and in cell environment), **N-15-M**, **E-11-F**, **Q-14-R** and **A-17-E** emerged as the most active peptides. For this reason, these four peptides were used for further analysis. In particular, the mechanism of action of the selected bioactive peptides, involved in the protective effects against oxidative stress in Caco-2 cells, was investigated. We focused on Keap1/Nrf2 pathway because it is the main regulatory system in oxidative stress conditions. In fact, when an oxidative imbalance occur, Keap1 and Nrf2 dissociate and Nrf2 translocates to the nucleus where it can bind ARE, promoting the overexpression of antioxidant enzymes such as glutathione reductase (GR), NADPH quinone oxidoreductase (NQO1), superoxide dismutase (SOD1) and thioredoxin reductase 1 (TrxR1). Therefore, to understand the involvement of Keap1/Nrf2 pathway, the translocation of Nrf2 from the cytosol to the nucleus was considered in cells treated with **N-15-M**, **E-11-F**, **Q-14-R** and **A-17-E** for 24 h. As result, **N-15-M**, **Q-14-R** and **A-17-E** increased the levels of Nrf2 present in the nucleus (Figure 3) suggesting that they activate the Keap1/Nrf2 system. Subsequently, as the amount of Nrf2 in the nucleus increased, we observed also an increase of antioxidant enzymes gene expression. To this purpose, GR, TrxR1, NQO1 and SOD1 gene expression was measured in Caco-2 cells treated with the four peptides for 24 h and again **N-15-M**, **Q-14-R** and **A-17-E** were able to increase the gene expression levels of the antioxidant enzymes (Figure 4) and the consequent protein expression (Figure 5) estimated with WB analysis. Moreover, TrxR1 and GR enzymatic activities were measured in cells treated in the same conditions and **N-15-M** and **Q-14-R** increased the activity of the tested antioxidant enzymes (Figure 6). In order to confirm our observations, molecular docking analysis between the structure of Keap1 and the four peptides was performed (Figure 7). The results showed that **N-15-M**, **Q-14-R** and **A-17-E**, but not **E-11-F**, interacted with Keap1 in the Kelch domain with specific amino acid residues, involved also in the binding between Keap1 and Nrf2 (Table 4). The Kelch repeats sequence of Keap1 (AA 327–609) is responsible for the binding to Nrf2 which participates with the DLG (AA 29–31) and ETGE (AA 79–82) motifs [21]. In particular, the ETGE motif guarantees a strong binding of Nrf2 to Keap1. Specific amino acids residues in the Kelch repeats (especially Arg380 and Arg415) facilitate the binding to the transcription factor. Our peptides are able to interact with Keap1 sequence with many of the amino acids involved in the binding to the ETGE motif. As apparent, **Q-14-R** interacts with Arg 380, Asn 382, Arg 415, Ser 508, Tyr 525 and Gln 530, while peptide **N-15-M** interacts with Arg 380, Asn 382, Arg 415, Tyr 525 and Ser 602. Furthermore, the bioactive peptides examined are able to interact with several other amino acids of the Kelch domain such as Arg 336, Asn 387, His 432, Gly 433, Ile 435, Gly 509, His 575 and Thr 576. Of note, molecular docking approach showed that **E-11-F** did not interact with Keap1.

The overall results suggested that the antioxidant effects highlighted in the cells treated with **N-15-M**, **Q-14-R** and **A-17-E** were due to the interaction of the bioactive peptides with the Keap1 pocket, which causes the disruption of the binding with Nrf2 and the subsequent activation of the signaling cascade. All these findings were in agreement with our previous results [28].

Finally, we studied the capability of these peptides to cross the intestinal barrier. Using the Transwell® technique, we administered the four peptides to differentiated Caco-2 cells in the apical compartment (Figure 8). After 10 and 120 min the apical and basolateral compartments were collected and analyzed by RP-HPLC and mass spectrometry. We observed that an appreciable amount of peptides were able to reach the basolateral compartment partly with modifications as showed by the mass spectrometry analysis (Figure 8). Table 5 reports in detail each peptide and breakdown fragments. More specifically, **N-15-M** and **E-11-F** showed the best intestinal barrier crossing capacity. In fact, the

0.13% and 0.21% of these peptides reached the basolateral compartment, respectively. On the other hand, **Q-14-R** and **A-17-E** underwent a slight fragmentation by the brush border peptidases and only the 0.02% and 0.05%, respectively, reached the basolateral compartment. This observation leads to think that the peptides ingested orally can reach the blood circulation and, if not cleaved, they can exert their beneficial effects in many organs and tissues.

5. Conclusions

New peptides identified from fermented milk were synthesized and analyzed in vitro and in a cellular model for their antioxidant properties. Four of these peptides, **N-15-M**, **E-11-F**, **Q-14-R** and **A-17-E**, were selected for their great protective effects against the action of oxidative stress induced by TbOOH both in the rescue of the viability and in the inhibition of ROS production. The selected bioactive peptides were further studied in order to better understand the mechanism of action of their antioxidant properties. The main conclusion, highlighted by the obtained results, was that the observed protective effects against oxidative stress of the antioxidant fermented milk-derived bioactive peptides were mostly due to the activation of Keap1/Nrf2 pathway.

Supplementary Materials: The following are available online at http://www.mdpi.com/2076-3921/9/2/117/s1, Figure S1: Fraction 6 uptake from Caco-2 cell monolayer. Cells were incubated in the presence of fraction 6 (150 μg) and the analysis of Apical (AP) and basolateral (BL) compartments was performed at the indicated time. Figure S2: Alignments between the reference proteins and the peptides identified by Proteome Discoverer and Mascot search. Oxidized methionine residues are indicated in lowercase (m); #PSM values are indicated in brackets near to each peptide sequence. The alignments are reported separated for each reference protein. Table S1: Files from ORBITRAP analysis of fraction 6.

Author Contributions: Conceptualization: M.P.R. and O.M.; samples production: E.F. and M.B.; extraction and purification of peptides: F.T., L.M. and S.F.; MS/MS analysis: G.A. and F.F.; peptides synthesis: S.F. and O.M.; experiment in cell cultures: F.T., L.M., A.F., V.S. and M.P.R.; molecular docking analysis: A.G.; data curation: F.T., F.F. and L.M.; writing—original draft preparation: M.P.R., O.M., A.B., F.T. and F.F.; writing—review and editing: all authors. All authors have read and agreed to the published version of the manuscript.

Funding: This research received no external funding.

Acknowledgments: The authors wish to thank the Cassa di Risparmio di Padova e Rovigo Holding (Cariparo) and Veneto Banca Holding for the acquisition of the LTQ-Orbitrap XL mass spectrometer and the MALDI-TOF/TOF mass spectrometer, respectively. In addition, the authors wish to thank Tito Calì for the suggestions and Real-Time PCR facilities.

Conflicts of Interest: The authors declare no conflict of interest.

References

1. Şanlier, N.; Gökcen, B.B.; Sezgin, A.C. Health benefits of fermented foods. *Crit. Rev. Food Sci. Nutr.* **2019**, *59*, 506–527. [CrossRef] [PubMed]
2. Rezac, S.; Kok, C.R.; Heermann, M.; Hutkins, R. Fermented Foods as a Dietary Source of Live Organisms. *Front. Microbiol.* **2018**, *9*. [CrossRef] [PubMed]
3. Savijoki, K.; Ingmer, H.; Varmanen, P. Proteolytic systems of lactic acid bacteria. *Appl. Microbiol. Biotechnol.* **2006**, *71*, 394–406. [CrossRef]
4. Shu, G.; Shi, X.; Chen, L.; Kou, J.; Meng, J.; Chen, H. Antioxidant Peptides from Goat Milk Fermented by Lactobacillus casei L61: Preparation, Optimization, and Stability Evaluation in Simulated Gastrointestinal Fluid. *Nutrients* **2018**, *10*, 797. [CrossRef] [PubMed]
5. Solieri, L.; Rutella, G.S.; Tagliazucchi, D. Impact of non-starter lactobacilli on release of peptides with angiotensin-converting enzyme inhibitory and antioxidant activities during bovine milk fermentation. *Food Microbiol.* **2015**, *51*, 108–116. [CrossRef] [PubMed]
6. Pihlanto, A. Lactic Fermentation and Bioactive Peptides. In *Lact. Acid Bact.—R Food Health Livest. Purp.*; InTech: Rijeka, Croatia, 2013; pp. 309–332. [CrossRef]
7. Bourdichon, F.; Casaregola, S.; Farrokh, C.; Frisvad, J.C.; Gerds, M.L.; Hammes, W.P.; Harnett, J.; Huys, G.; Laulund, S.; Ouwehand, A.; et al. Food fermentations: Microorganisms with technological beneficial use. *Int. J. Food Microbiol.* **2012**, *154*, 87–97. [CrossRef]

8. Vargas-Bello-Pérez, E.; Márquez-Hernández, R.I.; Hernández-Castellano, L.E. Bioactive peptides from milk: animal determinants and their implications in human health. *J. Dairy Res.* **2019**, *86*, 136–144. [CrossRef]
9. Dziuba, B.; Dziuba, M. Milk proteins-derived bioactive peptides in dairy products: molecular, biological and methodological aspects. *Acta Sci. Pol. Technol. Aliment.* **2014**, *13*, 5–26. [CrossRef]
10. Pihlanto, A. Antioxidative peptides derived from milk proteins. *Int. Dairy J.* **2006**, *16*, 1306–1314. [CrossRef]
11. Sánchez, A.; Vázquez, A. Bioactive peptides: A review. *Food Qual. Saf.* **2017**, *1*, 29–46. [CrossRef]
12. Toldrá, F.; Reig, M.; Aristoy, M.-C.; Mora, L. Generation of bioactive peptides during food processing. *Food Chem.* **2018**, *267*, 395–404. [CrossRef] [PubMed]
13. Lorenzo, J.M.; Munekata, P.E.S.; Gómez, B.; Barba, F.J.; Mora, L.; Pérez-Santaescolástica, C.; Toldrá, F. Bioactive peptides as natural antioxidants in food products—A review. *Trends Food Sci. Technol.* **2018**, *79*, 136–147. [CrossRef]
14. Li, Z.; Jiang, A.; Yue, T.; Wang, J.; Wang, Y.; Su, J. Purification and identification of five novel antioxidant peptides from goat milk casein hydrolysates. *J. Dairy Sci.* **2013**, *96*, 4242–4251. [CrossRef] [PubMed]
15. Karami, Z.; Akbari-adergani, B. Bioactive food derived peptides: a review on correlation between structure of bioactive peptides and their functional properties. *J. Food Sci. Technol.* **2019**, *56*, 535–547. [CrossRef]
16. Bindoli, A.; Rigobello, M.P. Principles in Redox Signaling: From Chemistry to Functional Significance. *Antioxid. Redox Signal.* **2012**, *18*, 1557–1593. [CrossRef]
17. Kurutas, E.B. The importance of antioxidants which play the role in cellular response against oxidative/nitrosative stress: current state. *Nutr. J.* **2016**, *15*, 71. [CrossRef]
18. Kensler, T.W.; Wakabayashi, N.; Biswal, S. Cell Survival Responses to Environmental Stresses Via the Keap1-Nrf2-ARE Pathway. *Annu. Rev. Pharmacol. Toxicol.* **2007**, *47*, 89–116. [CrossRef]
19. Tonelli, C.; Chio, I.I.C.; Tuveson, D.A. Transcriptional Regulation by Nrf2. *Antioxid. Redox Signal.* **2017**, *29*, 1727–1745. [CrossRef]
20. Baird, L.; Dinkova-Kostova, A.T. The cytoprotective role of the Keap1-Nrf2 pathway. *Arch. Toxicol.* **2011**, *85*, 241–272. [CrossRef]
21. Dinkova-Kostova, A.T.; Kostov, R.V.; Canning, P. Keap1, the cysteine-based mammalian intracellular sensor for electrophiles and oxidants. *Arch. Biochem. Biophys.* **2017**, *617*, 84–93. [CrossRef]
22. Tonolo, F.; Moretto, L.; Folda, A.; Scalcon, V.; Bindoli, A.; Bellamio, M.; Feller, E.; Rigobello, M.P. Antioxidant Properties of Fermented Soy during Shelf Life. *Plant Foods Hum. Nutr.* **2019**, *74*, 287–292. [CrossRef]
23. Fields, G.B.; Noble, R.L. Solid phase peptide synthesis utilizing 9-fluorenylmethoxycarbonyl amino acids. *Int. J. Pept. Protein Res.* **1990**, *35*, 161–214. [CrossRef] [PubMed]
24. Carpino, L.A.; Imazumi, H.; El-Faham, A.; Ferrer, F.J.; Zhang, C.; Lee, Y.; Foxman, B.M.; Henklein, P.; Hanay, C.; Mügge, C.; et al. The Uronium/Guanidinium Peptide Coupling Reagents: Finally the True Uronium Salts. *Angew. Chem. Int. Ed.* **2002**, *41*, 441–445. [CrossRef]
25. Tonolo, F.; Moretto, L.; Ferro, S.; Folda, A.; Scalcon, V.; Sandre, M.; Fiorese, F.; Marin, O.; Bindoli, A.; Rigobello, M.P. Insight into antioxidant properties of milk-derived bioactive peptides in vitro and in a cellular model. *J. Pept. Sci.* **2019**, *25*. [CrossRef] [PubMed]
26. Tonolo, F.; Sandre, M.; Ferro, S.; Folda, A.; Scalcon, V.; Scutari, G.; Feller, E.; Marin, O.; Bindoli, A.; Rigobello, M.P. Milk-derived bioactive peptides protect against oxidative stress in a Caco-2 cell model. *Food Funct.* **2018**, *9*, 1245–1253. [CrossRef] [PubMed]
27. Yao, J.; Ge, C.; Duan, D.; Zhang, B.; Cui, X.; Peng, S.; Liu, Y.; Fang, J. Activation of the Phase II Enzymes for Neuroprotection by Ginger Active Constituent 6-Dehydrogingerdione in PC12 Cells. *J. Agric. Food Chem.* **2014**, *62*, 5507–5518. [CrossRef]
28. Tonolo, F.; Folda, A.; Cesaro, L.; Scalcon, V.; Marin, O.; Ferro, S.; Bindoli, A.; Rigobello, M.P. Milk-derived bioactive peptides exhibit antioxidant activity through the Keap1-Nrf2 signaling pathway. *J. Funct. Food* **2019**. [CrossRef]
29. Lowry, O.H.; Rosebrough, N.J.; Farr, A.L.; Randall, R.J. Protein Measurement with the Folin Phenol Reagent. *J. Biol. Chem.* **1951**, *193*, 265–275.
30. Kurcinski, M.; Jamroz, M.; Blaszczyk, M.; Kolinski, A.; Kmiecik, S. CABS-dock web server for the flexible docking of peptides to proteins without prior knowledge of the binding site. *Nucleic Acids Res.* **2015**, *43*. [CrossRef]
31. Dominguez, C.; Boelens, R.; Bonvin, A.M.J.J. HADDOCK: A Protein-Protein Docking Approach Based on Biochemical or Biophysical Information. *J. Am. Chem. Soc.* **2003**, *125*, 1731–1737. [CrossRef]

32. Van Zundert, G.C.P.; Rodrigues, J.P.G.L.M.; Trellet, M.; Schmitz, C.; Kastritis, P.L.; Karaca, E.; Melquiond, A.S.J.; van Dijk, M.; de Vries, S.J.; Bonvin, A.M.J.J. The HADDOCK2.2 Web Server: User-Friendly Integrative Modeling of Biomolecular Complexes. *J. Mol. Biol.* **2016**, *428*, 720–725. [CrossRef] [PubMed]
33. Abraham, M.J.; Murtola, T.; Schulz, R.; Páll, S.; Smith, J.C.; Hess, B.; Lindahl, E. GROMACS: High performance molecular simulations through multi-level parallelism from laptops to supercomputers. *SoftwareX* **2015**, *1–2*, 19–25. [CrossRef]
34. Krissinel, E.; Henrick, K. Inference of Macromolecular Assemblies from Crystalline State. *J. Mol. Biol.* **2007**, *372*, 774–797. [CrossRef] [PubMed]
35. Pettersen, E.F.; Goddard, T.D.; Huang, C.C.; Couch, G.S.; Greenblatt, D.M.; Meng, E.C.; Ferrin, T.E. UCSF Chimera—A visualization system for exploratory research and analysis. *J. Comput. Chem.* **2004**, *25*, 1605–1612. [CrossRef] [PubMed]
36. Minkiewicz, P.; Iwaniak, A.; Darewicz, M. BIOPEP-UWM Database of Bioactive Peptides: Current Opportunities. *Int. J. Mol. Sci.* **2019**, *20*, 5978. [CrossRef] [PubMed]
37. Lo, S.-C.; Li, X.; Henzl, M.T.; Beamer, L.J.; Hannink, M. Structure of the Keap1:Nrf2 interface provides mechanistic insight into Nrf2 signaling. *EMBO J.* **2006**, *25*, 3605–3617. [CrossRef] [PubMed]

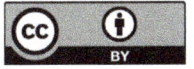

© 2020 by the authors. Licensee MDPI, Basel, Switzerland. This article is an open access article distributed under the terms and conditions of the Creative Commons Attribution (CC BY) license (http://creativecommons.org/licenses/by/4.0/).

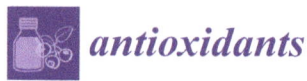

Article

Anti-Atherosclerotic Effect of *Hibiscus* Leaf Polyphenols against Tumor Necrosis Factor-alpha-Induced Abnormal Vascular Smooth Muscle Cell Migration and Proliferation

Cheng-Chung Chou [1], Chi-Ping Wang [2,3], Jing-Hsien Chen [2,4,*] and Hui-Hsuan Lin [2,4,*]

[1] Laboratory Medicine, Antai Medical Care Corporation Antai Tian-Sheng Memorial Hospital, Pingtung County 928, Taiwan; s109017@yahoo.com.tw
[2] Department of Clinical Laboratory, Chung Shan Medical University Hospital, Taichung City 0201, Taiwan; cshb015@csh.org.tw
[3] Department of Nutrition, Chung Shan Medical University, Taichung City 40201, Taiwan
[4] Department of Medical Laboratory and Biotechnology, Chung Shan Medical University, Taichung City 40201, Taiwan
* Correspondence: cjh0828@csmu.edu.tw (J.-H.C.); linhh@csmu.edu.tw (H.-H.L.); Tel.: +886-424-730-022 (ext. 12195) (J.-H.C.); +886-424-730-022 (ext. 12410) (H.-H.L.)

Received: 2 November 2019; Accepted: 3 December 2019; Published: 5 December 2019

Abstract: The proliferation and migration of vascular smooth muscle cells (VSMCs) are major events in the development of atherosclerosis following stimulation with proinflammatory cytokines, especially tumor necrosis factor-alpha (TNF-α). Plant-derived polyphenols have attracted considerable attention in the prevention of atherosclerosis. *Hibiscus* leaf has been showed to inhibit endothelial cell oxidative injury, low-density lipoprotein oxidation, and foam cell formation. In this study, we examined the anti-atherosclerotic effect of *Hibiscus* leaf polyphenols (HLPs) against abnormal VSMC migration and proliferation in vitro and in vivo. Firstly, VSMC A7r5 cells pretreated with TNF-α were demonstrated to trigger abnormal proliferation and affect matrix metalloproteinase (MMP) activities. Non-cytotoxic doses of HLPs abolished the TNF-α-induced MMP-9 expression and cell migration via inhibiting the protein kinase PKB (also known as Akt)/activator protein-1 (AP-1) pathway. On the other hand, HLP-mediated cell cycle G0/G1 arrest might be exerted by inducing the expressions of p53 and its downstream factors that, in turn, suppress cyclin E/cdk2 activity, preventing retinoblastoma (Rb) phosphorylation and the subsequent dissociation of Rb/E2F complex. HLPs also attenuated reactive oxygen species (ROS) production against TNF-α stimulation. In vivo, HLPs improved atherosclerotic lesions, and abnormal VSMC migration and proliferation. Our data present the first evidence of HLPs as an inhibitor of VSMC dysfunction, and provide a new mechanism for its anti-atherosclerotic activity.

Keywords: proliferation; migration; vascular smooth muscle cells; atherosclerosis; tumor necrosis factor-alpha; *Hibiscus* leaf polyphenols

1. Introduction

Atherosclerosis is considered a chronic inflammatory process and involves a complex pathophysiological effect, including endothelial dysfunction, low-density lipoprotein (LDL) oxidation, foam cell formation, and vascular smooth muscle cell (VSMC) proliferation and migration at different stages of this disease [1,2]. Elevated plasma LDL concentration contributes to the initiation of atherosclerosis [3]. Oxidized LDL triggers endothelial cells to release chemokines in contribution to recruitment of monocytes, resulting in the transformation of the lipid-laden macrophages into foam cells [3]. In the lesion progression, these activated macrophages still secrete proinflammatory cytokines, especially tumor necrosis factor-alpha (TNF-α), which enhances VSMC migration and proliferation [1,3]. Subsequently, VSMC transforms and proliferates into foam cells, and thus the accumulation of foam cells leading to fatty streaks results in the formation of atherosclerotic plaques [2]. Thus, inhibition of abnormal VSMC migration and proliferation is an attractive strategy for clinical therapy of atherosclerosis and restenosis after percutaneous coronary interventions.

VSMC is normally quiescent, but upon vascular injury, it transforms into a more synthetic phenotype with progressively increasing capacity for activation, proliferation, and migration [1,4]. In the atherosclerotic process, VSMC migrates from the media to the intima, forms the neointima progressively with abundant levels of extracellular matrix (ECM) proteins, and then eventually leads to plaque formation [2]. Identification of key proteins involved in the process, such as matrix metalloproteinases (MMPs), is vital for understanding atherosclerosis and devising new therapies. MMPs are a subfamily of the metzincin superfamily of endogenous proteinases that break down components of ECM. Among them, the gelatinases (MMP-2 and MMP-9) degrade efficiently native collagen types IV and laminin, and promote a VSMC migratory phenotype [5]. Moreover, the gene expression of MMPs is majorly regulated by the transcriptional factors, such as activator protein-1 (AP-1) or nuclear factor-kappaB (NF-κB) through the serine/threonine protein kinase PKB (also known as Akt) or extracellular signal-regulated kinase (ERK) pathways, or by the MMP protein activators or inhibitors. One review study concluded that oxidative stress could enhance MMP activity and expression [6], and recent studies further indicate that MMP-mediated ECM remodeling is modulated by reactive oxygen species (ROS) [7]. Hence, MMPs and their regulatory signaling have been considered as promising targets for anti-atherosclerotic agents [8].

In arterial media, VSMC is at low proliferative indices (<0.05%) and remains in the G0/G1 phase of the cell cycle [4]. However, VSMC re-enters into the cell cycle from the quiescent state to proliferate under the stimulation of several cytokines in pathological processes, which plays an important role in the development of atherosclerosis [1]. VSMC begins to divide in response to cytokines, exits the G1 phase, and then enters the S phase. During the G1/S transition, cyclin D1/cyclin-dependent kinase (cdk) 4 and cyclin E/cdk2 complexes are required. The complexes participate in the hyperphosphorylation of retinoblastoma (Rb) tumor suppressor, leading phosphorylated Rb (p-Rb) to release E2F transcription factor, allowing the cells to progress into S phase [9]. The kinase activities of these cyclin/cdk complexes are regulated by cdk inhibitors (cki), including p16, p21, and p27. The gatekeeper of the mammalian cell cycle, p53, plays a key role in controlling G0/G1 arrest through its downstream factor, such as p21 [10].

Previous studies have reported that *Hibiscus* leaf, an edible part of *H. sabdariffa* Linne (*Malvaceae*) [11], possesses hypoglycemic [12], hypolipidemic [13,14], and antioxidant [13,15] effects, as demonstrated by various experimental models (Table S1). For the standardization of each extract, our studies also indicated that (−)-epicatechin gallate (ECG; 16.5 ± 5.6%) was identified to be present in the highest level in *Hibiscus* leaf polyphenols (HLPs), followed by ellagic acid (EA; 10.31 ± 3.43%) and catechin (Cat; 7.4 ± 2.6%), and traces of only quercetin (Que; 0.8 ± 0.4%) and ferulic acid (FA; 0.7 ± 0.3%) were detected (Table S2) [14]. In this regard, the aqueous and methanol extracts of *H. sabdariffa* leaves showed anti-atherogenic effects in hyperlipidemia animals induced by cholesterol [11,12], and inhibited foam cell formation, as well as protected endothelial cells from injury in vitro [11,16]. Our recent studies also revealed that *Hibiscus* leaf aqueous extract, due to its high content in polyphenols, has apoptotic and anti-migratory effects on prostate cancer cells [17,18]. However, little information is available on the isolation and characterization of a polyphenolic extract of *H. sabdariffa* leaves. In the present study, HLP was partially characterized by biochemical and spectroscopic assays, and evaluated for the ability to inhibit TNF-α-stimulated VSMC dysfunction.

Many studies have indicated that plant-derived polyphenols have various pharmacological and biological effects, such as antioxidant, anti-inflammatory, anti-hyperlipidemia, anti-diabetes, anti-atherogenic, and anti-tumor abilities [19]. Furthermore, although the protective effects of HLPs on endothelial cells and macrophages have been demonstrated previously, the in vivo function and the molecular target of HLPs on VSMC remain to be elucidated in cardiovascular microenvironment. Using a model of VSMC exposed to TNF-α and the well-established atherosclerotic rabbit experiment, to our knowledge, this is the first report revealing the TNF-α-antagonist potential of HLPs in vitro and in vivo.

2. Materials and Methods

2.1. Preparation of HLP and Detection of Polyphenolic Compounds

One hundred grams of *H. sabdariffa* L. (Malvaceae) dried leaves, obtained from Taitung City, Taitung Country, Taiwan, were extracted three times with methanol (300 mL) at 50 °C for 3 h, and the samples were filtered after each extraction. The methanol was evaporated under reduced pressure, and the residue was dissolved in 500 mL of distilled water at 50 °C and extracted with 200 mL of hexane to remove pigments. The aqueous phase was extracted three times with 180 mL of ethyl acetate, and the solvent was removed from the extract with a vacuum rotary evaporator. The residue was re-dissolved in 250 mL of distilled water and was lyophilized to obtain about 2.5 g of HLP. The polyphenolic components of HLP were further analyzed as follows. All reagents and pure compounds were purchased from Sigma-Aldrich Chemical Co. (St. Louis, MO, USA). Total phenolic acid content was determined by the Folin-Ciocalteau method [20] using gallic acid (GA) as a standard. To start, 0.1 mg of HLP was first dissolved in a tube with 1 mL of distilled water, and 0.5 mL of Folin-Ciocalteu reagent (2 N) was added and mixed thoroughly. After 3 min, 3 mL of Na_2CO_3 solution (2%) was added, and the mixture was allowed to stand for 15 min. The absorbance of the mixture at 750 nm was measured on a spectrophotometer (Beckman Coulter DU 730, Brea, CA, USA). The concentration of total flavonoid was assayed according to the Jia method [21]. A standard curve using rutin (Rut) was also prepared. Next, 0.5 mL of HLP (1 mg/mL) was diluted with 1.25 mL of distilled water. Afterwards, 75 µL of $NaNO_2$ solution (5%) was added to the mixture. After an interval of 6 min, 150 µL of $AlCl_3·6H_2O$ solution (10%) was added, and the mixture was allowed to stand for another 5 min. Then, 0.5 mL of NaOH (1 M) and 2.5 mL of distilled water were added. The solution was mixed, and the absorbance was immediately measured against the prepared control at 510 nm. The polyphenolic components of HLP were confirmed by high performance liquid chromatography (HPLC) system using a Hewlett-Packard Vectra 436/33 N system with a diode array detector (all from Waters Corp., Milford, MA, USA). The HLP was filtered through a 0.45 µm filter disc, and then 20 µL of HLP was injected onto a 5 µm RP-18 column (4.6 × 150 mm i.d.; Phenomenex, Inc., Torrance, CA, USA). The mobile phase contained two solvents, including solvent A (formic acid/water = 10:90) and solvent B (formic acid/acetonitrile/water = 10:30:60), run by a linear gradient method at room temperature as follows: From 10% solvent B to 40% solvent B (flow rate = 1.0 mL/min) over 25 min. The chromatography was monitored at 240 and 345 nm, and an ultraviolet (UV) spectrum (Beckman Coulter Inc., Brea, CA, USA) was collected to confirm peak purity. The HPLC analysis of 10 kinds of standard polyphenols showed the retention times (RT) as follows: GA (4.58 min), protocatechuic acid (PCA, 7.50 min), Cat (9.39 min), ECG (11.21 min), EA (13.29 min), Rut (14.01 min), p-coumaric acid (CA, 14.44 min), FA (15.28 min), Que (21.57 min), and naringenin (Nar, 24.48 min), respectively. Consistent with our previous study [16], the yield of HLP was approximately 25.0%, and polyphenols were indeed present in HLP (Table S2).

2.2. Cell Culture

A rat VSMC cell line A7r5 was purchased from the Bioresource Collection and Research Center. A7r5 cells were cultured in Dulbecco's modified Eagle's medium (DMEM) supplemented with 10% fetal bovine serum, 1% penicillin-streptomycin mixed antibiotics, 1% glutamine, and 1.5 g/L sodium bicarbonate (all regents from Hyclone, Logan, Utah, USA). All cell cultures were maintained at 37 °C under 95% moisturized air with 5% CO_2. Before cell treatments, A7r5 cells were seeded onto each 60 mm Petri dish (Corning Inc, Corning, NY, USA) at a density of 10^5 for 24 h. For induction of

VSMC dysfunction, A7r5 cells at 70% confluence were serum-starved for 24 h and treated with TNF-α (10 ng/mL; Sigma-Aldrich, St Louis, MO, USA) for 24 h.

2.3. 3-(4,5-Dimethylthiazol-Zyl)-2,5-Diphenyltetrazolium Bromide (MTT) Assay

A7r5 cells were seeded onto each 24-well plate (Corning Inc, Corning, NY, USA) at a density of 10^5 cells/mL, and treated with various concentrations of TNF-α (0–20 ng/mL) alone or TNF-α (10 ng/mL) in combination with HLP (0–1.0 mg/mL) for 24 or 48 h. Thereafter, the medium was changed, MTT (0.1 mg/mL, Sigma, St. Louis, MO, USA) was added for next 4-h incubation. The viable cell number was directly proportional to the formazan production, which was solubilized in isopropanol and detected at 563 nm with a spectrophotometer. The MTT assay was used to evaluate the effect of TNF-α alone or TNF-α and/or HLP on cell viability, and to determine the non-cytotoxic doses of HLP, as described by Chen et al. [16].

2.4. Gelatin Zymography Protease Assay

The activities of MMP-2 and MMP-9 in the serum-free conditioned medium were evaluated by gelatin zymography according to a previously described method by Huang et al. [22]. In short, samples were prepared with standard sodium dodecyl sulfate (SDS)-gel loading buffer containing 0.01% SDS (Sigma-Aldrich, St Louis, MO, USA). The prepared samples (25 μg total protein) were not boiled before loading, but subjected to electrophoresis on 8% SDS polyacrylamide gels (1.0-mm-thick, acrylamide/bis-acrylamide = 30/1.2) containing 0.1% gelatin (Sigma-Aldrich, St Louis, MO, USA). After electrophoresis, the gel was washed twice with 100 mL distilled water containing 2% Triton X-100 (Sigma-Aldrich, St Louis, MO, USA) on a shaker for 30 min at room temperature to remove SDS, and incubated in 100 mL reaction buffer (0.02% NaN_3, 10 mM $CaCl_2$ and 40 mM Tris-HCl (pH 8.0)) at 37 °C for 12 h. The gel was further stained with Coomassie brilliant blue R-250 dye (Abcam plc, Cambridge, UK) followed by destaining with methanol/acetic acid/water (50:75:875, $v/v/v$).

2.5. Real-Time Reverse Transcription Polymerase Chain Reaction (RT-PCR)

Total RNAs were extracted using a TRIzol reagent (Invitrogen, Life Technologies, Carlsbad, CA, USA) according to the manufacturer's instructions, as described by Chiu et al. [18]. In general, the mRNA levels were analyzed by quantitative real-time RT-PCR using a Bio-Rad iCycler system (Bio-Rad, Hercules, CA, USA), and normalized to the housekeeping gene, β-actin. The sequences of primers (MDBio Inc., Taipei, Taiwan) used in the experiments are listed in Table S3.

2.6. Protein Isolation and Western Blotting

The preparation of cytosolic and nuclear fractions of the cells was performed using the Nuclear and Cytoplasmic Extraction Reagent Kit (Thermo Scientific, Rockford, IL, USA), described by Chiu et al. [18]. In brief, the harvested cells were washed with phosphate-buffered saline (PBS) and incubated on ice in Reagent A for 2 min. Reagent B was added, and the mixture was further incubated on ice for 5 min. Reagent C was added, and the contents were mixed by inverting the tube several times, followed by centrifugation (700× g) at 4 °C for 10 min. The supernatant (cytosol) was collected and centrifuged (12,000× g) at 4 °C for 15 min. Then, the nuclear pellet was washed twice with wash buffer (10 mM Tris-HCl (pH 7.5), 0.4% Nonidet P-40, and 10 mM KCl) to remove non-lysed cells. A protease inhibitor cocktail (Bio-Rad Labs., Hercules, CA, USA) was added to all solutions before use. Western blot analysis was carried out according to a previously described method by Chen et al. [16]. Whole cell lysate was prepared using sample buffer containing 2% SDS, 10% glycerol, 5% β-mercaptoethanol, and 50 mM Tris-HCl (pH 6.8), and then extracted using sonication. Equal amounts of proteins were separated by 8–15% SDS–polyacrylamide gels and transferred to nitrocellulose membranes (Bio-Rad Labs., Hercules, CA, USA). In order to block non-specific binding, the nitrocellulose membranes were incubated with 5% nonfat dry milk for 1–2 h at 4 °C, and then overnight with polyclonal first antibodies against MMP-2, MMP-9, p-Akt, Akt, p-ERK, ERK, c-Jun, c-Fos, NF-κB, p-p53, p53, p21, p27, p16, PCNA (proliferating cell nuclear antigen), E2F, and p-Rb were from Santa Cruz Biotech (CA, USA). In the subsequent day, the blots were incubated with the appropriate horseradish peroxidase-conjugated secondary antibodies (goat anti-rabbit IgG or goat anti-mouse IgG), from Sigma-Aldrich (St Louis, MO, USA), for 1 h, and detection was performed using an enhanced chemiluminescence (ECL) reagent (Amersham, Arlington Heights, IL, USA). The cytosolic and nuclear protein were respectively determined by Western blotting using anti-β-actin and anti-C23 antibodies, purchased from Santa Cruz Biotechnology Inc. (Santa Cruz, CA, USA), as loading controls. Protein level was quantified by densitometry using FUJIFILM-Multi Gauge V2.2 software (Fujifilm, Kyoto, Japan).

2.7. AP-1 and NF-κB Binding Assay

DNA-binding activities of AP-1 and NF-κB in nuclear extracts were assayed by electrophoretic mobility shift assay (EMSA) with biotin-labeled double-stranded AP-1 or NF-κB oligonucleotides (MDBio Inc., Taipei, Taiwan), as described by Chiu et al. [18]. EMSA was carried out by using the Lightshift kit from Pierce (Rockford, IL, USA). Binding reactions containing 10 μg of nuclear extracts, 1 μg poly (dI·dC), 12.5 μg poly-L-lysine, 2 pmol of oligonucleotide probe, and 2 μL of 10× binding buffer were incubated for 20 min at room temperature. Protein-DNA complexes were separated by electrophoresis on a 6% non-denaturing acrylamide gel, transferred to positively charged nylon membranes (Millipore, Bedford, MA, USA), and then UV cross-linked. Gel shifts were visualized with a streptavidin-horseradish peroxidase followed using chemiluminescent detection.

2.8. Wound-Healing Migration Assay

To study the possibility that HLP alter migration of VSMC-treated TNF-α, the cell medium was replaced with serum-containing medium following the treatments of TNF-α (10 ng/mL) in the absence or presence various concentrations (0, 0.01, 0.05, and 0.10 mg/mL) of HLP, and the monolayers were wounded using scraping with a 20-μL pipette tip. At the indicated times (0, 24, and 48 h) after scraping, the above-treated cells were washed twice in PBS (pH 7.4). The cells were photographed using a phase-contrast microscope (Olympus, Tokyo, Japan) [23].

2.9. Boyden Chamber Invasion Assay

To test the effect of HLP on the in vitro invasiveness of VSMC-treated TNF-α, a modified Boyden chamber (Neuro Probe, Cabin John, MD, USA) invasion assay coating with a layer of Matrigel (25 mg/50 mL; Sigma-Aldrich, St Louis, MO, USA) was used [23], and was applied to polycarbonate membrane filters with an 8.0 μm pore size (Nucleopore, Pleasanton, CA, USA). Afterwards, the membrane was fixed with methanol, and then stained with 10% Giemsa (Sigma-Aldrich, St Louis, MO, USA). The image of cells invaded through the membrane was capture and counted under the light microscope.

2.10. Cell Growth Curve Analysis

VSMC was seeded into a 6-well culture plate at a density of 7×10^4 cells/mL, and then incubated with TNF-α (10 ng/mL) in the absence or presence various concentrations (0, 0.2, and 0.5 mg/mL) of HLP for 24 h. The cell numbers were further counted using the Corning Cell Counter with a reusable glass counting chamber (Corning Inc, Corning, NY, USA) each day for 2 days. On the basis of the mean number of cells in these wells, the growth curves were formed.

2.11. Bromodeoxyuridine (BrdU) Cell Proliferation Assay

To identify the cells in S phase of cell cycle, the BrdU cell proliferation assay (Oncogene, Cambridge, MA, USA) was carried out according to the manufacturer's manual. In brief, A7r5 cells were seeded into a 96-well plate (4×10^3 cells/well) and grown in DMEM medium supplemented with 5% FBS overnight. The cells were rinsed once with serum-free medium, and then treated with TNF-α (10 ng/mL) in the presence or absence of various concentrations (0.2 and 0.5 mg/mL) of HLP in serum-free medium for 24 h. In most of the experiments, pulse labeling of synthesized DNA was used. For this, the BrdU label was added 1 h before the experimental end. The cells were fixed, denatured, and probed with anti-BrdU antibody. Absorbance was determined at dual wavelengths of 450 and 540 nm in a microplate reader system (Bio-Rad Labs., Hercules, CA, USA). Proliferative value (BrdU incorporation) was expressed as a percentage of absorbance of the treated cells to the absorbance of the non-treated control cells. The BrdU incorporation of the control group was set to 100%.

2.12. Cell Cycle Analysis by DNA Content

The quantification of cell cycle distribution was examined using a FACScan laser flow cytometer (Becton Dickinson, San Jose, CA, USA). The VSMC was treated with TNF-α (10 ng/mL) in the absence or presence various concentrations (0.2 and 0.5 mg/mL) of HLP for 24 h; collected, rinsed with PBS twice; fixed in 70% ethanol at −20 °C overnight; and then stained with propidium iodide (PI) solution (20 µg/mL of PI, 20 µg/mL of RNase A, and 0.1% Triton X-100; all chemicals from Sigma-Aldrich, St Louis, MO, USA) for 20 min in the dark at room temperature. Each phase of cell cycle was presented as the cell number versus the DNA content as indicated by the intensity of fluorescence, and gated into subG1, G0/G1, S, and G2/M phases with CELLQuest Version 3.3 software (Becton Dickinson, San Jose, CA, USA).

2.13. Immunoprecipitation

For detection of protein-protein interaction, immunoprecipitation was carried out. In short, 500 µg of protein from cell lysates was precleared with protein A–agarose beads (Pierce Biotechnology, Rockford, IL, USA), followed by immunoprecipitation using polyclonal antibodies against cdk2 or E2F, purchased from Santa Cruz Biotechnology Inc. (Santa Cruz, CA, USA). Immune complexes were harvested with protein A, and immunoprecipitated proteins were then assayed by Western blotting, as above. Immunodetection was performed using polyclonal anti-cyclin E or anti-Rb antibodies (Santa Cruz Biotechnology Inc., Santa Cruz, CA, USA).

2.14. Intracellular ROS Assay

The fluorescent probe, dichlorofluorescin diacetate (DCFH-DA), purchased from Enzo Life Sciences Inc. (Farmingdale, NY, USA), was used to determine the effect of HLP on intracellular ROS generation by TNF-α stimulation. In brief, the confluent A7r5 cells in the 6-well plates at 10^5 cells/well were treated with TNF-α (10 ng/mL) in the absence or presence various concentrations (0.2 and 0.5 mg/mL) of HLP for 24 h. After removing the treated cells from the wells, the cells were incubated with 2 µM of DCFH-DA at 37 °C for 30 min. The fluorescence intensity of intracellular ROS production was evaluated at an excitation and emission wavelength of 485 and 530 nm, respectively, using Muse™ Cell Analyzer (EMD Millipore Corporation, Merck Life Sciences, KGaA, Darmstadt, Germany). Values were expressed relative to the fluorescence signal of the control.

2.15. Evaluation of Atherosclerotic Lesions In Vivo

New Zealand white male rabbits weighing between 1800 and 2200 g were randomly divided into five experimental groups as follows: Group I, normal control group (Purina Lab Diet 5031); group II, high-fat diet (HFD); group III, HFD with 0.5% HLP group (HFD + 0.5% HLP); group IV, HFD with 1% HLP group (HFD + 1% HLP); and group V, normal diet with 1% HLP group (cytotoxicity group of HLP). The rabbits in groups II, III, and IV were fed on a HFD containing 95.7% standard Purina Chow (Purina Mills Inc., Louis, MI, USA), 1.3% cholesterol, and 3% lard oil (Sigma-Aldrich, St Louis, MO, USA) for 25 weeks to induce the atherosclerotic process., In groups III, IV, and V, the rabbits were treated with oral feeding 0.5% or 1% HLP at the same time. The dose regimen for these groups was based on a previous study published by Chiu et al. [18]. For the care and use of laboratory animals, the use of all rabbits was reviewed and approved by Chung Shan Medical

University animal care committee according to the guidelines of the Institutional Animal Care and Use Committee (IACUC approval number: 893). After 25 weeks of supplementation, aortic arches from each rabbit were collected and then stained with hematoxylin and eosin (H & E) for the pathological analysis. Serum was also collected and stored at −80 °C until measurements of serum biochemical parameters and TNF-α using a cytoscreen immunoassay kit (BioSource International, Camarillo, CA, USA). For immunohistochemistry (IHC), commercial monoclonal anti-alpha smooth muscle actin (α-SMA, a marker of VSMC migration), obtained from Santa Cruz Biotechnology Inc. (Santa Cruz, CA, USA), and anti- PCNA (a marker of VSMC proliferation) were used for target detection in the paraffin-embedded tissues.

2.16. Statistical Analysis

In vitro data are reported as means ± standard deviation (SD) of three independent experiments. The in vivo effect of each treatment was analyzed from 6 rabbits ($n = 6$) in each group. Statistical significances of difference throughout this study were evaluated by one-way analysis of variance (ANOVA). $p < 0.05$ was considered statistically significant.

3. Results

3.1. Non-Cytotoxic Doses of HLP Inhibits TNF-α-Induced Cell Viability Loss and MMP Activation

A7r5 cell viability was investigated following incubation with a range of concentrations (from 1 to 20 ng/mL) of TNF-α for 24 h, and it was found that TNF-α at low concentrations (lower than 10 ng/mL) dose-dependently increased the cell viability. However, above the dose of 10 ng/mL, TNF-α reduced about 10% of cell viability (Figure 1a). Because MMPs break down components of ECM, which is a crucial role in the process of VSMC migration [7,8], the effect of TNF-α on MMP activities was then tested by gelatin zymography in serum-free conditioned medium to identify the contribution of MMP-2 or MMP-9 to the pro-migratory ability of TNF-α. As shown in Figure 1b, MMP-9 activity was tremendously increased by TNF-α in a concentration-dependent manner, whereas MMP-2 activity was less affected. According to the results, to provide a maximum dynamic range for quantifying the VSMC proliferative and pro-migratory responses, cell incubation with 10 ng/mL of TNF-α for 24 h was chosen in all subsequent experiments.

In our previous study, HLP at concentrations of > 0.05 mg/mL was demonstrated to be an antioxidant agent, as tested by its 1,1-diphenyl-2-picrylhydrazyl (DPPH) scavenging effect and ability to inhibit LDL oxidation in standard antioxidant evaluation [14], as shown in Table S4. Next, a preliminary screening was performed to study the effect of HLP alone (Figure S1) or together with TNF-α at 10 ng/mL (Figure 1c) on A7r5 cell growth for 24 h, using the MTT assay. The viability of A7r5 was significantly decreased by 0.25, 0.50, and 1.0 mg/mL of HLP in the absence or presence of TNF-α in a dose-dependent manner, when receptively compared to the control and TNF-α alone group. In order to study whether HLP is an inhibitor of cell migration and MMP-9 activation in the TNF-α-treated VSMC, the effect of HLP on A7r5 cell viability by MTT assay, showing cell growth, was significantly altered by the treatments of above the dose of HLP at 0.25 mg/mL, and was excluded in further studies (Figure 1c). In subsequent experimental migration research, the concentration range was used to avoid the influence of cell viability on the observed parameters. As shown in Figure 1d, it is worth noting the TNF-α-induced increase in MMP-9 activity was significantly inhibited in the cells incubated with the combinations of TNF-α together with this dose range of HLP (between 0.01 and 0.10 mg/mL).

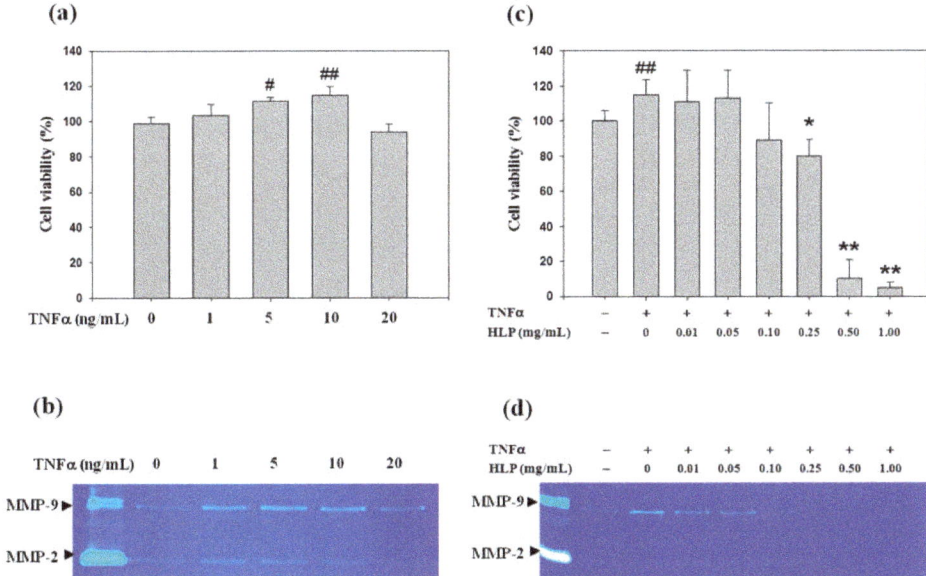

Figure 1. Effect of tumor necrosis factor-alpha (TNF-α) or/and *Hibiscus* leaf polyphenol (HLP) on cell viability and matrix metalloproteinase (MMP) activities in vascular smooth muscle cells (VSMCs). (**a**) A7r5 cells were treated with various concentrations (0–20 ng/mL) of TNF-α for 24 h. Cell viability was analyzed by MTT assay. (**b**) A7r5 cells in serum-free medium were treated with various concentrations of TNF-α for 24 h. The culture medium of cells after treatment was subjected to gelatin zymography to analyze the MMP activity. (**c**) A7r5 cells were treated with TNF-α (10 ng/mL) in the absence or presence of various concentrations (0.01, 0.05, 0.10, 0.25, 0.50 and 1.00 mg/mL) of HLP for 24 h. Cell viability was analyzed by MTT assay. The quantitative data are presented as mean ± standard deviation (SD) (n = 3) from three independent experiments. # p < 0.05, ## p < 0.01 compared with the control. * p < 0.05, ** p < 0.01 compared with the TNF-α group. (**d**) A7r5 cells in serum-free medium were treated with TNF-α in the absence or presence of various concentrations of HLP for 24 h. The culture medium of cells after treatment was subjected to gelatin zymography to analyze the MMP activity. The result is representative of at least three independent experiments. +, added; −, non-added.

3.2. HLP Downregulated TNF-α-Increased Protein and mRNA Levels of MMPs

To understand further the downregulatory effects of HLP on the TNF-α-activated MMP-9, Western blotting was performed. As shown in Figure 2a, TNF-α elevated the protein levels of MMP-2 and MMP-9, and TNF-α together with the indicated concentrations of HLP (0.01, 0.05, and 0.10 mg/mL) caused a marked decreased level of MMP-9, but not MMP-2. The HLP-mediated decrease in the protein level of MMP-9 coincided well with its mRNA level, as evidenced by quantitative RT-PCR results (Figure 2b), indicating that HLP might downregulate the expression of MMP-9 majorly, but that of MMP-2 partially, at the transcriptional level.

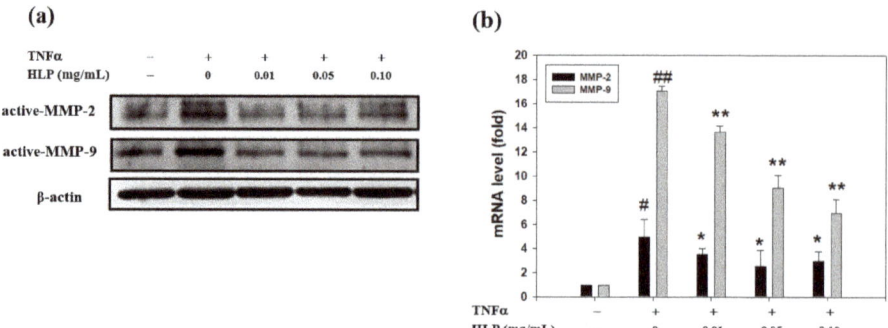

Figure 2. Effect of HLP on TNF-α-induced protein and mRNA levels of MMPs in VSMCs. A7r5 cells were treated with TNF-α (10 ng/mL) in the absence or presence of various concentrations (0, 0.01, 0.05, and 0.10 mg/mL) of HLP for 24 h. (**a**) Western blot analysis and (**b**) real-time quantitative RT-PCR of protein and mRNA levels of MMP-2 and MMP-9 in the treated cells. β-actin was served as an internal control of protein level. The quantitative data are presented as mean ± SD (n = 3) from three independent experiments. # p < 0.05, ## p < 0.01 compared with the control. * p < 0.05, ** p < 0.01 compared with the TNF-α group. +, added; −, non-added.

3.3. HLP Inhibits TNF-α-Induced Akt/AP-1 Signaling

MAPK and Akt have been shown to be involved in MMP-9 induction in various tumor types and migratory cell phenotypes [5,23]. To examine whether the activities of these protein kinases are downregulated by HLP, we analyzed their phosphorylation in A7r5 cells after being exposed to 10 ng/mL of TNF-α in the presence or absence of HLP at the indicated concentrations for 24 h. Immunoblot analysis with anti-phospho-specific antibodies was then performed. As shown in Figure 3a, the TNF-α-induced phosphorylated level of Akt was tremendously reduced by HLP in a concentration-dependent manner, whereas that of ERK was little affected. MMP-9 promoter was shown to have several transcription-factor-binding motifs, including binding sites for AP-1 and NF-κB [23], indicating that the AP-1 and NF-κB signal pathway may play a key role in the regulation of MMP-9 expression. Therefore, whether HLP could interfere the translocation of AP-1 or NF-κB into the nucleus in TNF-α-stimulated VSMC by immunoblotting analysis of the nucleus extracts prepared from the treated cells was then tested. The data in Figure 3b demonstrate that stimulation with 10 ng/mL of TNF-α for 24 h induced significantly the nuclear levels of c-Jun, c-Fos, and NF-κB (p65), compared to that of the control group. After exposure to TNF-α for 24 h, HLP treatments inhibited nuclear levels of c-Jun and c-Fos, components of transcription factor AP-1, in a dose-dependent manner, with the higher concentrations (0.10 mg/mL) being more effective. In contrast, there was no noticeable change in the translocation of nuclear NF-κB in the same condition of HLP treatments. Furthermore, to confirm that HLP could affect the DNA-binding activities of the translocated AP-1 and NF-κB in the TNF-α model VSMC, EMSA was carried out. The nuclear extracts of the above-treated cells were incubated with a DNA probe specific for AP-1, and the binding was analyzed by mobility shift (Figure 3c). A decrease in the DNA binding activity of AP-1 (left panel), but not NF-κB (right panel), was presented in the cells treated with TNF-α in the presence of HLP at various concentrations for 24 h.

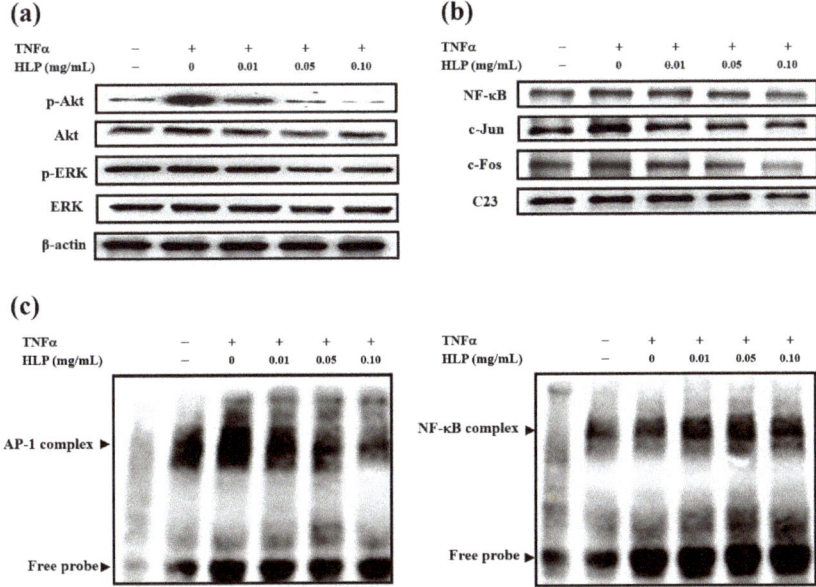

Figure 3. Effect of HLP on TNF-α-induced Akt/AP-1 signaling in VSMCs. A7r5 cells were treated with TNF-α (10 ng/mL) in the absence or presence of various concentrations (0, 0.01, 0.05 and 0.10 mg/mL) of HLP for 24 h; (**a**) the cytoplasmic fraction was analyzed for the expressions of p-Akt, Akt (protein kinase PKB, also known as Akt), p-ERK, and ERK (extracellular signal-regulated kinase), and (**b**) the nuclear fraction was analyzed for the expressions of NF-κB, c-Jun, and c-Fos, two components of activator protein-1 (AP-1). These protein levels were determined by Western blotting. β-actin and C23 served as a cytoplasmic and nuclear internal control, respectively. (**c**) The nuclear extracts were analyzed for AP-1 (left panel) and NF-κB (right panel) DNA-binding activities using biotin-labeled AP-1 and NF-κB specific oligonucleotide by electrophoretic mobility shift assay (EMSA). Lane 1 represents nuclear extracts incubated with unlabeled oligonucleotide (free probe) to confirm the specificity of binding. Results are representative of at least three independent experiments. +, added; −, non-added.

3.4. HLP Inhibits TNF-α-Induced Abnormal VSMC Migration

To evaluate whether HLP reversed A7r5 cells from the TNF-α stimulation, a set of well-established and classical methods, wound-healing and Boyden chamber assays, was used to determine VSMC migration. The effect of HLP on abnormal VSMC migration was analyzed by wound-healing assay, in which A7r5 cells were induced to migrate by physical wounding of cells plated on fibronectin-precoated 6-well plates. Under light microscopy, an apparent and gradual increase of cells in the denude zone was observed at the cells exposed to TNF-α more than control for 24 and 48 h (Figure 4a). A7r5 cells treated with TNF-α, together with the indicated doses of HLP, showed a reduced capacity to heal the wounded area, compared to the TNF-α alone. The quantitative results demonstrate that HLP could dose- and time-dependently inhibit TNF-α-stimulated VSMC migration. Subsequently, the effect of HLP on VSMC invasion was examined by a Boyden chamber coated with Matrigel under light microscopy. After a 24-h incubation period, TNF-α promoted a marked increase in the amount of cell invasion. The results further show that the number of cells invaded to the lower chamber was significantly reduced by HLP treatments. The data in Figure 4b indicate that such decrease was dose-dependent, with a 70% decrease when the TNF-α model cells were treated with HLP at 0.01 mg/mL. Therefore, it is possible that the anti-VSMC migratory/invasive effect of HLP was conducted by inactivating Akt/AP-1, subsequently leading to a reduction in MMP-9 expression and activation in TNF-α stimulation.

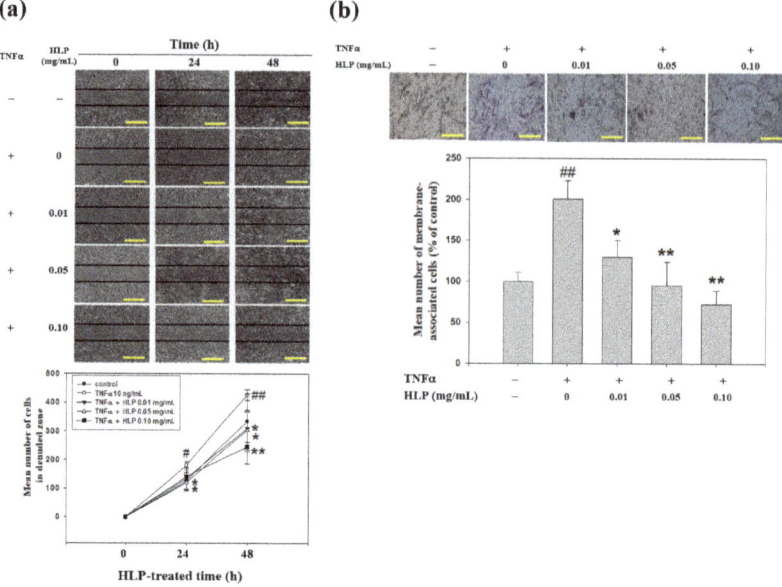

Figure 4. Effect of HLP on TNF-α-induced A7r5 cell motility and invasion. (**a**) Monolayers of A7r5 cells treated with TNF-α (10 ng/mL) in the absence or presence of various concentrations (0, 0.01, 0.05 and 0.10 mg/mL) of HLP were scraped and the number of cells in the denuded zone was photographed and quantified after indicated times (0, 24, and 48 h). Quantitative assessment of the mean number of cells in the denuded zone was presented as mean ± SD (n = 3) from three independent experiments. (**b**) A7r5 cells were treated with TNF-α in the absence or presence of various concentrations of HLP for 24 h. Invasion assay was performed using Boyden chamber. Representative photomicrographs of the membrane-associated cells were assayed by Giemsa stain. The purple parts indicate the membrane-associated cells. "% of control" denotes the mean number of cells in the membrane expressed as a proportion of that control group. Images were taken at 200× magnification; scale bar, 30 μm. The quantitative data are presented as mean ± SD (n = 3) from three independent experiments. # p < 0.05, ## p < 0.01 compared with the control. * p < 0.05, ** p < 0.01 compared with the TNF-α group. +, added; −, non-added.

3.5. HLP Inhibits TNF-α-Induced Abnormal VSMC Proliferation

In the following experiment, the cytotoxic effect of HLP at dosages above 0.10 mg/mL and TNF-α (10 ng/mL) was also detected using cell growth curve analysis. As shown in Figure 5a, the TNF-α-induced proliferation of A7r5 cells under the uses of TNF-α and HLP at 0.2 and 0.5 mg/mL was significantly lower than that under TNF-α alone. Importantly, the cell growth curve confirmed the anti-proliferative effect was more pronounced when HLP at the doses of > 0.10 mg/mL were used in the TNF-α-exposed cells. We then investigated whether the HLP effect against TNF-α was attributed by induction of cell death or/and inhibition DNA synthesis. For this purpose, the level of DNA synthesis through BrdU incorporation in the treated cells grown under low-serum conditions was measured. As shown in Figure 5b, TNF-α caused an increase in BrdU incorporation, and TNF-α together with higher doses of HLP had a marked decreased level in BrdU incorporation.

To further hypothesize that HLP may be involved in the VSMC cell death, flow cytometry was used to examine whether the number of hypodiploid cells (apoptotic cells), which are stained less intensely with PI dye, can be unequivocally detected in the subG1 phase (left panel, Figure 5c). When A7r5 cells were treated with TNF-α at 10 ng/mL in the presence of HLP at 0.2 mg/mL for 24 h, it was not observed that an apparent accumulation of cells in the subG1 phase. Here, the cell cycle distribution of

TNF-α-treated VSMC affected by HLP was also evaluated. The 24-h TNF-α-stimulated cells showed a marked increase in S phase with fewer cells in G0/G1 phase, after TNF-α alone compared with control. When compared with the TNF-α alone group, the combination group had fewer cells in S phase and more cells in G0/G1 phase, indicating the 24-h HLP treatments could significantly lead to cell cycle block at G0/G1 phase in a dose-dependent manner (right panel, Figure 5c). In addition, when the cells were exposed to 0.5 mg/mL of HLP, a concomitant time-dependent slight and significant increase in apoptotic rates, compared to the TNF-α-treated group, was observed. Since the combination of HLP (0.2 mg/mL) and TNF-α (10 ng/mL) has the best antagonistic action of cell cycle regulation, the doses of combination were selected for further mechanistic studies of anti-VSMC proliferation, especially in G0/G1 arrest.

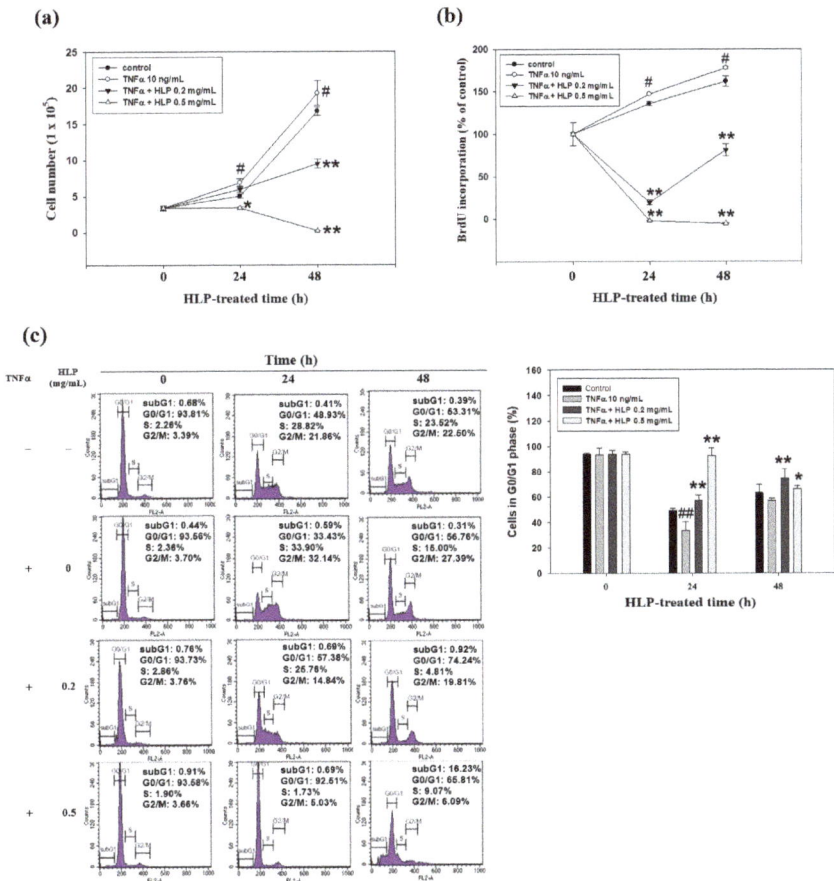

Figure 5. Effect of HLP on TNF-α-treated A7r5 cell growth curve, DNA synthesis, and cell cycle progression. A7r5 cells were treated with TNF-α (10 ng/mL) in the absence or presence of various concentrations (0, 0.2 and 0.5 mg/mL) of HLP for indicated time (0, 24 and 48 h). (**a**) The cell growth curve was evaluated using the Corning Cell Counter. (**b**) DNA synthesis was assayed by BrdU assay. (**c**) Cell cycle distribution was detected by flow cytometery. Quantitative assessment of the percentage of the cells in the cell cycle distribution (subG1, G0/G1, S, and G2/M phase) was indicated by PI dye. The proportion of cells in G0/G1 phase was quantitatively presented as mean ± SD (n = 3) of three independent experiments ± SD. # p < 0.05, ## p < 0.01 compared with the control. * p < 0.05, ** p < 0.01 compared with the TNF-α group. +, added; −, non-added.

3.6. HLP Induces Cell Cycle Arrest in the Present of TNF-α

To investigate further the mechanism of the effect HLP on cell cycle arrest at G0/G1 phase, A7r5 cells treated with TNF-α (10 ng/mL) in the presence or absence of HLP (0.2 mg/mL) for 24 and 48 h were subjected to immunoblot analysis. We first analyzed the expressions of phospho-p53 (p-p53), p53, and cki, including p16, p21, and p27. Among them, p-p53, p21, and p27 levels were significantly induced by a 24-h HLP treatment (Figure 6a). To further investigate whether the inhibitory effect of HLP on TNF-α occurred because it blocked A7r5 cell cycle progression, the changes in protein levels of PCNA, E2F, and p-Rb, regulators of cell cycle G0/G1 arrest, were also studied (Figure 6b). Stimulation with TNF-α at 10 ng/mL for not only 24 h, but also 48 h, promoted time-dependently the expressions of PCNA, E2F, and p-Rb, compared to the receptive control group. After exposure to TNF-α for 48 h, the HLP treatment significantly inhibited three expressions (Figure 6b).

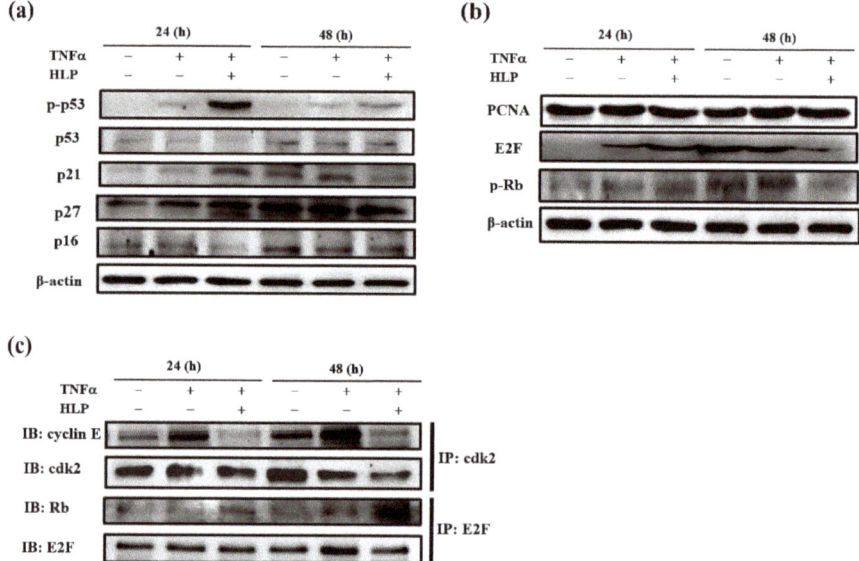

Figure 6. Effect of HLP on TNF-α-regulated the expressions of cell cycle regulatory proteins in VSMCs. A7r5 cells were treated with TNF-α (10 ng/mL) in the absence or presence of 0.2 mg/mL of HLP for 24 and 48 h. The protein levels of cdi, including p-p53, p53, p21, p27, and p16 (**a**), anti-proliferating cell nuclear antigen (PCNA), E2F, and p-Rb (**b**) were determined by Western blotting. β-actin was served as an internal control. (**c**) The expressions of cyclin E/cdk2 and Rb/E2F complexes were further analyzed. The cell extracts were immunoprecipitated (IP) with cdk2 or E2F. The precipitated complexes were examined for immunoblotting (IB) using anti-cyclin E or Rb antibody. Results are representative of at least three independent experiments. +, added; −, non-added.

Using immunoprecipitation, we confirmed that the addition of TNF-α upregulated the formation of cyclin E/cdk2 complex without noticeable change in cyclin D/cdk4 complex (data not shown) in A7r5 cells at 24 to 48 h, but HLP reversed the increases (line 1, Figure 6c). Moreover, there was a more significant increase in expression of Rb/E2F complex in the TNF-α combined with HLP treatments group (Figure 6c). As shown in Figure 6c (line 3), an increase in Rb/E2F complex was correlated with a decrease in p-Rb at 48 h of cell cycle (line 3, Figure 6b). The HLP-increased expression of Rb/E2F complex prevented the release of E2F transcription factor, and then reduced the transcription of the genes required for the cell cycle progression (Figure 6b,c). These data show that HLP regulated the association of cyclin E/cdk2, and Rb/E2F, inducing the cell cycle arrest at G0/G1 phase of A7r5 cells in the presence of TNF-α.

3.7. HLP Reduced Atherosclerotic Lesions, and the Abnormal Migration and Proliferation of VSMC in a Rabbit Model

Oxidant stress is a major cause of VSMC dysfunction and inflammation through various pathways [6,7]. To investigate the antioxidant action of HLP resulting from VSMC dysfunction, the ROS generation (DCF fluorescence) following the HLP treatments in the TNF-α-stimulated cells was examined (left panel, Figure 7a). The results showed that TNF-α significantly increased the fluorescence of intracellular ROS generation at not only 24 h, but also 48 h, whereas HLP at 0.2 mg/mL inhibited production of intracellular ROS (right panel, Figure 7a), implicating its antioxidant effects. In the same condition, the inhibitory effect of HLP on the amount of hydrogen peroxide (H_2O_2), the major form of ROS, was similar to the result of ROS production upon TNF-α stimulation (Figure S2). Collectively, these results suggest that cyclin E/cdk2-dependent Rb phosphorylation and Akt/AP-1/MMP-9 signaling pathway mediated the in vitro action of HLP against to TNF-α-induced ROS production, controlling the balance of VSMC proliferation and migration (Figure 7b).

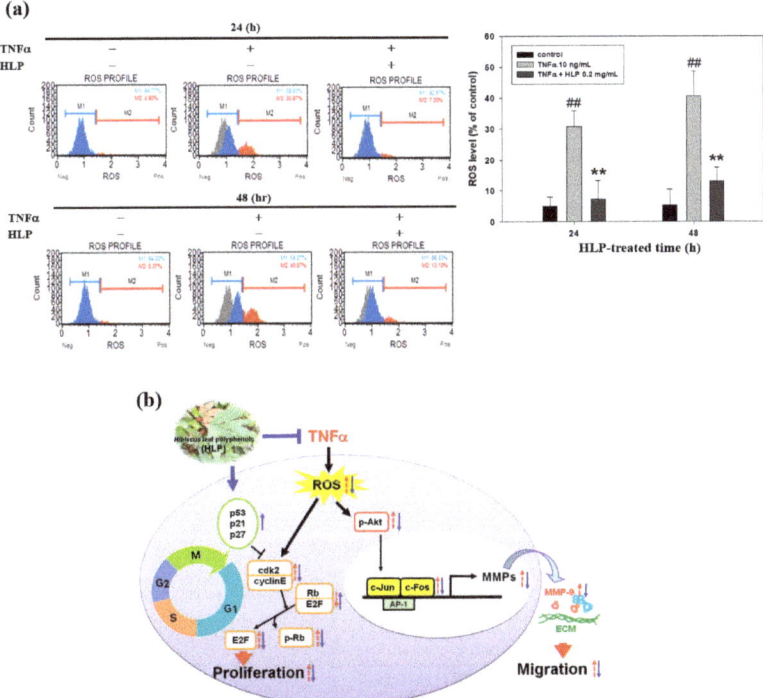

Figure 7. Effect of HLP on TNF-α-induced ROS production in VSMC. (**a**) A7r5 cells were treated with TNF-α (10 ng/mL) in the absence or presence of 0.2 mg/mL of HLP for 24 and 48 h. The treated cells were then labeled with fluorescent probe, dichlorofluorescin diacetate (DCFH-DA), and reactive oxygen species (ROS) production was measured using Muse™ Cell Analyzer. M1: DCF-negative cells. M2: DCF-positive cells. The results are presented as mean ± SD (n = 3) from three independent experiments. ## $p < 0.01$ compared with the control. ** $p < 0.01$ compared with the TNF-α group. +, added; −, non-added. (**b**) Schematic representation of TNF-α-antagonist potential of HLP on VSMCs. TNF-α induces intracellular ROS production, leading cell migration and proliferation through Akt/AP-1/MMP-9 signaling and cyclin E/cdk2-mediated Rb phosphorylation in A7r5 cells. HLP functions against TNF-α via downregulation of Akt/MMP-9 and upregulation of p53 signals that subsequently inhibit VSMC migration and proliferation. Red arrows represent the changes in response to TNF-α stimulation; blue arrows represent changes in TNF-α-exposed VSMCs receiving HLP intervention.

3.8. HLP Reduced Atherosclerotic Lesions and the Abnormal Migration and Proliferation of VSMC in a Rabbit Model

Because abnormal VSMC migration and proliferation contribute significantly in the pathogenesis of cardiovascular diseases, improvements in VSMC dysfunction will prevent the development of atherosclerosis [24]. For the clinical use of HLP for atherosclerosis, we investigated the HLP effect against VSMC dysfunction, using an atherosclerotic rabbit model. As shown in Figure 8a,b, HLP can significantly reduce the elevation of the concentrations of serum triglycerides (TG), total cholesterol (CHO), and LDL cholesterol (LDL-c) (Figure 8a), and the ratio of LDL-c and high-density lipoprotein cholesterol (HDL-c) (Figure 8b) enhanced by a HFD treatment. Past reports have shown that the decrease of LDL-c/HDL-c ratio, not just the LDL-c level alone, is of a lot of importance for reducing the atheroma burden [24,25]. In addition, the serum level of TNF-α was also significantly reduced after HFD-fed rabbits were treated with HLP (Figure 8c), confirming that HLP has a TNF-α antagonistic effect. Our study showed, in addition to possessing benefits to serum lipids, HLP can effectively decrease serum LDL/HDL ratio and TNF-α level, thus improving atherosclerosis.

To evaluate the in vivo atheroprotective effect of HLP against the extent of atherosclerosis in the aorta, the area of fatty region in the atherosclerotic lesions was analyzed using oil Red-O staining. The data in Figure 8d reveal that the subintimal lipid deposition in the HFD-treated rabbits was improved after HLP treatment. In addition, IHC staining indicated the expressions of α-SMA (upper panel) and PCNA (lower panel), served receptively as markers of VSMC migration and proliferation, were showed in the intima of atherosclerotic lesions from aortic roots of the rabbits treated with HFD (Figure 8e). As shown in Figure 8e, VSMC dysfunction was significantly observed in the atherosclerotic lesions in the HFD-treated rabbits, but very few expressions of α-SMA and PCNA in the HFD plus HLP-fed rabbits, which was consistent with the HLP-reduced the cell migration and proliferation in TNF-α-treated A7r5 cells in vitro (Figures 4 and 5). In the treatment process, HLP administration did not have any adverse effects on body weight or liver and renal function, compared to those of control (data not shown). Additionally, Western blotting of tissue extracts in the aortic arch showed the expressions of active-MMP-9, p-Akt, and E2F were markedly decreased, but the phosphorylation of p53 was increased in the group of HFD plus HLP, when compared with HLP or HFD-fed groups (Figure 8f). These results indicate that HLP can significantly improve VSMC dysfunction of HFD-treated rabbits by inhibiting cell migratory and proliferative signal pathways in vivo, as well as in vitro (Figure 8g).

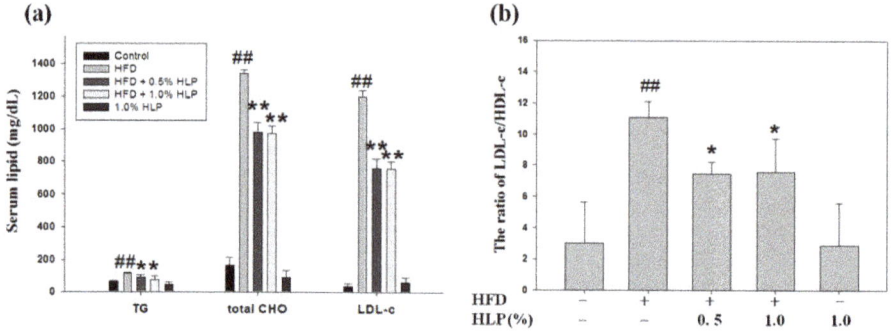

Figure 8. *Cont.*

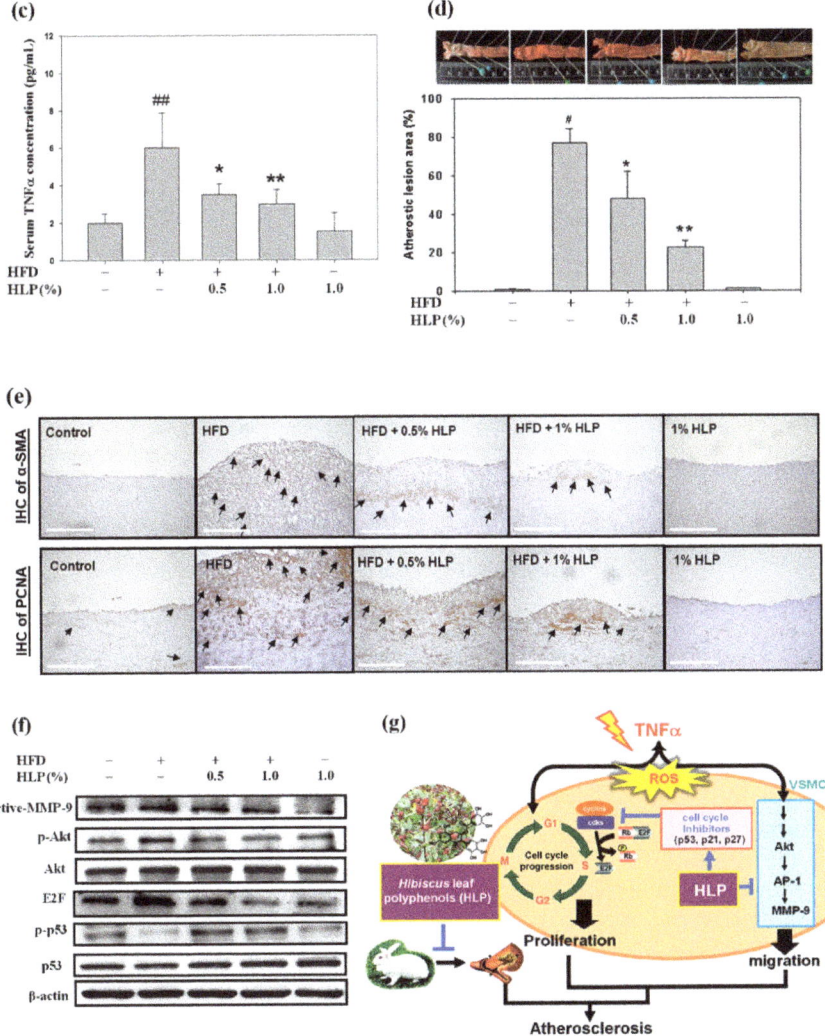

Figure 8. Effect of HLP on atherosclerotic lesions, and VSMC migration and proliferation in vivo. Among five groups, New Zealand white rabbits fed on a high-fat diet (HFD) were divided into three groups. At the same time, two of the groups were orally treated with HLP at a dose of 0.5% or 1.0%. These rabbits were sacrificed after 25 weeks. The serum levels of triglycerides (TG), total cholesterol (CHO), low-density lipoprotein cholesterol (LDL-c) (**a**), ratio of LDL-c/ high-density lipoprotein cholesterol (HDL-c) (**b**), and TNF-α (**c**) were determined by ELISA assays. The results are presented as mean ± SD from one independent experiment. # $p < 0.05$, ## $p < 0.01$ compared with the control. * $p < 0.05$, ** $p < 0.01$ compared with the HFD group. The aortic arches were collected for (**d**) oil red O stain, (**e**) immunohistochemistry (IHC) staining of α-SMA (upper panel), PCNA (lower panel). Images were taken at 400× magnification; scale bar, 50 μm. (**f**) Western blot analysis of MMP-9, p-Akt, Akt, E2F, p-p53, and p53 protein expressions was carried out with the tissue extracts from them. β-actin was served as an internal control. Results are representative of at least three independent experiments. +, added; −, non-added. (**g**) Overview of pathways for the proposed mechanism of HLP-induced inhibition of atherosclerosis in rabbits and VSMC migration/proliferation.

4. Discussion

H. sabdariffa Linne (*Malvaceae*), an attractive plant believed to be native to African countries, is cultivated in both Southern and Eastern Taiwan [26]. The calyces of the plant are typically used in foods and beverages, such as jam, jellies, and teas [15,26]. Previous studies have shown that various extracts of calyces of *H. sabdariffa* L., including *H. sabdariffa* aqueous extracts (HSEs), *H. sabdariffa* anthocyanins (HAs), and its polyphenol-rich extracts (HPEs), have been reported to exhibit a wide variety of activities against hypertension, inflammation, liver disorders, diabetes, cancer, atherosclerosis, and other metabolic syndromes [26]. While the focus has been on the calyx, the leaves of this plant are also consumed as a leafy vegetable in many countries [15]. The *Hibiscus* leaf has been also reported to exert many biologic effects, including antioxidant [13,15], anti-hyperlipidemic [13,14], anti-cancer [17,18], anti-atherosclerotic [11,16], and anti-inflammatory [15] activities, as shown in Table S1. Our recent studies have indicated that HLP, a methanol extract of *Hibiscus* leaf, is rich in polyphenols [16], including ECG and other polyphenols (Cat, EA, Que, and FA; Table S2). In the literature, ECG-enriched HLP exhibited to inhibit ox-LDL uptake and lipid-laden foam cell formation, promoted cholesterol efflux [16], and reduced ox-LDL-mediated endothelial cell injury and apoptosis [11], so HLP was expected to have potential as an anti-atherogenic agent. ECG, one of the major tea catechins, plays an important protective role in the cardiovascular system, and has been reported to possess anti-atherogenic properties in in vitro and in vivo studies [27]. It has been shown that the anti-atherosclerotic effect of Cat is associated with their antioxidant, anti-hypertensive, hypolipidaemic, and anti-mutagenic effects [28]. These Cat have been indicated to suppress the LDL oxidation and the foam cell formation in in vivo atherosclerotic lesions [27], and MMP-2 activities in cell culture supernatant of pulmonary VSMC [29]. Previous studies have indicated that EA, a polyphenolic compound present in berries, scavenged free radicals and improved lipid peroxidation [30]. According to the past and present works, the findings cooperatively show the anti-atherosclerotic activities of HLP may be contributed by their biological properties of these polyphenolic components.

In the comparison of components between both extracts, polyphenolic extracts from flowers (HPE) and leaves (HLP) of *H. sabdariffa* L., the total flavonoid content of HPE and HLP was estimated to near to 20% and 75%, respectively, via Jia method [16,22]. The results show the polyphenolic extract of *Hibiscus* leaves exhibited an about 3.8-fold content of flavonoids compared to that of its flowers. In addition to the above, HLP seems to possess stronger protective properties from VSMC dysfunction than HPE [22], including the inhibitory effects on MMP expression and cell migration (Figures 2 and 4). Huang et al. demonstrated that HPE at the doses of 0.01 and 0.10 mg/mL reduced high glucose-stimulated cell migration about 30% and 80%, respectively, by measuring the wound-healing assay [22]. In this study, above the dose of HLP at 0.01 mg/mL could completely reverse the TNF-α-increased proportion of cell migration (Figure 4a). These data suggest that HLP could exert the anti-migratory effect at lower doses than HPE.

Atherosclerosis is a multistep and chronic inflammatory process that involves interactions between various soluble mediators, endothelial cells, monocytes, and VSMCs. Monocyte-derived growth factors and cytokines further affect the vascular wall by stimulating VSMC migration and proliferation [31]. The inflammatory cytokine TNF-α has been shown to play a vital role in the disruption of the vascular circulation, and its increased expression induces the production of ROS, resulting in endothelial cell injury and VSMC dysfunction [32]. The blockade of TNF-α has been demonstrated to improve cardiovascular morbidity and mortality in chronic inflammatory disease [33]. The model of TNF-α-stimulated VSMCs has been applied to mimic the VSMC dysfunction during atherosclerotic development [31]. Therefore, the atheroprotective effects of HLP were investigated in a model of VSMCs exposed to TNF-α in vitro. The extract, at a concentration in a range of 0.01–0.10 mg/mL, possessed inhibitory effects on VSMC migration, as evidenced by the results of the decreased activities and expressions of MMPs, the levels of key migratory proteins, and the wound-healing and invasive abilities of VSMCs (Figures 1d and 2, Figures 3 and 4). The effect of the higher concentrations (>0.10 mg/mL) showed that it repressed cell growth and DNA synthesis, as well as enhanced cell apoptosis (Figure 5). Similarly, Won et al. reported that the mechanisms of catechins action against cardiovascular diseases include the inhibition of VSMC proliferation [34]. Further studies have also indicated that many polyphenols prevented atherosclerosis through inhibiting proliferation and/or inducing apoptosis of VSMC [35]. The findings of this study reveal, for the first time, the protective effects of HLP on this model, examined in each test, provide bifunctional results of HLP. Therefore, it is convincing that HLP could potentially be used in the treatment of atherosclerosis.

As mentioned above, the migration of VSMCs from medial to intima contributes to the formation of atherosclerosis [2]. MMPs, a family of proteinases, promote ECM degradation, which, in turn, facilitates cell migration. Activated Akt induced AP-1, which is required for the production of MMPs [36]. However, upon TNF-α stimulation, the mechanism(s) mediating MMP activation and the MMP-regulated downstream signals have yet to be clarified. TNF-α promoted VSMC chemotaxis via Akt and MAPK activation, as reported by Chan et al. [31]. The Akt antagonist PTEN was also shown to be involved in VSMC migration [37]. Consistent with previous reports, this study confirmed that it is therefore possible that HLP inhibits TNF-α-stimulated MMP-9 activation by downregulating Akt/AP-1 pathway, and subsequently prevents VSMC migration. Furthermore, previous studies have indicated that oxidative stress modulated by ROS promotes VSMC dysfunction developing atherosclerosis and also induces MMP-mediated ECM remodeling and cell cycle progression [6,7,38]. In this study, TNF-α increased the production of intracellular ROS, especially of the H_2O_2 level, and this might influence the overall signaling pathways of VSMC migration/proliferation. In this regard, HLP attenuated ROS generation against TNF-α stimulation (Figure 7), and it might contribute to MMP inhibition and cell cycle regulation by HLP. Further investigations are needed to clarify this issue. Consistent with previous reports and our past results, as shown in Table S4, this study confirmed that HLP possesses strong antioxidant ability in inhibiting the VSMC dysfunction and atherosclerotic development.

Next, to study the mechanism(s) of HLP-inhibited VSMC proliferation, the regulation of cell cycle arrest was examined. VSMCs begin to divide in response to mitogens and enter the S phase upon vascular injury [9]. Cdks, working in conjunction with their activating subunits (cyclins), provide the driving force for cell cycle transitions [34]. The kinase activities of these cyclin/cdk complexes are regulated by cdi, including Ink4 proteins (p16, p18, and p19) and Cip/Kip proteins (p21, p27, and p57), and their upstream factor, the gatekeeper of mammalian cell cycle, p53 [10,39]. As expected, HLP treatments induced a G0/G1 phase growth arrest by inducing the cki-mediated cell cycle regulation (Figure 6). In addition, PCNA expression is increased in unstable atherosclerotic plaque [40]; moreover, PCNA is highly expressed in human VSMCs [41]. Consistent with previous reports, our studies showed that TNF-α significantly reduced A7r5 cell growth and increased PCNA expression (Figure 6b). Further data demonstrate a marked and dose-dependent reduction in neointimal expression of PCNA after fed with HLP in HFD-treated rabbits (Figure 8e), indicating that HLP ameliorates atherosclerosis by reducing PCNA expression, both in vitro and in vivo.

5. Conclusions

In conclusion, the findings of this study are schematically presented in Figure 8g. TNF-α generally induces ROS production, which influences Akt/AP-1/MMP-9 signaling and cyclin E/cdk2-mediated phosphorylation of Rb, leading to participation in abnormal VSMC migration and proliferation. Conversely, HLP is speculated to play a role in TNF-α antagonist, which contributes to inhibiting ROS generation and VSMC dysfunction. Because our in vitro data demonstrate that HLP inhibited TNFα-induced VSMC migration and proliferation, in vivo results indicate that HLP can effectively improve HFD-promoted atherosclerosis in rabbits via decreasing TNF-α secretion to confirm the anti-atherosclerotic effect of HLP (Figure 8a–d). As shown in Figure 8, HLP can pleiotropically inhibit rabbit atherosclerosis by reducing serum lipid levels, inflammation, atheroscletic lesion, and VSMC migration/proliferation via downregulation of Akt/MMP-9 and upregulation of p53 signals. Taken together, our findings indicate the anti-TNF-α effects of HLP on VSMC could likely contribute to its protection against atherosclerosis and other cardiovascular disorders.

Supplementary Materials: The following are available online at http://www.mdpi.com/2076-3921/8/12/620/s1: Table S1. Biological activities of *Hibiscus* leaf in previous studies; Table S2. Polyphenolic compound content (in %) in methanol extracts of *Hibiscus* leaf; Table S3. Sequences of primers used in RT-PCR; Table S4. Antioxidant capacity of HLP in standard antioxidant evaluation; Figure S1. Effect of HLP alone on cell viability in VSMCs; Figure S2. Effect of HLP on TNF-α-induced H_2O_2 production in VSMC.

Author Contributions: Conceptualization, J.-H.C. and H.-H.L.; methodology, C.-C.C. and C.-P.W.; formal analysis, C.-C.C. and C.-P.W.; writing—original draft preparation, C.-C.C.; writing—review and editing, J.-H.C. and H.-H.L.; supervision, J.-H.C. and H.-H.L.; project administration, H.H.L.; funding acquisition, C.-C.C.

Funding: This work was supported by a grant from the Antai Medical Care Corporation Antai Tian-Sheng Memorial Hospital (CSMU-TSMH-106-03), Pingtung County, Taiwan.

Conflicts of Interest: The authors declare no conflicts of interest.

References

1. Ross, R. Atherosclerosis-an inflammatory disease. *N. Engl. J. Med.* **1999**, *340*, 115. [CrossRef] [PubMed]
2. Glass, C.K.; Witztum, J.L. Atherosclerosis. The road ahead. *Cell* **2001**, *104*, 503. [CrossRef]
3. Lusis, A.J. Atherosclerosis. *Nature* **2000**, *407*, 233. [CrossRef] [PubMed]
4. Braun-Dullaeus, R.C.; Mann, M.J.; Dzau, V.J. Cell cycle progression: New therpeutic target for vascular proliferative disease. *Circulation* **1998**, *98*, 82. [CrossRef] [PubMed]
5. Mason, D.P.; Kenagy, R.D.; Hasenstab, D.; Bowen-Pope, D.F.; Seifert, R.A.; Coats, S.; Hawkins, S.M.; Clowes, A.W. Matrix metalloproteinase-9 overexpression enhances vascular smooth muscle cell migration and alters remodeling in the injured rat carotid artery. *Circ. Res.* **1999**, *85*, 1179. [CrossRef] [PubMed]
6. Hopkins, P.N. Molecular biology of atherosclerosis. *Physiol. Rev.* **2013**, *93*, 1317. [CrossRef]
7. Balzan, S.; Lubrano, V. LOX-1 receptor: A potential link in atherosclerosis and cancer. *Life Sci.* **2018**, *198*, 79. [CrossRef]
8. Newby, A.C. Matrix metalloproteinase inhibition therapy for vascular diseases. *Vascul. Pharmacol.* **2012**, *56*, 232. [CrossRef]
9. Lee, B.; Kim, C.H.; Moon, S.K. Honokiol causes the p21WAF1-mediated G(1)-phase arrest of the cell cycle through inducing p38 mitogen activated protein kinase in vascular smooth muscle cells. *FEBS Lett.* **2006**, *580*, 5177. [CrossRef]
10. Vidal, A.; Koff, A. Cell-cycle inhibitors: Three families united by a common cause. *Gene* **2000**, *247*, 1. [CrossRef]
11. Chen, J.H.; Lee, M.S.; Wang, C.P.; Hsu, C.C.; Lin, H.H. Autophagic effects of *Hibiscus sabdariffa* leaf polyphenols and epicatechin gallate (ECG) against oxidized LDL-induced injury of human endothelial cells. *Eur. J. Nutr.* **2017**, *56*, 1963–1981. [CrossRef] [PubMed]
12. Sachdewa, A.; Nigam, R.; Khemani, L.D. Hypoglycemic effect of *Hibiscus rosa sinensis* L. leaf extract in glucose and streptozotocin induced hyperglycemic rats. *Indian J. Exp. Biol.* **2001**, *39*, 284. [PubMed]
13. Ochani, P.C.; D'Mello, P. Antioxidant and antihyperlipidemic activity of *Hibiscus sabdariffa* Linn. leaves and calyces extracts in rats. *Indian J. Exp. Biol.* **2009**, *47*, 276. [PubMed]
14. Gosain, S.; Ircchiaya, R.; Sharma, P.C.; Thareja, S.; Kalra, A.; Deep, A.; Bhardwaj, T.R. Hypolipidemic effect of ethanolic extract from the leaves of *Hibiscus sabdariffa* L. in hyperlipidemic rats. *Acta. Pol. Pharm.* **2010**, *67*, 179–184. [PubMed]
15. Zhen, J.; Villani, T.S.; Guo, Y.; Qi, Y.; Chin, K.; Pan, M.H.; Ho, C.T.; Simon, J.E.; Wu, Q. Phytochemistry, antioxidant capacity, total phenolic content and anti-inflammatory activity of *Hibiscus sabdariffa* leaves. *Food Chem.* **2016**, *190*, 673. [CrossRef] [PubMed]
16. Chen, J.H.; Wang, C.J.; Wang, C.P.; Sheu, J.Y.; Lin, C.L.; Lin, H.H. *Hibiscus sabdariffa* leaf polyphenolic extract inhibits LDL oxidation and foam cell formation involving up-regulation of LXRα/ABCA1 pathway. *Food Chem.* **2013**, *141*, 397. [CrossRef]
17. Lin, H.H.; Chan, K.C.; Sheu, J.Y.; Hsuan, S.W.; Wang, C.J.; Chen, J.H. *Hibiscus sabdariffa* leaf induces apoptosis of human prostate cancer cells in vitro and in vivo. *Food Chem.* **2012**, *132*, 880. [CrossRef]
18. Chiu, C.T.; Chen, J.H.; Chou, F.P.; Lin, H.H. *Hibiscus sabdariffa* Leaf Extract Inhibits Human Prostate Cancer Cell Invasion via Down-Regulation of Akt/NF-kB/MMP-9 Pathway. *Nutrients* **2015**, *7*, 5065–5087. [CrossRef]

19. Meng, J.M.; Cao, S.Y.; Wei, X.L.; Gan, R.Y.; Wang, Y.F.; Cai, S.X.; Xu, X.Y.; Zhang, P.Z.; Li, H.B. Effects and Mechanisms of Tea for the Prevention and Management of Diabetes Mellitus and Diabetic Complications: An Updated Review. *Antioxidants* **2019**, *8*, 170. [CrossRef]
20. Lakenbrink, C.; Lapczynski, S.; Maiwald, B.; Engelhardt, U.H. Flavonoids and other polyphenols in consumer brews of tea and other caffeinated beverages. *J. Agric. Food Chem.* **2000**, *48*, 2848. [CrossRef]
21. Jia, Z.; Tang, M.; Wu, J. The determination of flavonoid contents in mulberry and their scavenging effects on superoxides radicals. *Food Chem.* **1999**, *64*, 555. [CrossRef]
22. Huang, C.N.; Chan, K.C.; Lin, W.T.; Su, S.L.; Wang, C.J.; Peng, C.H. *Hibiscus sabdariffa* inhibits vascular smooth muscle cell proliferation and migration induced by high glucose—A mechanism involves connective tissue growth factor signals. *J. Agric. Food Chem.* **2009**, *57*, 3073. [CrossRef] [PubMed]
23. Chan, K.C.; Ho, H.H.; Huang, C.N.; Lin, M.C.; Chen, H.M.; Wang, C.J. Mulberry leaf extract inhibits vascular smooth muscle cell migration involving a block of small GTPase and Akt/NF-kappaB signals. *J. Agric. Food Chem.* **2009**, *57*, 9147. [CrossRef] [PubMed]
24. Rivard, A.; Andrés, V. Vascular smooth muscle cell proliferation in the pathogenesis of atherosclerotic cardiovascular diseases. *Histol. Histopathol.* **2000**, *15*, 557. [CrossRef]
25. Choi, S.H.; Chae, A.; Miller, E.; Messig, M.; Ntanios, F.; DeMaria, A.N.; Nissen, S.E.; Witztum, J.L.; Tsimikas, S. Relationship between biomarkers of oxidized low-density lipoprotein, statin therapy, quantitative coronary angiography, and atheroma: volume observations from the REVERSAL (Reversal of Atherosclerosis with Aggressive Lipid Lowering) study. *J. Am. Coll. Cardiol.* **2008**, *52*, 24. [CrossRef]
26. Lin, H.H.; Chen, J.H.; Wang, C.J. Chemopreventive properties and molecular mechanisms of the bioactive compounds in *Hibiscus sabdariffa* Linne. *Curr. Med. Chem.* **2011**, *18*, 1245. [CrossRef]
27. Hayek, T.; Fuhrman, B.; Vaya, J.; Rosenblat, M.; Belinky, P.; Coleman, R.; Elis, A.; Aviram, M. Reduced progression of atherosclerosis in apolipoprotein E-deficient mice following consumption of red wine, or its polyphenols quercetin or catechin, is associated with reduced susceptibility of LDL to oxidation and aggregation. *Arterioscler. Thromb. Vasc. Biol.* **1997**, *17*, 2744. [CrossRef]
28. Ikeda, I.; Imasato, Y.; Sasaki, E.; Nakayama, M.; Nagao, H.; Takeo, T.; Yayabe, F.; Sugano, M. Tea catechins decrease micellar solubility and intestinal absorption of cholesterol in rats. *Biochim. Biophys. Acta* **1992**, *1127*, 141. [CrossRef]
29. Chowdhury, A.; Nandy, S.K.; Sarkar, J.; Chakraborti, T.; Chakraborti, S. Inhibition of pro-/active MMP-2 by green tea catechins and prediction of their interaction by molecular docking studies. *Mol. Cell. Biochem.* **2017**, *427*, 111. [CrossRef]
30. Laranjinha, J.; Vieirra, O.; Almeida, L.; Madeira, V. Inhibition of metmyoglobin/H2O2-dependent low density lipoprotein lipid peroxidation by naturally occurring phenolic acid. *Biochem. Pharmacol.* **1996**, *51*, 395. [CrossRef]
31. Chan, K.C.; Yu, M.H.; Lin, M.C.; Huang, C.N.; Chung, D.J.; Lee, Y.J.; Wu, C.H.; Wang, C.J. Pleiotropic effects of acarbose on atherosclerosis development in rabbits are mediated via upregulating AMPK signals. *Sci. Rep.* **2016**, *6*, 38642. [CrossRef] [PubMed]
32. Zhang, H.; Park, Y.; Wu, J.; Chen, X.P.; Lee, S.; Yang, J.; Dellsperger, K.C.; Zhang, C. Role of TNF-alpha in vascular dysfunction. *Clin Sci* **2009**, *116*, 219. [CrossRef] [PubMed]
33. Nishida, K.; Okada, Y.; Nawata, M.; Saito, K.; Tanaka, Y. Induction of hyperadiponectinemia following long-term treatment of patients with rheumatoid arthritis with infliximab (IFX), an anti-TNF-alpha antibody. *Endocr. J.* **2008**, *55*, 213. [CrossRef] [PubMed]
34. Won, S.M.; Park, Y.H.; Kim, H.J.; Park, K.M.; Lee, W.J. Catechins inhibit angiotensin II-induced vascular smooth muscle cell proliferation via mitogen-activated protein kinase pathway. *Exp. Mol. Med.* **2006**, *38*, 525. [CrossRef]
35. Ekshyyan, V.P.; Hebert, V.Y.; Khandelwal, A.; Dugas, T.R. Resveratrol inhibits rat aortic vascular smooth muscle cell proliferation via estrogen receptor dependent nitric oxide production. *J. Cardiovasc. Pharmacol* **2007**, *50*, 83. [CrossRef]
36. Tseng, H.C.; Lee, I.T.; Lin, C.C.; Chi, P.L.; Cheng, S.E.; Shih, R.H.; Hsiao, L.D.; Yang, C.M. IL-1β promotes corneal epithelial cell migration by increasing MMP-9 expression through NF-κB- and AP-1-dependent pathways. *PLoS ONE* **2013**, *8*, e57955. [CrossRef]
37. Huang, J.; Kontos, C.D. Inhibition of vascular smooth muscle cell proliferation, migration, and survival by the tumor suppressor protein PTEN. *Arterioscler. Thromb. Vasc. Biol.* **2002**, *22*, 745. [CrossRef]

38. Choi, E.S.; Yoon, J.J.; Han, B.H.; Jeong, D.H.; Kim, H.Y.; Ahn, Y.M.; Eun, S.Y.; Lee, Y.J.; Kang, D.G.; Lee, H.S. Samul-Tang Regulates Cell Cycle and Migration of Vascular Smooth Muscle Cells against TNF-α Stimulation. *Evi Based Complement Alterna Med.* **2018**, *2018*, 1024974. [CrossRef]
39. Jacks, T.; Weinberg, R.A. Cell-cycle control and its watchman. *Nature* **1996**, *381*, 643. [CrossRef]
40. Lavezzi, A.M.; Milei, J.; Grana, D.R.; Flenda, F.; Basellini, A.; Matturri, L. Expression of c-fos, p53 and PCNA in the unstable atherosclerotic carotid plaque. *Int. J. Cardiol.* **2003**, *92*, 59. [CrossRef]
41. Pickering, J.G.; Weir, L.; Jekanowski, J.; Kearney, M.A.; Isner, J.M. Proliferative activity in peripheral and coronary atherosclerotic plaque among patients undergoing percutaneous revascularization. *J. Clin. Invest.* **1993**, *91*, 1469. [CrossRef] [PubMed]

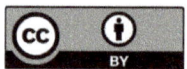 © 2019 by the authors. Licensee MDPI, Basel, Switzerland. This article is an open access article distributed under the terms and conditions of the Creative Commons Attribution (CC BY) license (http://creativecommons.org/licenses/by/4.0/).

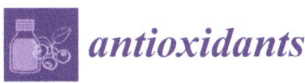

Article

Rosmarinus officinalis Essential Oil Improves Scopolamine-Induced Neurobehavioral Changes via Restoration of Cholinergic Function and Brain Antioxidant Status in Zebrafish (*Danio rerio*)

Luminita Capatina [1], Razvan Stefan Boiangiu [1], Gabriela Dumitru [1], Edoardo Marco Napoli [2], Giuseppe Ruberto [2], Lucian Hritcu [1,*] and Elena Todirascu-Ciornea [1]

1 Department of Biology, Faculty of Biology, Alexandru Ioan Cuza University of Iasi, 700506 Iasi, Romania; capatina.luminita@yahoo.com (L.C.); boiangiu.razvan@yahoo.com (R.S.B.); gabriela.dumitru@uaic.ro (G.D.); ciornea@uaic.ro (E.T.-C.)
2 Institute of Biomolecular Chemistry, National Research Council ICB-CNR, 95126 Catania, Italy; edoardo.napoli@icb.cnr.it (E.M.N.); giuseppe.ruberto@icb.cnr.it (G.R.)
* Correspondence: hritcu@uaic.ro; Tel.: +40-232201666

Received: 10 December 2019; Accepted: 8 January 2020; Published: 10 January 2020

Abstract: *Rosmarinus officinalis* L. is a traditional herb with various therapeutic applications such as antibacterial, antioxidant, anti-inflammatory, antidepressant, and anticholinesterase activities, and can be used for the prevention or treatment of dementia. In the present study, we tested whether *Rosmarinus officinalis* L. could counteract scopolamine-induced anxiety, dementia, and brain oxidative stress in the zebrafish model and tried to find the underlying mechanism. *Rosmarinus officinalis* L. essential oil (REO: 25, 150, and 300 µL/L) was administered by immersion to zebrafish (*Danio rerio*) once daily for eight days while scopolamine (100 µM) treatment was delivered 30 min before behavioral tests. The antidepressant and cognitive-enhancing actions of the essential oil in the scopolamine zebrafish model was measured in the novel tank diving test (NTT) and Y-maze test. The chemical composition was identified by Gas chromatograph–Mass spectrometry (GC-MS) analysis. The brain oxidative status and acetylcholinesterase (AChE) activity was also determined. REO reversed scopolamine-induced anxiety, memory impairment, and brain oxidative stress. In addition, a reduced brain AChE activity following the administration of REO in scopolamine-treated fish was observed. In conclusion, REO exerted antidepressant-like effect and cognitive-enhancing action and was able to abolish AChE alteration and brain oxidative stress induced by scopolamine.

Keywords: *Rosmarinus officinalis*; essential oil; scopolamine; anxiety; memory; oxidative stress

1. Introduction

Alzheimer's disease (AD) is a progressive neurodegenerative disorder, particularly affecting the cerebral cortex and hippocampus, leading to memory impairment. AD pathological hallmarks include extracellular accumulation of insoluble forms of amyloid-β, aggregation of the microtubule protein tau in neurofibrillary tangles in neurons, as well as the reduction in levels of acetylcholine [1,2].

Among various descriptive hypotheses regarding the cause of AD, the cholinergic hypothesis was the first proposed to explain AD based on the findings that a loss of cholinergic activity is commonly observed in the brains of AD patients [1]. In addition, this theory implied utilizing acetylcholinesterase inhibitors (AChEIs), which reversed memory deficits in AD patients. AChEIs could diminish memory impairment in AD patients by inhibiting the degradation of acetylcholine [3]. Currently, for the treatment of mild to moderate AD, three AChEIs are used: donepezil, rivastigmine, and galantamine [4]. Moreover, it has been reported that the daily living ability of AD patients subjected to rivastigmine and galantamine medications is better than those treated with donepezil [5]. AD is additionally associated with neuropsychiatric symptoms such as depression, anxiety, and apathy [6]. Oxidative stress is involved in age-related diseases and the pathological processes of neurodegenerative diseases, including AD [7].

Presently, there is no remedy for dementia-related afflictions, and existing medicines do not give satisfactory enhancements. Moreover, there are different side effects related to existing treatment. Herbal-based compounds could be a great source of anti-AD agents [8].

Although numerous studies have been performed to elucidate the effects of *Rosmarinus officinalis* extract on cognitive function in rodents [9–11], there is no such study conducted in zebrafish. Zebrafish exhibit complex cognition comparable to that seen in mammals [12,13], and there are behavioral tasks protocols based on rodent protocols such as active or passive avoidance test [14], Y-maze test [15], and T-maze test [16] for zebrafish. In zebrafish, scopolamine, a muscarinic acetylcholine receptor blocker, has been characterized to induce amnestic effects and is used in combination with nootropic and cognitive-enhancing drugs to study memory processes [17].

Supporting data demonstrate different biological effects of *Rosmarinus officinalis* L. Nematolahi et al. [18] demonstrated that *Rosmarinus officinalis* reduced memory-deficits, anxiety, and depression, and improved sleep quality in university students. Naderali et al. [9] reported that *Rosmarinus officinalis* extract improved memory deficits and mitigated neuronal degeneration induced by kainic acid in the rat hippocampus, due to its antioxidant profile. In addition, Karim et al. [10], by molecular docking and in vivo approaches, demonstrated anti-amnesic effects of nepitrin isolated from *Rosmarinus officinalis* on scopolamine-induced memory impairment in mice. Song et al. [11] demonstrated that a rat model of repetitive mild traumatic brain injury subjected to *Rosmarinus officinalis* extract exhibited improvement of cognitive deficits mediated by its antioxidant and anti-inflammatory profile.

The biological activities of the *Rosmarinus officinalis* could be related to the presence of volatile compounds, such as α-pinene, eucalyptol, and camphor, and phenolic compounds, such as carnosol, carnosic acid, and rosmarinic acid, with proved antioxidant, antibacterial, antifungal, anti-inflammatory, anti-AD, antidepressant and anxiolytic effects [18,19]. Therefore, the present study was designed to characterize the chemical components of the *Rosmarinus officinalis* essential oil (REO) and to evaluate the effects on anxiety, memory performance, and brain antioxidant status in a scopolamine-induced a zebrafish model of amnesia.

2. Materials and Methods

2.1. Essential Oil and Chemical Material

REO from biological cultivations was manufactured and kindly supplied by Flora Srl (Pisa, Italy), batch number 171861. Pure standards of essential oil compounds (see Table 1) were purchased from Sigma-Aldrich Chemical Co. and Fluka Chemie.

2.2. Gas Chromatograph–Mass Spectrometry (GC-MS) Analysis

A Gas Chromatograph (Shimadzu GC-17A, Shimadzu, Milan, Italy) with Flame Ionization Detector (GC-FID) equipped with a 15 m × 0.1 mm × 0.1 mm capillary column (Supelco SPB^{TM}-5, Merk KGaA, Darmstadt, Germany) was used. The operating condition followed those previously published [20]: 60 °C for 1 min, 60–280 °C at 10 °C/min, and then 280 °C for 1 min; injector temperature, 250 °C; and detector temperature, 280 °C with helium as carrier gas (1 mL/min). GC-MS analyses were performed with the same column and operative conditions mentioned above. Mass spectrometer parameters were the same as those previously published [21]. Component identification was based on comparison of their retention indexes with those relative to a mix of C_9–C_{22} n-alkanes, computer matching of spectral MS data, and fragmentation patterns with those in libraries [22,23], and co-injections with authentic samples (see Table 1).

2.3. Animals

In total, 50 adult (sex ratio was about 50:50 male:female, 3–4-month old, and 3–4 cm in length), wild-type short-fin strain zebrafish (*Danio rerio*) purchased from an authorized commercial dealer (Pet Product S.R.L., Bucharest, Romania) were used in the present study and acclimated for at least two weeks before experiments. Fish were fed twice daily with Norwin Norvitall flake (Norwin, Gadstrup, Denmark). Animals were randomly divided into groups of 10 fish/24 L housing tanks filled with unchlorinated water under a 14 h/10 h light/dark cycle. The water within the tanks was constantly aerated (7.20 mg O_2/L) using Tetra*tec*® air pumps (Tetra, Melle, Germany) and filtrated to avoid the accumulation of organic toxins. The water parameters were kept in the following ranges: pH 7.5, conductivity 500 µS, ammonium concentration < 0.004 ppm, and temperature 26 ± 1 °C. For the behavior studies, acclimated zebrafish were randomly assigned into the control, the scopolamine (Sco, 100 µM, Sigma-Aldrich, Darmstadt, Germany), and three REO treatment groups (25, 150, and 300 µL/L). The doses of the essential oil were chosen with reference to previous reports [24]. REO (25, 150, and 300 µL/L) was administered individually by immersion to zebrafish (*Danio rerio*) through transferring into 500 mL glass for 1 h, once daily for eight days, whereas scopolamine (100 µM) treatment was delivered individually by transferring into a 500 mL glass, 30 min before behavioral tests. The control group was immersed only in unchlorinated water. The working protocol (as summarized in Figure 1) was approved by the local board of ethics for animal experimentation (No. 15309/2019) and fully complied with the Directive 2010/63/EU of the European Parliament and of the Council of 22 September 2010 on the protection of animals. Efforts were made to reduce animal suffering and the number of animals utilized.

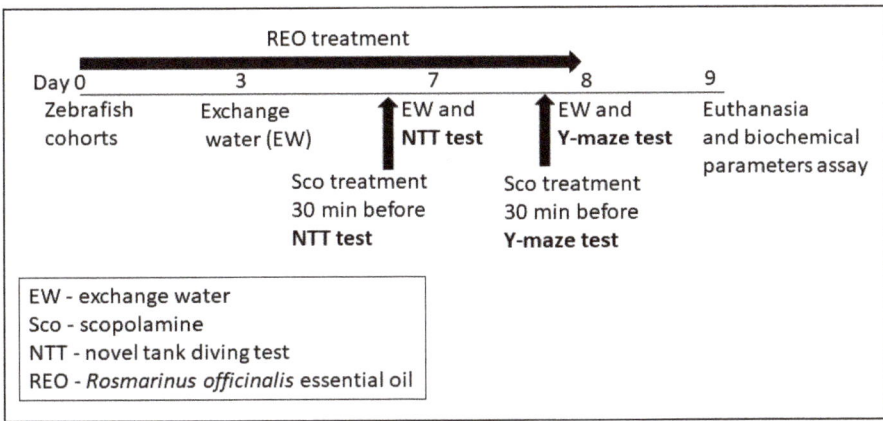

Figure 1. Scheme of the working protocol.

2.4. Behavioral Analysis

2.4.1. Novel Tank Diving Test (NTT)

NTT is a specific test used for assessing anxiety in zebrafish, as described by Cachat et al. [25]. The trapezoidal tank (1.5 L) used measured 15.2 cm (height) × 27.9 cm (top) × 22.5 cm (bottom) × 7.1 cm (width), equally divided into two horizontal sections (top and bottom). After 60 min of REO treatment, the animals were placed individually within the test tank without acclimatization, and swimming behavior was recorded for 6 min. The animals were recorded with a Logitech HD Webcam C922 Pro Stream camera (Logitech, Lausanne, Switzerland) placed 30 cm away from the tank and the videos were analyzed using ANY-Maze® software (Stoelting CO, Wood Dale, IL, USA). The following parameters were registered: the number of entries in the top/bottom zone of the tank, total distance traveled in the tank (m), and average velocity (m/s).

2.4.2. Y-Maze Test

Spatial memory and the response to novelty in zebrafish was assessed using the Y-maze task [26]. The position in the Y-maze task was considered an index of memory [27]. The apparatus consisted of a Y-maze glass aquarium with three arms (25 cm long, 8 cm wide, and 15 cm high), filled with 3 L of the same water used in the home aquarium. Visible geometric shapes such as squares, circles, and triangles were placed on the external Y-maze walls. The Y-maze arms were arbitrarily assigned: (i) the start arm, where fish began to investigate (always open); (ii) the novel arm, which was obstructed during the first trial, but open during the second trial; and (iii) the other arm (constantly open). The Y-maze center (neutral zone) was not counted in the analysis. The assignment comprised of two trials separated by 1 h to evaluate the response to novelty and spatial memory. During the first trial (training, 5 min), 60 min of REO treatment, the fish could investigate only two arms of the Y-maze (the start and the other arm), whereas the third arm (the novel arm) was obstructed. For the second trial, each fish was individually introduced into the start arm and free access to all three arms for 5 min to assess the response to novelty. Behavioral activity was analyzed using ANY-Maze® software (Stoelting CO, Wood Dale, IL, USA) and with a Logitech HD Webcam C922 Pro Stream camera (Logitech, Lausanne, Switzerland) placed above the Y-maze tank. The following measures were recorded: time spent in each arm to assess short-term spatial memory and, for the locomotory activity total, distance traveled (m) and turn angle (°) were assessed.

2.5. Biochemical Parameters Assay

After the recording of behavioral data, zebrafish were euthanized (10 min immersion in ice water, 2–4 °C) until loss of opercular motions [28], and their brains were isolated for biochemical parameters assay. The brains were gently homogenized in ice 0.1 M potassium phosphate buffer (pH 7.4), 1.15% KCl with Potter Homogenizer (Cole-Parmer, Vernon Hills, IL, USA). The resulted homogenate was centrifuged at $960 \times g$ for 15 min. The supernatant was used for the estimation of acetylcholinesterase (AChE), superoxide dismutase (SOD), catalase (CAT), glutathione peroxidase (GPX) specific activities, and malondialdehyde (MDA) level following the methods described in detail by Dumitru et al. [29]. Estimation of protein content was done through a bicinchoninic acid (BCA) protein assay kit (Sigma-Aldrich, Darmstadt, Germany) [30].

2.6. Statistical Analysis

Data are expressed as mean ± standard error of the mean (S.E.M). Results were analyzed by one-way analysis of variance (ANOVA) followed by Tuckey's post hoc multiple comparison test, considering treatment as a factor. Differences were considered significant at $p < 0.05$. GraphPad Prism 8.0 (GraphPad Software, Inc., San Diego, CA, USA) was used to perform statistical analyses and to produce graphics. Correlation among the behavioral scores, enzymatic activities, and lipid peroxidation was estimated by the Pearson correlation coefficient (r).

3. Results and Discussion

3.1. The Chemical Composition of the Essential Oil

The chemical composition of the REO was identified by GC-MS analysis (Figure 2) and is presented in Table 1. Seventy-seven chemicals, corresponding to 73.48% of the total oil, were identified in the REO. The most abundant chemical classes of the oil components were monoterpene hydrocarbons (40.14%), followed by oxygenated monoterpenes (26.44%), sesquiterpene hydrocarbons (4.74%), and other compounds (2.16%). The major components of the REO were eucalyptol (26.02%), α-pinene (19.89%), camphor (16.71%), camphene (8.67%), β-myrcene (3.97%), β-caryophyllene (3.11%), borneol (2.50%), and limonene (2.16%). Our results are supported by Bouyahya et al. [31], who reported eucalyptol (23.673%), camphor (18.743%), borneol (15.46%), and α-pinene (14.076%) as the major chemical components of the REO. In addition, Elyemni et al. [32] reported the presence of eucalyptol

(32.18%), camphor (16.20%), α-pinene (15.82%), camphene (9.16%), and α-terpineol (7.36%) in the chemical composition of the REO. Based on these studies, our essential oil exhibits a chemical composition commensurate to those reported by other authors who presume its memory-enhancing and antioxidant activity.

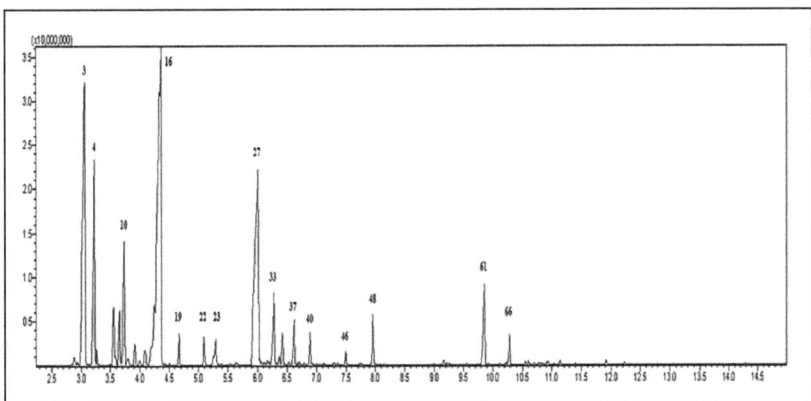

Figure 2. Gas chromatography-mass spectrometry (GC–MS) profile of the *Rosmarinus officinalis* essential oil (numbers refer to Table 1).

Table 1. Chemical composition of *Rosmarinus officinalis* essential oil [a].

No.	KI [b]	Compound	%
		Monoterpene hydrocarbons	40.14
1	920	Tricyclene	0.32
2	925	α-Thujene	0.09
3	934	α-Pinene [c]	19.89
4	949	Camphene	8.67
5	953	Thuja-2.4(10)-diene	0.33
6	972	Sabinene	0.02
7	975	β-Pinene [c]	1.56
10	988	β-Myrcene	3.97
12	1001	α-Phellandrene	0.63
13	1008	α-Terpinene	0.15
14	1015	*p*-Cymene	0.68
15	1024	Limonene [c]	2.16
17	1037	*cis*-β-Ocimene	0.16
18	1047	*trans*-β-Ocimene	0.04
19	1058	γ-Terpinene	0.74
22	1087	Terpinolene	0.75

Table 1. Cont.

No.	KI [b]	Compound	%
		Oxygenated monoterpenes	26.44
16	1033	Eucalyptol [c]	26.02
20	1070	cis-Sabinene hydrate	0.01
21	1075	cis-Linalool oxide	0.01
23	1098	Linalool	1.10
24	1109	endo-Fenchol	0.02
25	1115	exo-Fenchol	0.06
26	1125	α-Campholenal	0.14
27	1148	Camphor [c]	16.71
28	1151	Camphene hydrate	0.04
29	1155	Menthone	0.03
30	1158	Isopulegol	0.03
31	1162	trans-Pinocamphone	0.07
32	1164	Pinocarvone	0.07
33	1168	Borneol	2.50
34	1175	cis-Pinocamphone	0.17
35	1178	Terpinen-4-ol	0.78
36	1186	p-Cymen-8-ol	0.08
37	1191	a-Terpineol	1.38
38	1198	Myrtenol	0.10
39	1204	trans-Dihydro Carvone	0.06
40	1210	Verbenone	1.18
41	1221	trans-Carveol	0.01
42	1231	Linalyl formate	0.06
43	1242	cis-Dihydro Carvone	0.03
44	1244	Neral	0.01
45	1248	Carvone	0.03
46	1258	Linalyl acetate	0.35
47	1275	Geranial	0.01
48	1289	Bornyl acetate	1.10
49	1299	Thymol	0.01
50	1305	Carvacrol	0.03
51	1327	Piperitenone	0.02
52	1348	Eugenol	0.01
53	1361	Neryl acetate	0.01
54	1366	Linalyl isobutanoate	0.02
55	1376	α-ylangene	0.11
56	1380	α-Copaene	0.06
57	1384	Geranyl acetate	0.03
58	1403	Methyl eugenol	0.02

Table 1. Cont.

No.	KI [b]	Compound	%
		Sesquiterpenes	4.74
59	1410	α-Caryophyllene	0.01
60	1418	α-cis-Bergamotene	0.03
61	1425	β-Caryophyllene [c]	3.11
62	1433	β-Ylangene	0.02
63	1444	β-Bergamotene	0.01
64	1447	β-Copaene	0.02
65	1454	Aromadendrene	0.04
66	1459	α-Humulene	0.88
67	1480	γ-Muurolene	0.07
68	1484	α-Curcumene	0.09
69	1491	β-Selinene	0.02
70	1497	γ-Amorphene	0.06
71	1508	α-Muurolene	0.02
72	1510	β-Bisabolene	0.05
73	1518	γ-Cadinene	0.05
74	1527	δ-Cadinene	0.12
75	1543	α-Cadinene	0.01
76	1548	α-Calacorene	0.04
77	1589	Caryophyllene oxide	0.10
		Others	2.16
8	977	Octen-3-ol	0.37
9	982	3-Octanone	1.56
11	993	3-Octanol	0.23

[a] The numbering refers to the elution order, and values (relative peak area percent) represent averages of three determinations; [b] Retention Index (KI) relative to a standard mixture of n-alkanes on the SPB™-5 column; [c] co-elution with an authentic sample.

3.2. Effects on Anxiety-Like Behavior in NTT Test and on Y-Maze Response to Novelty and Spatial Memory

Figure 3 reports the effects of Sco (100 µM) and REO (25, 150, and 300 µL/L) treatment on anxiety-like behavior in the NTT test. Representative locomotion tracking pattern (Figure 3A) illustrates the differences in swimming traces among the top and bottom zones and shows that the Sco-treated group traveled a greater distance in the bottom zone, suggesting an anxiogenic profile. Additionally, Sco treatment increased the time spent in the bottom zone of the tank ($p < 0.0001$) (Figure 3B) along with decreasing the time spent in the top zone of the tank (Figure 3B) ($p < 0.0001$) as compared to control. Reducing the time spent in the top zone of the tank suggests the anxiogenic-like effect of Sco. Sco treatment produced a hypolocomotor effect, by decreasing total distance traveled ($p < 0.001$) (Figure 3C) and average velocity (i.e., magnitude and direction of zebrafish speed, $p < 0.01$) (Figure 3D) compared to control. By contrast, increasing the time spent in the top zone of the tank (Figure 3B) suggests the anxiolytic-like effect of REO. Moreover, treatment with REO prevents the anxiogenic-like effect of Sco, in a dose-dependent manner, as evidenced through increasing of total distance traveled ($p < 0.0001$) (Figure 3C) and average velocity ($p < 0.001$) (Figure 3D) as compared to Sco-alone treated fish.

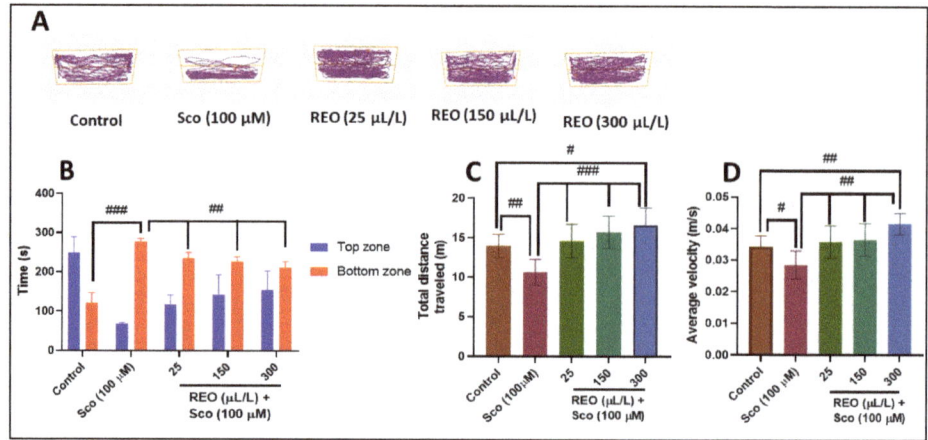

Figure 3. *Rosmarinus officinalis* essential oil (REO: 25, 150, and 300 μL/L) improved locomotion pattern and decreased anxiety in the NTT test. (**A**) Representative locomotion tracking pattern of the control, Sco (100 μM), and REO (25, 150, and 300 μL/L) treated groups. (**B**) The time spent by zebrafish in the top/bottom zone of the tank in different groups. (**C**) The total distance traveled by zebrafish in the tank in different groups. (**D**) The average velocity of zebrafish in the tank in different groups. Values are means ± S.E.M. ($n = 10$). For Tukey's post hoc analyses: (**B**) Control vs. Sco (100 μM): ### $p < 0.0001$, Sco vs. REO (25 μL/L): ## $p < 0.001$, Sco vs. REO (150 μL/L): ## $p < 0.001$, and Sco vs. REO (300 μL/L): ## $p < 0.001$; (**C**) Control vs. Sco (100 μM): ### $p < 0.0001$, Control vs. REO (300 μL/L): # $p < 0.01$, Sco vs. REO (25 μL/L): ### $p < 0.0001$, Sco vs. REO (150 μL/L): ### $p < 0.0001$, and Sco vs. REO (300 μL/L): ### $p < 0.0001$; and (**D**) Control vs. Sco (100 μM): # $p < 0.01$, Control vs. REO (300 μL/L): ## $p < 0.001$, Sco vs. REO (25 μL/L): ### $p < 0.0001$, Sco vs. REO (150 μL/L): ### $p < 0.0001$, and Sco vs. REO (300 μL/L): ### $p < 0.0001$.

Figure 4 shows the effects of Sco (100 μM) and REO (25, 150, and 300 μL/L) treatment on Y-maze response to novelty and spatial memory. Representative locomotion tracking pattern (Figure 4A) illustrates the differences in swimming traces among the Y-maze arms and shows that Sco treated group traveled a greater distance in the other arm, suggesting memory deficits. In addition, Sco administration significantly altered novel arm exploration ($p < 0.0001$) (Figure 4B) as compared to control zebrafish. The reduced percentage of time spent in novel arm suggests a memory impairment effect of Sco. The administration of Sco affects locomotion, as evidenced by the decreasing of total distance traveled ($p < 0.0001$) (Figure 4C) and turn angle ($p > 0.05$) (Figure 4D) compared to control. REO treatment significantly counters the Sco action induced hypolocomotion and memory deficits by improving the novel arm exploration ($p < 0.001$) (Figure 4B), while total distance traveled ($p < 0.01$) (Figure 4C) and turn angle ($p < 0.01$) (Figure 4D) was significantly increased at the high doses of REO (300 μL/L) as compared to Sco-alone treated zebrafish. Our results demonstrate that REO exhibited anxiolytic and memory-enhancing profile, which could be due to the presence of major active constituents shown in Table 1. The obtained results are in perfect agreement with those obtained by other groups that demonstrated anti-amnesic effects along with in vitro antioxidant and acetylcholinesterase and butyrylcholinesterase inhibition potential of *Rosmarinus officinalis* in scopolamine-induced memory impairment in mice [10]. Ozarowski et al. [33] demonstrated that *Rosmarinus officinalis* leaf extract improved long-term memory in rats, which can be partially explained by its inhibition of AChE activity in rat brain. Noori Ahmad Abadi et al. [34] reported that the hydroalcoholic extract of *Rosmarinus officinalis* L. leaf reduced anxiety in mice, probably due to the presence of flavonoids in this plant and their antioxidant property. Additionally, Abdelhalim et al. [35] attributed the anxiolytic effects of *Rosmarinus officinalis* with its effect on gamma-aminobutyric acid (GABA) receptors. Despite extensive knowledge about the effects of various *Rosmarinus officinalis* extracts on memory, anxiety, and AChE activity in the rodent brain, we demonstrated for the first time the cognitive-enhancing, anxiolytic, and antioxidant profile of REO in the scopolamine zebrafish model. Furthermore, our study demonstrated that zebrafish is rapidly becoming one of the main organisms in translational neuroscience research, successfully completing rodent models for the study of dementia-related conditions.

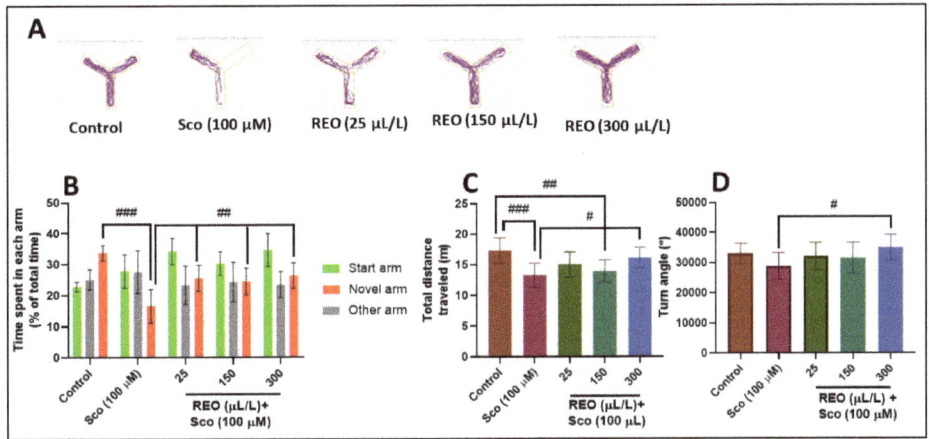

Figure 4. *Rosmarinus officinalis* essential oil (REO: 25, 150, and 300 µL/L) improved locomotion pattern and memory in the Y-maze test. (**A**) Representative locomotion tracking of the control, Sco (100 µM), and REO (25, 150, and 300 µL/L) treated groups. (**B**) The time spent in each arm (start, novel, and novel arms) in different groups. (**C**) The total distance traveled by zebrafish in the tank in different groups. (**D**) The turn angle of zebrafish in the tank in different groups. Values are means ± S.E.M. ($n = 10$). For Tukey's post hoc analyses: (**B**) Control vs. Sco (100 µM): ### $p < 0.0001$, Sco vs. REO (25 µL/L): ## $p < 0.001$, Sco vs. REO (150 µL/L): ## $p < 0.001$, and Sco vs. REO (300 µL/L): ## $p < 0.001$; (**C**) Control vs. Sco (100 µM): ### $p < 0.0001$, Control vs. Sco (100 µM): ## $p < 0.001$, and Sco vs. REO (300 µL/L): # $p < 0.01$; and (**D**) Sco vs. REO (300 µL/L): # $p < 0.01$.

3.3. Effects on AChE Activity

AChE decreases acetylcholine level and alleviates disease symptoms associated with the progressive loss of cholinergic function in AD [36]. Our results demonstrate that zebrafish subjected to Sco treatment exhibited increased AChE activity in the brain ($p < 0.0001$) as compared to the control group (Figure 5A). REO treatment significantly reduced AChE activity ($p < 0.0001$) in a dose-dependent manner, as compared to the Sco-treated group (Figure 5A). Thus, REO revealed an anti-AChE profile [19], which parallels improving memory parameters in zebrafish, as observed in NTT and Y-maze tests.

3.4. Effects on SOD, CAT, and GPX Specific Activities

Administration of Sco decreased the SOD specific activity ($p < 0.01$) (Figure 5B) in the zebrafish brain as compared to the control group, suggesting the augmentation in oxidative stress. REO significantly increase ($p < 0.0001$) (Figure 5B) the specific activity of SOD in the Sco-treated fish showing its promising antioxidant potential. CAT specific activity significantly decreased ($p < 0.01$) (Figure 5C) in Sco-exposed zebrafish as compared to the control group, whereas the administration of REO led to a significant increase ($p < 0.0001$) (Figure 5C) of CAT activity in the Sco-treated fish, supporting its antioxidant action. Moreover, GPX specific activity upon Sco administration leads to a significant decrease ($p < 0.0001$) (Figure 5D) as compared to the control group. REO treatment significantly restored this dramatic decrease in the Sco-treated fish showing prompt antioxidant potential. The results suggest that REO exhibits neuroprotective effects against oxidative stress, which is correlated with previously antioxidant properties of REO. Selmi et al. [37] reported that REO administration has significantly protected against alloxan-induced hepatic and renal oxidative stress due to the presence of phenolic and flavonoids compounds. Takayama et al. [38] demonstrated the antioxidant activity of REO against gastric damage induced by absolute ethanol in the rat. El-Hadary et al. [39] demonstrated antioxidant properties of REO against carbon tetrachloride-induced hepatotoxicity in rats mediated by phenolic compounds. Our results in accordance with the literature, suggesting the ability of REO to control brain oxidative damages by restoring the antioxidant enzyme activities.

3.5. Effects on MDA Level

The MDA level, an indicator of lipid peroxidation, was increased ($p < 0.001$) (Figure 5E) in the Sco-treated fish as compared to the control group. REO administration significantly reduced the MDA level ($p < 0.001$) (Figure 5E) to near the control level in Sco-treated fish.

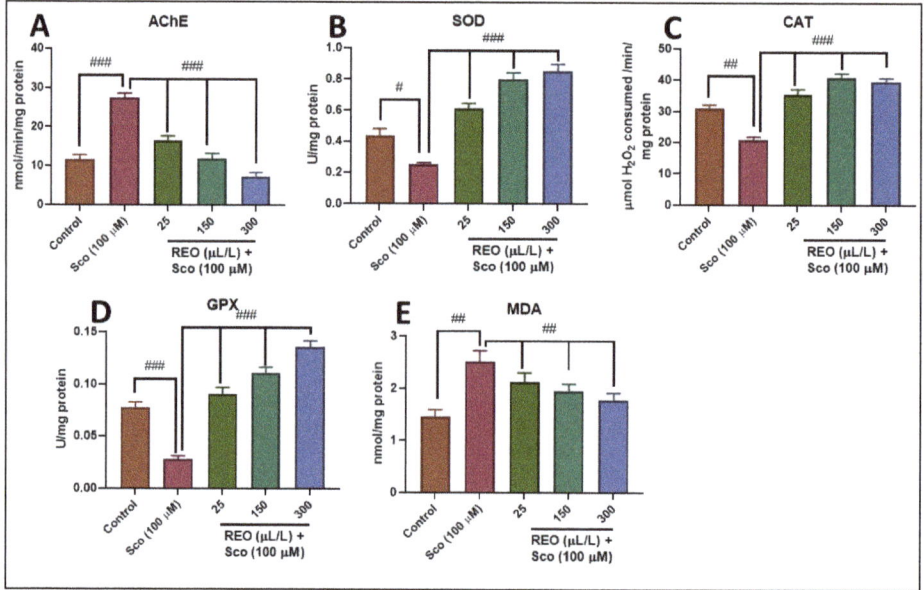

Figure 5. *Rosmarinus officinalis* essential oil (REO: 25, 150, and 300 µL/L) exhibited an anti-AChE effect and improved brain antioxidant status. The enzyme's specific activities: (**A**) AChE; (**B**) SOD; (**C**) CAT; (**D**) GPX; and (**E**) MDA level. Values are means ± S.E.M. ($n = 10$). For Tukey's post hoc analyses: (**A**) Control vs. Sco (100 µM): ### $p < 0.0001$, Sco vs. REO (25 µL/L): ### $p < 0.0001$, Sco vs. REO (150 µL/L): ### $p < 0.0001$, and Sco vs. REO (300 µL/L): ### $p < 0.0001$; (**B**) Control vs. Sco (100 µM): # $p < 0.01$, Sco vs. REO (25 µL/L): ### $p < 0.0001$, Sco vs. REO (150 µL/L): ### $p < 0.0001$, and Sco vs. REO (300 µL/L): ### $p < 0.0001$; (**C**) Control vs. Sco (100 µM): ## $p < 0.001$, Sco vs. REO (25 µL/L): ### $p < 0.0001$, Sco vs. REO (150 µL/L): ### $p < 0.0001$, and Sco vs. REO (300 µL/L): ### $p < 0.0001$; (**D**) Control vs. Sco (100 µM): ### $p < 0.0001$, Sco vs. REO (25 µL/L): ### $p < 0.0001$, Sco vs. REO (150 µL/L): ### $p < 0.0001$, and Sco vs. REO (300 µL/L): ### $p < 0.0001$; and (**E**) Control vs. Sco (100 µM): ## $p < 0.001$, Sco vs. REO (25 µL/L): ### $p < 0.0001$, Sco vs. REO (150 µL/L): ### $p < 0.0001$, and Sco vs. REO (300 µL/L): ### $p < 0.0001$.

Pearson correlation coefficient (r) was used to test the linear association among cognition, antioxidant enzymes, and lipid peroxidation (Figure 6). A high negative correlation for the time spent in the top zone of the tank vs. MDA ($n = 10$, $r = -0.863$, $p < 0.001$) (Figure 6A) and the time spent in novel arm vs. MDA ($n = 10$, $r = -0.737$, $p < 0.001$) (Figure 6B) was observed. The negative value of the

Pearson correlation coefficient indicates that the improvement of behavioral scores in specific tests such as NTT and Y-maze is well correlated with a low level of MDA, a marker of lipid peroxidation. In addition, strong negative correlations were evidenced by linear regression for AChE vs. the time spent in the top zone of the tank ($n = 10$, $r = -0.645$, $p < 0.001$) (Figure 6C) and AChE vs. the time spent in novel arm ($n = 10$, $r = -0.597$, $p < 0.01$) (Figure 6D). However, a positive significant correlation for AChE vs. MDA ($n = 10$, $r = 0.608$, $p < 0.01$) (Figure 6E) was noticed when linear regression was calculated. In this case, the negative and positive values of the Pearson correlation coefficient indicate that increasing behavioral scores is well correlated with decreasing of AChE activity and MDA level. Pérez-Fons et al. [40] demonstrated a relationship between the antioxidant capacity and effect of rosemary (*Rosmarinus officinalis* L.) polyphenols on membrane phospholipid order. By using the Pearson correlation coefficient (r) determination, we evidenced that improving memory performance in Sco-treated rats is related to increasing antioxidant enzyme activity along with a diminished level of lipid peroxidation, supporting REO neuroprotective profile. No significant correlation between biochemical parameters was observed.

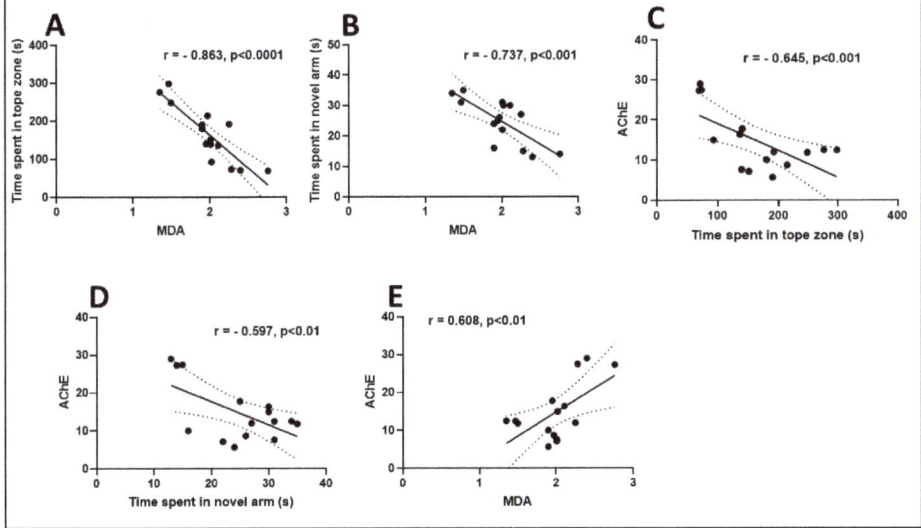

Figure 6. Correlation analyses between behavioral and biochemical parameters (Pearson's correlation, $n = 10$): (**A**) time spent in tope zone (s) vs. MDA; (**B**) time spent in novel arm (s) vs. MDA; (**C**) AChE vs. time spent in tope zone (s); (**D**) AChE vs. time spent in novel arm (s) and (**E**) AChE vs. MDA. Data expressed are time spent in the top zone (s), time spent in novel arm (s), AChE (nmol/min/mg protein), and MDA (nmol/mg protein).

4. Conclusions

This study showed that REO counteracts cognitive performance decrease and anxiety increase resulting from Sco treatment through a mechanism implying mitigation of brain oxidative stress and regulation of AChE activity.

Author Contributions: Conceptualization, L.H., L.C., and R.S.B.; Methodology, L.C., R.S.B., G.D., E.T.-C., E.M.N., and G.R.; Formal Analysis, L.C., R.S.B., G.D., and E.T.-C.; Investigation, L.C., R.S.B., G.D., and E.T.-C.; Writing—Original Draft Preparation, L.H., L.C., and R.S.B.; Writing—Review and Editing, L.H.; Supervision, L.H.; and Funding Acquisition, L.H. All authors have read and agreed to the published version of the manuscript.

Funding: This project was funded by the Ministry of Research and Innovation within Program 1—Development of the national RD system, Subprogram 1.2—Institutional Performance—RDI excellence funding projects, Contract No. 34PFE/19.10.2018.

Acknowledgments: The authors thank Tonia Strano for her skillful technical assistance for GC-MS analysis and Flora Srl for supplying the essential oil subject of this study.

Conflicts of Interest: The authors declare no conflict of interest.

References

1. Craig, L.A.; Hong, N.S.; Kopp, J.; McDonald, R.J. Reduced cholinergic status in hippocampus produces spatial memory deficits when combined with kainic acid induced seizure. *Hippocampus* **2008**, *18*, 1112–1121. [CrossRef] [PubMed]
2. Masters, C.L.; Bateman, R.; Blennow, K.; Rowe, C.C.; Sperling, R.A.; Cummings, J.L. Alzheimer's disease. *Nat. Rev. Dis. Prim.* **2015**, *1*, 15056. [CrossRef] [PubMed]
3. Liu, P.-P.; Xie, Y.; Meng, X.-Y.; Kang, J.-S. History and progress of hypotheses and clinical trials for Alzheimer's disease. *Signal Transduct. Target. Ther.* **2019**, *4*, 1–22. [CrossRef] [PubMed]
4. Doody, R.S.; Dunn, J.K.; Clark, C.M.; Farlow, M.; Foster, N.L.; Liao, T.; Gonzales, N.; Lai, E.; Massman, P. Chronic Donepezil Treatment Is Associated with Slowed Cognitive Decline in Alzheimer's Disease. *Dement. Geriatr. Cogn. Disord.* **2001**, *12*, 295–300. [CrossRef] [PubMed]
5. Bullock, R.; Touchon, J.; Bergman, H.; Gambina, G.; He, Y.; Rapatz, G.; Nagel, J.; Lane, R. Rivastigmine and donepezil treatment in moderate to moderately-severe Alzheimer's disease over a 2-year period. *Curr. Med. Res. Opin.* **2005**, *21*, 1317–1327. [CrossRef] [PubMed]
6. Lyketsos, C.G.; Carrillo, M.C.; Ryan, J.M.; Khachaturian, A.S.; Trzepacz, P.; Amatniek, J.; Cedarbaum, J.; Brashear, R.; Miller, D.S. Neuropsychiatric symptoms in Alzheimer's disease. *Alzheimer's Dement.* **2011**, *7*, 532–539. [CrossRef]
7. Tönnies, E.; Trushina, E. Oxidative Stress, Synaptic Dysfunction, and Alzheimer's Disease. *J. Alzheimer's Dis.* **2017**, *57*, 1105–1121. [CrossRef]
8. Jafarian, S.; Ling, K.-H.; Hassan, Z.; Perimal-Lewis, L.; Sulaiman, M.R.; Perimal, E.K. Effect of zerumbone on scopolamine-induced memory impairment and anxiety-like behaviours in rats. *Alzheimer's Dement.* **2019**, *5*, 637–643. [CrossRef]
9. Naderali, E.; Nikbakht, F.; Ofogh, S.; Rasoolijazi, H. The role of rosemary extract (40% carnosic acid) in degeneration of hippocampal neurons induced by kainic acid in the rat: The behavioral and histochemical approach. *J. Integr. Neurosci.* **2018**, *17*, 31–43. [CrossRef]
10. Karim, N.; Khan, I.; Abdelhalim, A.; Abdel-Halim, H.; Hanrahan, J.R. Molecular docking and antiamnesic effects of nepitrin isolated from *Rosmarinus officinalis* on scopolamine-induced memory impairment in mice. *Biomed. Pharmacother.* **2017**, *96*, 700–709. [CrossRef]
11. Song, H.; Xu, L.; Zhang, R.; Cao, Z.; Zhang, H.; Yang, L.; Guo, Z.; Qu, Y.; Yu, J. Rosemary extract improves cognitive deficits in a rats model of repetitive mild traumatic brain injury associated with reduction of astrocytosis and neuronal degeneration in hippocampus. *Neurosci. Lett.* **2016**, *622*, 95–101. [CrossRef] [PubMed]
12. Gerlai, R. Zebrafish and relational memory: Could a simple fish be useful for the analysis of biological mechanisms of complex vertebrate learning? *Behav. Process.* **2017**, *141*, 242–250. [CrossRef] [PubMed]
13. Meshalkina, D.A.; Kizlyk, M.N.; Kysil, E.V.; Collier, A.D.; Echevarria, D.J.; Abreu, M.S.; Barcellos, L.J.G.; Song, C.; Kalueff, A.V. Understanding zebrafish cognition. *Behav. Process.* **2017**, *141*, 229–241. [CrossRef] [PubMed]
14. Xu, X.; Scott-Scheiern, T.; Kempker, L.; Simons, K. Active avoidance conditioning in zebrafish (Danio rerio). *Neurobiol. Learn. Mem.* **2007**, *87*, 72–77. [CrossRef]
15. Aoki, R.; Tsuboi, T.; Okamoto, H. Y-maze avoidance: An automated and rapid associative learning paradigm in zebrafish. *Neurosci. Res.* **2015**, *91*, 69–72. [CrossRef]
16. Braida, D.; Ponzoni, L.; Martucci, R.; Sparatore, F.; Gotti, C.; Sala, M. Role of neuronal nicotinic acetylcholine receptors (nAChRs) on learning and memory in zebrafish. *Psychopharmacology* **2014**, *231*, 1975–1985. [CrossRef]
17. Hamilton, T.J.; Morrill, A.; Lucas, K.; Gallup, J.; Harris, M.; Healey, M.; Pitman, T.; Schalomon, M.; Digweed, S.; Tresguerres, M. Establishing zebrafish as a model to study the anxiolytic effects of scopolamine. *Sci. Rep.* **2017**, *7*, 15081. [CrossRef]

18. Nematolahi, P.; Mehrabani, M.; Karami-Mohajeri, S.; Dabaghzadeh, F. Effects of *Rosmarinus officinalis* L. on memory performance, anxiety, depression, and sleep quality in university students: A randomized clinical trial. *Complement. Ther. Clin. Pract.* **2018**, *30*, 24–28. [CrossRef]
19. Miraj, S. An evidence-based review on herbal remedies of *Rosmarinus officinalis*. *Der Pharm. Lett.* **2016**, *8*, 426–436.
20. Napoli, E.M.; Curcuruto, G.; Ruberto, G. Screening of the essential oil composition of wild Sicilian rosemary. *Biochem. Syst. Ecol.* **2010**, *38*, 659–670. [CrossRef]
21. Tuttolomondo, T.; Dugo, G.; Ruberto, G.; Leto, C.; Napoli, E.M.; Potortí, A.G.; Fede, M.R.; Virga, G.; Leone, R.; D'Anna, E.; et al. Agronomical evaluation of Sicilian biotypes of Lavandula stoechas L. spp. stoechas and analysis of the essential oils. *J. Essent. Oil Res.* **2015**, *27*, 115–124. [CrossRef]
22. Epa, N.; Mass, N.I.H.; Library, S.; Ei, V.Z.; Sparkman, J.A. NIST Standard Reference Database 1A. In *Natl. Inst. Stand. Technol. NIST*; 2004. Available online: https://www.nist.gov/system/files/documents/srd/NIST1aVer22Man.pdf (accessed on 9 December 2019).
23. Sparkman, O.D. Review. *J. Am. Soc. Mass Spectrom.* **2007**, *18*, 803–806. [CrossRef]
24. Dos Santos, A.C.; Junior, G.B.; Zago, D.C.; Zeppenfeld, C.C.; da Silva, D.T.; Heinzmann, B.M.; Baldisserotto, B.; da Cunha, M.A. Anesthesia and anesthetic action mechanism of essential oils of Aloysia triphylla and Cymbopogon flexuosus in silver catfish (Rhamdia quelen). *Vet. Anaesth. Analg.* **2017**, *44*, 106–113. [CrossRef] [PubMed]
25. Cachat, J.M.; Canavello, P.R.; Elkhayat, S.I.; Bartels, B.K.; Hart, P.C.; Elegante, M.F.; Beeson, E.C.; Laffoon, A.L.; Haymore, W.A.M.; Tien, D.H.; et al. Video-aided analysis of zebrafish locomotion and anxiety-related behavioral responses. *Neuromethods* **2011**, *51*, 1–14.
26. Cognato, G.d.P.; Bortolotto, J.W.; Blazina, A.R.; Christoff, R.R.; Lara, D.R.; Vianna, M.R.; Bonan, C.D. Y-Maze memory task in zebrafish (Danio rerio): The role of glutamatergic and cholinergic systems on the acquisition and consolidation periods. *Neurobiol. Learn. Mem.* **2012**, *98*, 321–328. [CrossRef]
27. Zanandrea, R.; Abreu, M.S.; Piato, A.; Barcellos, L.J.G.; Giacomini, A.C.V.V. Lithium prevents scopolamine-induced memory impairment in zebrafish. *Neurosci. Lett.* **2018**, *664*, 34–37. [CrossRef]
28. Batista, F.L.A.; Lima, L.M.G.; Abrante, I.A.; de Araújo, J.I.F.; Batista, F.L.A.; Abrante, I.A.; Magalhães, E.A.; de Lima, D.R.; Lima, M.d.C.L.; do Prado, B.S.; et al. Antinociceptive activity of ethanolic extract of Azadirachta indica A. Juss (Neem, Meliaceae) fruit through opioid, glutamatergic and acid-sensitive ion pathways in adult zebrafish (Danio rerio). *Biomed. Pharmacother.* **2018**, *108*, 408–416. [CrossRef]
29. Dumitru, G.; El-Nashar, H.A.S.; Mostafa, N.M.; Eldahshan, O.A.; Boiangiu, R.S.; Todirascu-Ciornea, E.; Hritcu, L.; Singab, A.N.B. Agathisflavone isolated from Schinus polygamus (Cav.) Cabrera leaves prevents scopolamine-induced memory impairment and brain oxidative stress in zebrafish (Danio rerio). *Phytomedicine* **2019**, *58*, 152889. [CrossRef]
30. Smith, P.K.; Krohn, R.I.; Hermanson, G.T.; Mallia, A.K.; Gartner, F.H.; Provenzano, M.D.; Fujimoto, E.K.; Goeke, N.M.; Olson, B.J.; Klenk, D.C. Measurement of protein using bicinchoninic acid. *Anal. Biochem.* **1985**, *150*, 76–85. [CrossRef]
31. Bouyahya, A.; Et-Touys, A.; Bakri, Y.; Talbaui, A.; Fellah, H.; Abrini, J.; Dakka, N. Chemical composition of *Mentha pulegium* and *Rosmarinus officinalis* essential oils and their antileishmanial, antibacterial and antioxidant activities. *Microb. Pathog.* **2017**, *111*, 41–49. [CrossRef]
32. Elyemni, M.; Louaste, B.; Nechad, I.; Elkamli, T.; Bouia, A.; Taleb, M.; Chaouch, M.; Eloutassi, N. Extraction of Essential Oils of *Rosmarinus officinalis* L. by Two Different Methods: Hydrodistillation and Microwave Assisted Hydrodistillation. *Sci. World J.* **2019**, *2019*. [CrossRef] [PubMed]
33. Ozarowski, M.; Mikolajczak, P.L.; Bogacz, A.; Gryszczynska, A.; Kujawska, M.; Jodynis-Liebert, J.; Piasecka, A.; Napieczynska, H.; Szulc, M.; Kujawski, R.; et al. *Rosmarinus officinalis* L. leaf extract improves memory impairment and affects acetylcholinesterase and butyrylcholinesterase activities in rat brain. *Fitoterapia* **2013**, *91*, 261–271. [CrossRef] [PubMed]
34. Noori Ahmad Abadi, M.; Mortazavi, M.; Kalani, N.; Marzouni, H.Z.; Kooti, W.; Ali-Akbari, S. Effect of Hydroalcoholic Extract of *Rosmarinus officinalis* L. Leaf on Anxiety in Mice. *J. Evid. Based Complement. Altern. Med.* **2016**, *21*, NP85–NP90. [CrossRef] [PubMed]
35. Abdelhalim, A.; Karim, N.; Chebib, M.; Aburjai, T.; Khan, I.; Johnston, G.A.R.; Hanrahan, J.R. Antidepressant, anxiolytic and antinociceptive activities of constituents from *Rosmarinus officinalis*. *J. Pharm. Pharm. Sci.* **2015**, *18*, 448–459. [CrossRef] [PubMed]

36. Li, S.M.; Mo, M.S.; Xu, P.Y. Progress in mechanisms of acetylcholinesterase inhibitors and memantine for the treatment of Alzheimer's disease. *Neuroimmunol. Neuroinflamm.* **2015**, *2*, 274–280.
37. Selmi, S.; Rtibi, K.; Grami, D.; Sebai, H.; Marzouki, L. Rosemary (*Rosmarinus officinalis*) essential oil components exhibit anti-hyperglycemic, anti-hyperlipidemic and antioxidant effects in experimental diabetes. *Pathophysiology* **2017**, *24*, 297–303. [CrossRef]
38. Takayama, C.; de-Faria, F.M.; de Almeida, A.C.A.; Dunder, R.J.; Manzo, L.P.; Socca, E.A.R.; Batista, L.M.; Salvador, M.J.; Souza-Brito, A.R.M.; Luiz-Ferreira, A. Chemical composition of *Rosmarinus officinalis* essential oil and antioxidant action against gastric damage induced by absolute ethanol in the rat. *Asian Pac. J. Trop. Biomed.* **2016**, *6*, 677–681. [CrossRef]
39. El-Hadary, A.E.; Elsanhoty, R.M.; Ramadan, M.F. In vivo protective effect of *Rosmarinus officinalis* oil against carbon tetrachloride (CCl4)-induced hepatotoxicity in rats. *PharmaNutrition* **2019**, *9*, 100151. [CrossRef]
40. Pérez-Fons, L.; GarzÓn, M.T.; Micol, V. Relationship between the Antioxidant Capacity and Effect of Rosemary (*Rosmarinus officinalis* L.) Polyphenols on Membrane Phospholipid Order. *J. Agric. Food Chem.* **2010**, *58*, 161–171. [CrossRef]

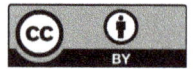

© 2020 by the authors. Licensee MDPI, Basel, Switzerland. This article is an open access article distributed under the terms and conditions of the Creative Commons Attribution (CC BY) license (http://creativecommons.org/licenses/by/4.0/).

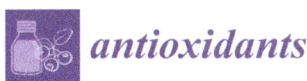

Review

The Effects and Mechanisms of Cyanidin-3-Glucoside and Its Phenolic Metabolites in Maintaining Intestinal Integrity

Jijun Tan [1], Yanli Li [1], De-Xing Hou [2] and Shusong Wu [1,*]

[1] Hunan Collaborative Innovation Center for Utilization of Botanical Functional Ingredients, College of Animal Science and Technology, Hunan Agricultural University, Changsha 410128, China; jijun995@outlook.com (J.T.); liyanli125@hotmail.com (Y.L.)
[2] The United Graduate School of Agricultural Sciences, Faculty of Agriculture, Kagoshima University, Kagoshima 890-0065, Japan; hou@chem.agri.kagoshima-u.ac.jp
* Correspondence: wush688@hunau.edu.cn

Received: 10 September 2019; Accepted: 8 October 2019; Published: 12 October 2019

Abstract: Cyanidin-3-glucoside (C3G) is a well-known natural anthocyanin and possesses antioxidant and anti-inflammatory properties. The catabolism of C3G in the gastrointestinal tract could produce bioactive phenolic metabolites, such as protocatechuic acid, phloroglucinaldehyde, vanillic acid, and ferulic acid, which enhance C3G bioavailability and contribute to both mucosal barrier and microbiota. To get an overview of the function and mechanisms of C3G and its phenolic metabolites, we review the accumulated data of the absorption and catabolism of C3G in the gastrointestine, and attempt to give crosstalk between the phenolic metabolites, gut microbiota, and mucosal innate immune signaling pathways.

Keywords: cyanidin-3-glucoside; phenolic metabolites; gut microbiota; signaling pathways; intestinal injury

1. Introduction

Anthocyanins belong to polyphenols, which are one kind of secondary metabolite with polyphenolic structure widely occurring in plants. They serve as key antioxidants and pigments that contribute to the coloration of flowers and fruits. Although anthocyanins vary in different plants, six anthocyanidins, including pelargonidins, cyanidins, delphinidins, peonidins, petunidins, and malvidins, are considered as the major natural anthocyanidins. Berries, such as red raspberry (*Rubus idaeus* L.), blue honeysuckle (*Lonicera caerulea* L.), and mulberry are used as folk medicine traditionally, and their extracts have been used in the treatment of disorders such as cardiovascular disease [1], obesity [2], neurodegeneration [3], liver diseases [4], and cancer [5], in recent years. Cyanidin-3-glucoside (C3G) is one of the most common anthocyanins naturally found in black rice, black bean, purple potato, and many colorful berries. C3G possesses strong antioxidant activity potentially due to the two hydroxyls on the B ring [6], as shown in Figure 1. Recent studies have suggested that C3G potentially exerts functions primarily through C3G metabolites (C3G-Ms) [7], and more than 20 kinds of C3G-Ms have been identified in serum by a pharmacokinetics study in humans [8]. Although the function and mechanism of C3G-Ms are still not clear, protocatechuic acid (PCA) [9–12], phloroglucinaldehyde (PGA) [1], vanillic acid (VA) [13–15], ferulic acid (FA) [16–19], and their derivates represent the main bioactive metabolites of C3G due to their antioxidant and anti-inflammatory properties.

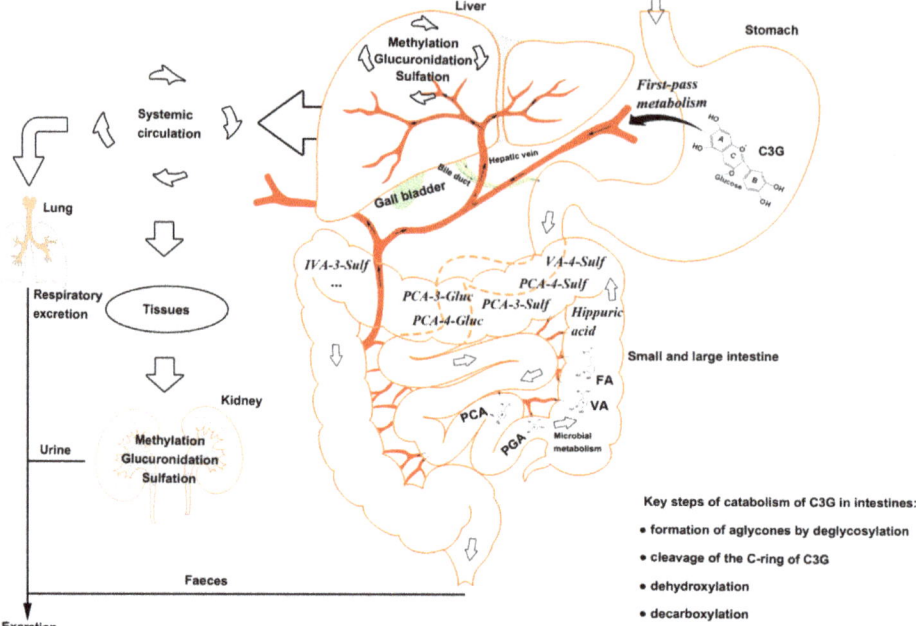

Figure 1. The catabolism process of cyanidin-3-glucoside (C3G) in an organism. C3G can be hydrolyzed to its aglycone by enzymes in the small intestine, and further degraded to phenolic compounds by gut microbiota. Microbial catabolism of C3G in the distal small intestine and large intestine is performed by the cleavage of the heterocyclic flavylium ring (C-ring), followed by dehydroxylation or decarboxylation to form multistage metabolites, which enter the liver and kidney by circulation. C3G, cyanidin-3-glucoside; FA, ferulic acid; PCA, protocatechuic acid; PGA, phloroglucinaldehyde; VA, vanillic acid.

2. Absorption and Catabolism of C3G in the Gastrointestine

Most of the anthocyanins remain stable in the stomach and upper intestine [20,21]. The stomach is considered as one of the predominant sites for anthocyanin and C3G absorption [22,23], although high concentration (85%) of anthocyanins has been found in the distal intestine [24]. There is potential for the first-pass metabolism of C3G in the stomach, that is, C3G can be effectively absorbed from the gastrointestinal tract and undergoes extensive first-pass metabolism, which can enter the systemic circulation as metabolites [25].

Anthocyanins are stable under acidic conditions but extremely unstable under alkaline conditions. The higher the pH is, the more colorless and substituent forms of anthocyanin are predominant [26]. The catabolism of C3G is mainly completed in the distal small intestine, such as ileum [22], and in the upper large intestine, such as the colon [27], with the decomposition by microbiota [28]. C3G can be hydrolyzed to their aglycones by enzymes in the small intestine, and further degraded to phenolic compounds by gut microbiota, in which microbial catabolism of C3G is performed by the cleavage of the heterocyclic flavylium ring (C-ring), followed by dehydroxylation or decarboxylation [29]. Subsequently, phase II metabolites and multistage metabolites (including bacterial metabolites) can enter the liver and kidney to form more methylate, gluronide, and sulfate conjugated metabolites by enterohepatic circulation and blood circulation (Figure 1).

3. Biological Functions of C3G-Ms

Only several C3G-Ms have shown potential biological function, although more than 20 kinds of C3G-Ms have been identified [8,30]. PCA and phloroglucinaldehyde (PGA) are considered as the major bioactive phenolic metabolites produced by phase I metabolism, which undergo cleavage of the C ring of C3G. PCA can increase the antioxidant capacity of cells potentially by increasing the activity of antioxidant enzymes, such as catalase (CAT) in hypertensive rats or arthritis-model rats [31,32], superoxide dismutase (SOD) [33], and glutathione peroxidase (GPx) in mice or macrophages [33–36], and thus attenuate lipid peroxidation. Meanwhile, PCA has been reported to inhibit the production of inflammatory mediators, such as interleukin (IL)-6, tumor necrosis factor-α (TNF-α), IL-1β, and prostaglandin E_2 (PGE_2) [37–39], potentially by suppressing the activation of nuclear factor-κB (NF-κB) and extracellular signal-regulated kinase (ERK) [33,38] in murine BV2 microglia cells and colitis-model mice. PGA has also shown an inhibitory effect on inflammation potentially by modulating the production of IL-1β, IL-6, and IL-10 [40] in human whole blood cultures, although there are few reports about the molecular mechanisms. Our previous studies have revealed that both PCA and PGA are capable to down-regulate the MAPK pathway, especially suppress the activation of ERK, and PGA can directly bind to ERK1/2 [41] in murine macrophages.

Phase II metabolites of C3G, such as PCA-3-glucuronide (PCA-3-Gluc), PCA-4-glucuronide (PCA-4-Gluc), PCA-3-sulfate (PCA-3-Sulf), PCA-4-sulfate (PCA-4-Sulf), VA, VA-4-sulfate (VA-4-Sulf), isovanillic acid (IVA), IVA-3-sulfate (IVA-3-Sulf), and FA, are mostly derived from PCA and PGA [1,8]. VA and FA represent the bioactive phenolic metabolites based on recent studies. VA may suppress the generation of reactive oxygen species (ROS) [42] and lipid peroxidation [32], potentially by increasing the activity of antioxidant enzymes such as SOD, CAT, and GPx [43,44], as well as the level of antioxidants such as vitamin E [43,44], vitamin C [43,44], and glutathione (GSH) [45] in mice, hamster, and diabetic hypertensive rats. Additionally, VA can inhibit the production of pro-inflammatory cytokines such as TNF-α, IL-6, IL-1β, and IL-33 by down-regulating caspase-1 and NF-κB pathways [45–47] in mice or mouse peritoneal macrophages and mast cells. FA has also been reported to attenuate both oxidative stress and inflammation potentially by suppressing the production of free radicals (ROS and NO in rats, rat intestinal mucosal IEC-6 cell, or murine macrophages) [48–50], enhancing Nrf2 expression and down-stream antioxidant enzymes (SOD and CAT in rats or swiss albino mice) [48,51], and inhibiting the activation of proinflammatory proteins (p38 and IκB in HUVEC cells) [52] and cytokines production, such as IL-18 in HUVEC cells [52], IL-1β in mice [53], IL-6 in obese rats [54], and TNF-α in mice [53]. However, both VA and FA showed a limited effect on the activation of MAPK pathway and production of inflammatory cytokines, such as monocyte chemoattractant protein-1 (MCP-1) and TNF-α in a high-fat diet-induced mouse model of nonalcoholic fatty liver disease [41]. Table 1 summarizes the biological functions of the main bioactive metabolites, including PCA, PGA, VA, and FA.

Table 1. Biological functions of C3G-Ms.

C3G-Ms	Biological Functions	Objects	Results
PCA	Antioxidant	Rats, mice, macrophages	Treatment with PCA increased T-AOC [31], catalase [33], SOD [33] and GPx [33–36] levels, but decreased ROS [35], MDA [31] and hydroperoxides [31] levels.
	Anti-inflammatory	Mice, macrophages	PCA decreased IL-6 [33,37,39], TNF-α [33,39], IL-1β [33,39] and PGE_2 production [39], and inhibited ERK, NF-κB p65 activation [33].
PGA	Anti-inflammatory	Mice, Human	PGA decreased serum levels of MCP-1 and TNF-α in high fat diet-induced mice [41]; PGA inhibited the production of IL-1β and IL-6 in human whole blood cultures after LPS stimulation, but no significant difference ($p > 0.01$) [40].

Table 1. Cont.

C3G-Ms	Biological Functions	Objects	Results
VA	Antioxidant	Hamsters, mice, rats	VA increased SOD [43,44], catalase [43,44], GPx [43,44], vitamin E [43,44], vitamin C [43,44] and GSH [43–45] levels.
	Anti-inflammatory	Rats, mice, macrophages	VA inhibited caspase-1, NF-κB and MAPKs activation [45–47], decreased production of COX-2, PGE$_2$ and NO [46], and reduced the levels of TNF-α [45,46], IL-6 [46,55], IL-1β [45] and IL-33 [45].
FA	Antioxidant	Rats, mice, IEC-6 cells	FA decreased the production of ROS [45–47], MDA [49], NO [49], enhanced SOD [48,49] and CAT [48,51] activity, and promoted the activation of Nrf2 [51].
	Anti-inflammatory	HUVEC cells, mice, rats	FA decreased the expression of caspase-1 [52], ICAM-1 [52], VCAM-1 [52], IL-18 [52], IL-1β [50,52–54], IL-6 [50,54], TNF-α [53], and inhibited the phosphorylation of p38 and IκB [52].

Notes: C3G-Ms, cyanidin-3-glucoside metabolites; CAT, catalase; COX-2, cyclooxygenase-2; ERK, extracellular signal-regulated kinase; FA, ferulic acid; GSH, glutathione; ICAM-1, intercellular adhesion molecule-1; LPS, lipopolysaccharide; MAPKs, mitogen-activated protein kinases; MCP-1, monocyte chemoattractant protein-1; MDA, malondialdehyde; NF-κB, nuclear factor-κB; NO, nitric oxide; PCA, protocatechuic acid; PGA, phloroglucinaldehyde; PGE2, prostaglandin E2; ROS, reactive oxygen species; T-AOC, total antioxidant capacity; VA, vanillic acid; VCAM-1, vascular cell adhesion molecule-1; SOD, superoxide dismutase; TNF-α, tumor necrosis factor-α.

4. Crosstalk between Gut Microbiota and C3G&C3G-Ms

Bacteria can use phenolic compounds as substrates to obtain energy [56,57] and to form fermentable metabolites which can exert bioactive functions similar to parent anthocyanins [58], and thus, gut microbiota play an important role in the metabolism of anthocyanins and the secondary phenolic metabolites after the removal of anthocyanins' sugar moiety [59].

PCA has already been proven as the gut microbiota metabolite of C3G [60], as *Lactobacillus* and *Bifidobacterium* have the maximum ability to produce the β-glucosidase so that anthocyanins are transformed to PCA [61]. *Lactobacillus* and *Bifidobacterium* are also observed to produce p-coumaric acid and FA under different carbon sources [57,62], while *Bacillus subtilis* and *Actinomycetes* are involved in the bioconversion of VA to guaiacol [63].

On the other hand, anthocyanins are capable of modulating the growth of special intestinal bacteria [24] and increasing microbial abundances [64]. Anthocyanins have been reported to increase the relative abundance of beneficial bacteria such as *Bifidobacterium* and *Akkermansia*, which are believed to be closely related to anti-inflammatory effects [24,65]. Monofloral honey from *Prunella Vulgaris*, rich in PCA, VA, and FA, showed protective effects against dextran sulfate sodium-induced ulcerative colitis in rats potentially through restoring the relative abundance of *Lactobacillus* [66]. Our previous studies also found that the *Lonicera caerulea* L. berry rich in C3G could attenuate inflammation potentially through the modulation of gut microbiota, especially the ratio of *Firmicutes* to *Bacteroidetes* in a mouse model of experimental non-alcoholic fatty liver disease [67]. Nevertheless, another study revealed that propolis rich in PCA, VA, and FA could suppress intestinal inflammation in a rat model of dextran sulfate sodium-induced colitis potentially by reducing the population of *Bacteroides* spp [68]. This may be because of the inhibitory and lethal effects on pathogenic bacteria by anthocyanins and their metabolites. PCA has been reported to inhibit the growth of *E. coli*, *P. aeruginosa*, and *S. aureus* [69]. VA can decrease the cucumber rhizosphere total bacterial *Pseudomonas* and *Bacillus spp.* community by changing their compositions [70]. FA is identified as highly effective against the growth of *Botrytis cinerea* isolated from grape [71]. Table 2 shows the microbial species that can biotransform C3G&C3G-Ms and the bacteriostasis effects of C3G-Ms.

The mechanisms underlying the anti-microbial effect of anthocyanins are not clear yet. Ajiboye et al. have pointed out that PCA may induce oxidative stress in gram-negative bacteria [69], that is, PCA can combine with O_2 to form $\bullet O^{2-}$, which attacks the polyunsaturated fatty acid components of the membrane to cause lipid peroxidation, and attacks the thiol group of protein to cause protein oxidation. To be more precise, $\bullet O^{2-}$ can be continually produced by autoxidation of PCA and semiquinone oxidation through the inhibition of NADH-quinone oxidoreductase (NQR) and succinate-quinone oxidoreductase (SQR). Although SOD converts $\bullet O^{2-}$ to H_2O_2, which can be finally changed to H_2O and O_2 by catalase, excessive H_2O_2 produces $\bullet OH$ during the Fenton reaction ($Fe^{2+} \rightarrow Fe^{3+}$), and $\bullet OH$ attacks the base of DNA and results in DNA breakage. In addition, the suppression of NQR and SQR may lead to ATP depletion. Finally, bacterial death could be induced by lipid peroxidation, protein oxidation, DNA breakage, and ATP depletion. (Figure 2).

Table 2. Crosstalk between C3G&C3G-Ms and microorganism.

Microbial Species	Features	Bioconversion	Bacteriostasis
Lactobacillus (L. paracasei, B. lactis and B. dentium) and Bifidobacterium	Gram-positive anaerobes	C3G and cyanidin 3-rutinoside →PCA [60,61]	PCA—|E. coli, P. aeruginosa and S. aureus [69]
Lactobacillus (L. acidophilus K1) and Bifidobacterium (B. catenulatum KD 14, B. longum KN 29 and B. animalis Bi30)	Gram-positive anaerobes	Methyl esters of phenolic acids →FA [57,62]	FA—|Botrytis cinerea [71]
Bacillus subtilis and Actinomycetes (Streptomyces sp. A3, Streptomyces sp. A5 and Streptomyces sp. A13)	Gram-positive facultative anaerobes	VA→guaiacol [63]	VA—|Pseudomonas and Bacillus spp. [70]

Notes: →, generate; —\|, inhibit.

Given these, interactions between C3G&C3G-Ms and gut microbiota can improve the bioavailability of C3G. C3G&C3G-Ms potentially ameliorate micro-ecological dysbiosis by inhibiting gram-negative bacteria. But it is worth noting that a few studies have demonstrated that the over-consumption of polyphenols had significant negative effects on reproduction and pregnancy [72–74]. Although it is inexplicit whether there is a correlation with the changes of gut microbiota composition, the negative effects of polyphenols-mediated modulation of gut microbiota should be focused on.

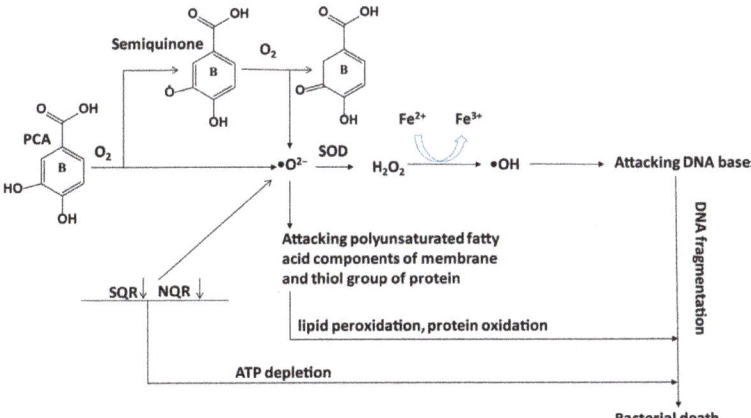

Figure 2. Potential mechanisms underlying the lethal effect of PCA on gram-negative bacteria. Autoxidation of PCA and semiquinone oxidation through the inhibition of NADH-quinone oxidoreductase (NQR) and succinate-quinone oxidoreductase (SQR) can cause ATP depletion and produce $\bullet O^{2-}$, which attacks the polyunsaturated fatty acid components of the membrane to cause lipid peroxidation and attacks the thiol group of protein to cause protein oxidation. Although SOD converts $\bullet O^{2-}$ to H_2O_2, which can be finally changed to H_2O and O_2 by catalase, excessive H_2O_2 produces $\bullet OH$ during the Fenton reaction ($Fe^{2+} \rightarrow Fe^{3+}$), and $\bullet OH$ attacks DNA bases to cause DNA fragmentation. Ultimately, lipid peroxidation, protein oxidation, DNA fragmentation, and ATP depletion induce bacterial death. PCA, protocatechuic acid; SOD, superoxide dismutase.

5. The Potential Mechanisms of C3G&C3G-Ms against Intestinal Injury

Multiple studies have shown that C3G&C3G-Ms have an essential role in intestinal health [55,75,76]. The potential mechanisms of C3G&C3G-Ms against intestinal injury are considered as they act in a synergistic manner between the antioxidant, anti-inflammatory, and anti-apoptosis function.

5.1. Antioxidant

The protective effect of C3G&C3G-Ms against intestinal injury is largely based on their antioxidant ability. On the one hand, C3G, along with its bioactive phenolic metabolites, including PCA, VA, and FA, can up-regulate the antioxidant enzyme system, such as increasing the activities of manganese-dependent superoxide dismutase (MnSOD) [34] and GSH [34,77]. On the other hand, they can also down-regulate the pro-oxidant system, such as decrease the expression of cyclooxygenase-2 (COX-2) [77,78] and inducible nitric oxide synthase (iNOS) [77,78], and thus, decreasing the production of free radicals, including ROS [79] and reactive nitrogen species (RNS) [78]. Our previous study has shown that the *Lonicera caerulea* L. berry rich in C3G may enhance the expression of nuclear factor (erythroid-derived 2)-like 2 (Nrf2) and MnSOD during the earlier response in LPS-induced macrophages [80].

Nrf2 is a transcription factor with a basic leucine zipper (bZIP) that regulates the expression of antioxidant enzymes. Under normal conditions, Nrf2 is kept in ubiquitination by Cullin 3 and Kelch like-ECH-associated protein 1 (KEAP1), which facilitates ubiquitination of Nrf2. In this regard, Nrf2 forms a virtuous cycle so that it does not come into the nucleus to bind with the antioxidant response element (ARE) to modulate the transcription of down-stream genes. Once upon oxidative stress, Nrf2 can be released from KEAP1 to enter the nucleus with the disruption of cysteine residues in KEAP1 [81], or the activation of protein kinase C (PKC) [82], extracellular signal-regulated kinase (ERK) or p38 MAPKs [83], GSK-3β [84], and phosphoinositide 3-kinase (PI3K) [85]. In the nucleus, Nrf2 binds with ARE and other bZIP proteins (like small Maf) to induce down-stream genes to transcribe.

The bioactive phenolic metabolites of C3G have also been reported to activate Nrf2. PCA may increase the activities of glutathione reductase (GR) and glutathione peroxidase (GPx) by the c-Jun NH_2-terminal kinase (JNK)-mediated Nrf2 pathway in murine macrophages, as silencing of the JNK gene expression can attenuate the PCA-induced nuclear accumulation of Nrf2 [86]. FA potentially induces the expression of Nrf2 and HO-1 via the activation of the PI3K/Akt pathway, as the specific PI3K/Akt inhibitor can suppress FA-induced Nrf2 and HO-1 expression, and block the FA-induced increase in occludin and ZO-1 protein expression in rat intestinal epithelial cells [49]. The potential mechanisms underlying the C3G-Ms induced expression of Nrf2 is summarized in Figure 3.

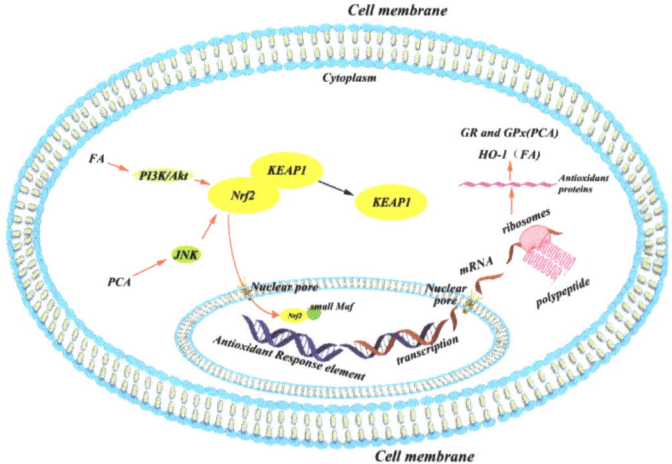

Figure 3. Potential mechanisms underlying the C3G-Ms regulated Nrf2 system. PCA and FA may induce the nuclear translocation of Nrf2 via JNK and PI3K/Akt pathways, respectively. FA, ferulic acid; GPx, glutathione peroxidase; GR, glutathione reductase; JNK, c-Jun NH_2-terminal kinase; KEAP1, Kelch like-ECH-associated protein 1; Nrf2, nuclear factor (erythroid-derived 2)-like 2; PCA, protocatechuic acid; PI3K, phosphatidylinositol 3-Kinase.

5.2. Anti-Inflammatory

Endotoxin produced by dysbacteriosis is considered as the major trigger of inflammation in intestines [87,88]. When gram-negative bacteria such as *Escherichia coli* and *Salmonella* predominate in gut, bacterial lipopolysaccharide (LPS) can form a complex called LPS binding proteins (LBP) to be associated with pattern recognition receptors (CD14) which locate on the cell membrane, and then activate toll-like receptors (TLRs), such as the TLR4 pathway, to induce inflammatory reactions in different types of cells, such as epithelial cells and immune cells [24]. TLR4 dimerizes itself and induces two major pathways, the myeloid differentiation factor 88 (MyD88)-dependent pathway and MyD88-independent pathway. In the dependent pathway, MyD88-induced phosphorylation of interleukin receptor-associated kinases 1 (IRAK1) and IRAK4 can activate the tumor necrosis-associated factor 6 (TRAF-6) adapter protein, which forms a complex with the enzymes that activate transforming growth factor beta-activated kinase-1 (TAK1) during ubiquitination. Then TAK1 induces the phosphorylation of the inhibitor kinase complex (IKKβ), which further induces the decoupling of NFκB in the dimer of NFκBp50 and NFκBp65 by degrading its inhibitory protein IκB. Finally, NFκB enters the nucleus and modulates the expression of a series of inflammatory cytokine genes [24].

Overexpression of inflammatory cytokines largely influences the expression of epithelial tight junctions (TJs) such as zonula occludens-1 (ZO-1), occludin, and claudin [89,90], which increase cellular permeability and give more access for LPS to enter cells [91,92]. The pro-inflammatory cytokines, like TNF-α, IFN-γ, and IL-1β, can induce an increase in intestinal TJ permeability potentially through the activation of myosin light chain kinase (MLCK), which appeared to be an important pathogenic mechanism contributing to the development of intestinal inflammation [93]. Another factor that aggravates intestinal inflammation is that macrophages can be recruited to adhere and infiltrate into inflammatory sites through chemokines and intercellular adhesion molecule-1 (ICAM-1), which is largely increased by the activation of the NF-κB signaling pathway [94] among several cell types including leukocytes, endothelial cells, and macrophages [95].

In addition to the influence on gut microbiota, the inhibitory effect of anthocyanins on epithelial inflammation is another important factor that acts against intestinal injury [64,76]. Ferrari et al. have demonstrated that the main protective effect of C3G in chronic gut inflammatory diseases is derived from the selective inhibition of the NF-κB pathway in epithelial cells [76]. Our previous studies have also shown that the *Lonicera caerulea* L. berry rich in C3G can inhibit LPS-induced inflammation potentially through TAK1-mediated mitogen-activated protein kinase (MAPK) and NF-κB pathways in an LPS-induced mouse paw edema and macrophage cell model [80]. Although the metabolites of C3G are complicated, recent studies have revealed that phenolic metabolites identified in blood circulation, such as PCA, PGA, VA, and FA, may modulate inflammatory signaling pathways. PCA, VA, and FA can suppress the production of ICAM-1, and thus, alleviate inflammatory infiltration and damage in vascular endothelial cells [52,96]. In a mouse colitis model, PCA can decrease both mRNA levels and protein concentration of Sphingosine kinases (SphK), which induces the phosphorylation of sphingosine to form sphingosine-1-phosphate (S1P), but increase the expression of S1P lyase (S1PL) which irreversibly degrade S1P, and thus, inhibit SphK/S1P pathway-mediated activation of the NF-κB pathway through S1P receptors (S1PR) [33]. The main mechanism of VA on inflammation is that it can down-regulate the MAPK pathway by suppressing the phosphorylation of ERK, JNK, and p38 [47]. It is reported that FA may prevent macrophages from responding to LPS, potentially through target myeloid differentiation factor 88 (MyD88) mediated pro-inflammatory signaling pathways [50,97], while other studies suggested that FA may increase the expression of TJs, such as occludin and ZO-1 via regulating HO-1 expression to prevent LPS enter the cells [52]. In our previous studies, both C3G and its phenolic metabolites showed inhibitory effects on LPS-activated inflammatory pathways in macrophages, and C3G can directly bind to TAK1 and ERK1/2, while PGA, one of phase I metabolites, can also directly bind to ERK1/2 [41,80]. These studies suggest that C3G and its phenolic metabolites may attenuate both a primary and secondary inflammatory response and by inactivating pro-inflammatory pathways and enhancing cellular barrier function (Figure 4).

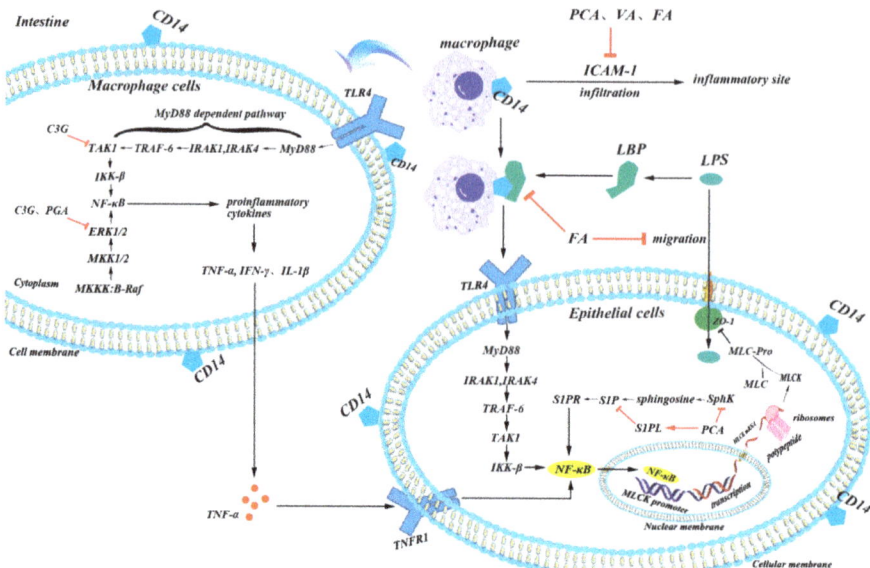

Figure 4. Potential mechanisms of C3G&C3G-Ms in attenuating intestinal inflammation. C3G and its phenolic metabolites mainly modulate inflammation by three ways, first, to suppress the production of chemotactic factors such as ICAM-1 and thus alleviate inflammatory infiltration, second, to down-regulate inflammatory pathways such as TAK1-mediated MAPK pathway and SphK/S1P mediated NF-κB pathway, finally, the down-regulated inflammatory pathways, and up-regulated antioxidant pathway, as mentioned in Figure 3, will maintain sufficient expression of tight junction proteins such as ZO-1 to promote normal intestinal barrier function, and thus prevent LPS from entering mucosal cells. C3G, cyanidin 3-glucoside; FA, ferulic acid; ICAM-1, intercellular adhesion molecule-1; PCA, protocatechuic acid; PGA, phloroglucinaldehyde; SphK, Sphingosine kinases; S1P, sphingosine-1-phosphate; TAK1, transforming growth factor beta-activated kinase-1; VA, vanillic acid.

5.3. Anti-Apoptosis

Under normal conditions, the homeostasis between apoptosis and proliferation of intestinal epithelial cells regulates the normal morphological structure and physiological function of the intestinal tract [98]. However, pathological factors, such as intestinal flora disorder, may induce local inflammation and subsequently, the infiltration of immune cells, such as leukocytes, that can be easily activated by microbial products causing the overproduction of RNS and ROS, which finally causes abnormal apoptosis among intestinal cells [34,99,100]. Although mechanisms underlying apoptosis are complicated, it has been considered that apoptosis is mainly mediated by two ways [101]. On the one hand, pro-apoptotic factors such as ROS may change mitochondrial permeability and induce the release of second mitochondria-derived activator of caspases (SMACs) into the cytoplasm to bind and inactivate the inhibitor of apoptosis proteins (IAPs) like Bcl-2 [102,103], which inhibit the activation of caspase and contribute to protecting intestinal epithelial cells from apoptosis [104]. On the other hand, increased mitochondrial permeability can also cause the release of cytochrome c (Cyto C), the inducer of apoptotic protease activating factor-1 (Apaf-1), through the mitochondrial apoptosis-induced channel (MAC), which is generally suppressed by Bcl-2 family proteins [105], to induce the production of caspase 9 and caspase 3 and promote apoptosis [105].

The effects of C3G on apoptosis are various in different cell models. It has been reported that C3G can potentially inhibit human colon cancer cell proliferation through promoting apoptosis and suppressing angiogenesis [106,107]. But in other normal cases, C3G showed the protective effects on gastrointestinal cells, as well as endothelial cells, and obviously inhibited apoptosis by regulating apoptosis associated proteins, such as reducing the cytoplasmatic levels in Bax [108] and inhibiting the expression of caspase-8 [109], caspase-9 [108], and caspase-3 [108,109] to attenuate gastrointestinal damage. The impacts of C3G-Ms on apoptosis are similar to C3G, and multiple studies have suggested that PCA [35,36,100] and FA [110,111] may act against apoptosis in various models, although other studies revealed that C3G-Ms (PCA, FA) might promote apoptosis of colorectal adenocarcinoma cells [112]. The mechanism of C3G-Ms against apoptosis is still unclear, but a recent study has shown that in addition to the direct quenching of ROS, PCA may inhibit the expression of pro-apoptotic Bax in mitochondria and subsequently, increase the ratio of Bcl-2/Bax to reduce the production of caspase 8, caspase 9, and caspase 3 in injured gastrointestinal mucosa (Figure 5) [36].

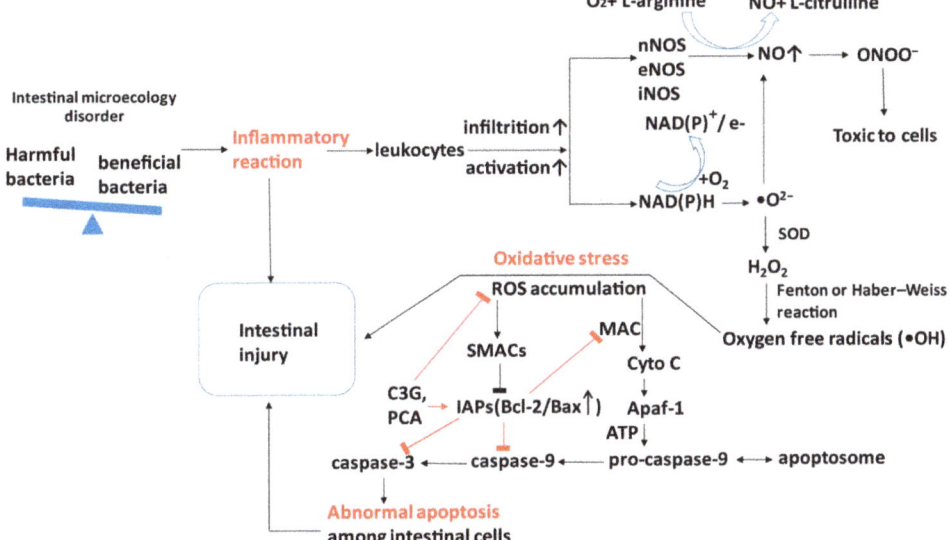

Figure 5. Potential mechanisms of C3G&C3G-Ms against apoptosis in intestinal epithelial cells. Intestinal flora disorder can induce the overproduction of pro-apoptotic factors such as ROS to increase mitochondrial permeability and cause the release of SMACs to bind and inactivate IAPs, such as Bcl-2. Since IAPs inhibit the activation of MAC and caspase to inhibit apoptosis, the inactivation of IAPs will induce the release of Cyto C through MAC, and subsequently induce the expression of Apaf-1 and caspase to cause apoptosis. C3G and its metabolites PCA can directly quench ROS and activate IAPs to inhibit the release of Cyto C and expression of caspases. Apaf-1, apoptotic protease activating factor-1; Cyto C, cytochrome C; C3G, cyanidin 3-glucoside; IAPs, inhibitor of apoptosis proteins; MAC, mitochondrial apoptosis-induced channel; PCA, protocatechuic acid; ROS, reactive oxygen species; SMACs, second mitochondria-derived activator of caspases.

6. Conclusions

Due to the strong antioxidant and anti-inflammatory properties, anthocyanins present in natural products offer great hope as an alternative therapy for chronic disorders, such as cardiovascular disease, fatty liver disease, inflammatory bowel disease, and glucose-lipid metabolism disorders. Maintaining the gut integrity plays an important role in the health-promoting functions of anthocyanins, as the intestinal tract is not only the main place for digestion and absorption of food but also the first defense barrier against external pathogens and stimulus. It is commonly believed that the degradation of anthocyanins in the gastrointestinal tract decreases their bioavailability; however, recent studies based on the microbiome and metabonomics have suggested that the interaction between natural bioactive compounds and gut microbiota may potentially increase health benefits. On the one hand, anthocyanins can modulate the gut microbiota composition through either bacteriostasis effect or as nutrients to promote the growth of specific microbes. On the other hand, gut microbiota may break down anthocyanins to form multiple metabolites, which are absorbed into the systemic circulation to exert positive or negative effects. Thus, understanding the interactions between anthocyanins and microorganisms, as well as the effects of anthocyanin-derived metabolites on cellular signaling pathways, is necessary for the rational use of anthocyanins. The breakdown of C3G in the gastrointestinal tract generates a series of secondary phenolic metabolites, which take up the main part of C3G-derived bioactive phenolics in circulation. Those metabolites, such as PCA, PGA, VA, and FA, not only regulate the gut microbiota potentially by their lethal effects on microorganisms but also affect the Nrf2-mediated antioxidant system and inflammatory pathways, such as the TAK1-mediated MAPK pathway and SphK/S1P mediated NF-κB pathway. Based on this, C3G and its metabolites improve the microenvironment and attenuate the oxidative stress and inflammation to reduce the cell death of enterocytes, which ultimately maintain intestinal integrity and function. However, species-specific microbial communities and their products affected by C3G and its bioactive metabolites, and how those products regulate signaling pathways and physiological responses are still not clear. Future studies based on multi-omics analysis will provide an insight into both the health benefits and negative effects of C3G and contribute to the rational use of this common natural anthocyanin.

Author Contributions: Writing—original draft preparation, J.T. and Y.L.; Writing—review and editing, S.W. and D.-X.H.; supervision, S.W.

Funding: The authors gratefully acknowledge the support from the National Natural Science Foundation of China (31772819), Hunan Provincial Natural Science Foundation for Distinguished Young Scholars (2019JJ30012), and Double-First-Class Construction Project of Hunan Province (kxk201801004).

Conflicts of Interest: The authors declare no conflicts of interest.

Abbreviations

ARE, antioxidant response element; bZIP, basic leucine zipper; CAT, catalase; COX-2, cyclooxygenase-2; C3G, cyanidin-3-glucoside; Cyto C, cytochrome c; ERK, extracellular signal-regulated kinase; FA, ferulic acid; GPx, glutathione peroxidase; GR, glutathione reductase; GSH, glutathione; IAPs, inhibitor of apoptosis proteins; ICAM-1, intercellular adhesion molecule-1; IKK, IκB kinases; IRAK, interleukin receptor-associated kinases; iNOS, inducible nitric oxide synthase; IVA, isovanillic acid; JNK, c-Jun NH2-terminal kinase; KEAP1, kelch like-ECH-associated protein 1; LBP, LPS binding proteins; LPS, lipopolysaccharide; MAC, mitochondrial apoptosis-induced channel; MAPK, mitogen-activated protein kinase; MDA, malondialdehyde; MLCK, myosin light chain kinase; MnSOD, manganese-dependent superoxide dismutase; MyD88, myeloid differentiation factor 88; NF-κB, nuclear factor-κB; NQR, NADH-quinone oxidoreductase; Nrf2, nuclear factor (erythroid-derived 2)-like 2; PCA, protocatechuic acid; PGA, phloroglucinaldehyde; PGE_2, prostaglandin E_2; PI3K, phosphoinositide 3-kinase; PKB, protein kinase B; PKC, protein kinase C; RNS, reactive nitrogen species; ROS, reactive oxygen species; SMACs, second mitochondria-derived activator of caspases; S1P, sphingosine-1-phosphate; S1PL, S1P lyase; S1PR, S1P receptors; SphK, sphingosine kinases; SQR, succinate-quinone oxidoreductase; TAK1, transforming growth factor beta activated kinase-1; T-AOC, total antioxidant capacity; TJs, tight junctions; TLR4, toll-like receptor 4; TNF-α, tumor necrosis factor-alpha; TRAF, tumor necrosis-associated factor; VA, vanillic acid; ZO-1, zonula occludens-1.

References

1. Amin, H.P.; Czank, C.; Raheem, S.; Zhang, Q.; Botting, N.P.; Cassidy, A.; Kay, C.D. Anthocyanins and their physiologically relevant metabolites alter the expression of IL-6 and VCAM-1 in CD40L and oxidized LDL challenged vascular endothelial cells. *Mol. Nutr. Food Res.* **2015**, *59*, 1095–1106. [CrossRef] [PubMed]
2. You, Y.; Yuan, X.; Liu, X.; Liang, C.; Meng, M.; Huang, Y.; Han, X.; Guo, J.; Guo, Y.; Ren, C.; et al. Cyanidin-3-glucoside increases whole body energy metabolism by upregulating brown adipose tissue mitochondrial function. *Mol. Nutr. Food Res.* **2017**, *61*, 1700261. [CrossRef] [PubMed]
3. Tremblay, F.; Waterhouse, J.; Nason, J.; Kalt, W. Prophylactic neuroprotection by blueberry-enriched diet in a rat model of light-induced retinopathy. *J. Nutr. Biochem.* **2013**, *24*, 647–655. [CrossRef] [PubMed]
4. Wu, S.; Yano, S.; Hisanaga, A.; He, X.; He, J.; Sakao, K.; Hou, D.-X. Polyphenols from *Lonicera caerulea* L. berry attenuate experimental nonalcoholic steatohepatitis by inhibiting proinflammatory cytokines productions and lipid peroxidation. *Mol. Nutr. Food Res.* **2017**, *61*, 1600858. [CrossRef] [PubMed]

5. Ferrari, D.; Speciale, A.; Cristani, M.; Fratantonio, D.; Molonia, M.S.; Ranaldi, G.; Saija, A.; Cimino, F. Cyanidin-3-O-glucoside inhibits NF-kB signalling in intestinal epithelial cells exposed to TNF-alpha and exerts protective effects via Nrf2 pathway activation. *Toxicol. Lett.* **2016**, *264*, 51–58. [CrossRef]
6. Rice-Evans, C.; Miller, N.; Paganga, G. Antioxidant properties of phenolic compounds. *Trends Plant Sci.* **1997**, *2*, 152–159. [CrossRef]
7. Bharat, D.; Ramos, R.; Cavalcanti, M.; Petersen, C.; Begaye, N.; Cutler, B.R.; Costa, M.M.A.; Ramos, R.K.L.G.; Ferreira, M.R.; Li, Y.; et al. Blueberry metabolites attenuate lipotoxicity-induced endothelial dysfunction. *Mol. Nutr. Food Res.* **2018**, *62*, 1700601. [CrossRef]
8. De Ferrars, R.M.; Czank, C.; Zhang, Q.; Botting, N.P.; Kroon, P.A.; Cassidy, A.; Kay, C.D. The pharmacokinetics of anthocyanins and their metabolites in humans. *Br. J. Pharmacol.* **2014**, *171*, 3268–3282. [CrossRef]
9. Ma, Y.; Chen, F.; Yang, S.; Chen, B.; Shi, J. Protocatechuic acid ameliorates high glucose-induced extracellular matrix accumulation in diabetic nephropathy. *Biomed. Pharmacother.* **2018**, *98*, 18–22. [CrossRef]
10. Jang, S.-A.; Song, H.S.; Kwon, J.E.; Baek, H.J.; Koo, H.J.; Sohn, E.-H.; Lee, S.R.; Kang, S.C. Protocatechuic acid attenuates trabecular bone loss in ovariectomized mice. *Oxidative Med. Cell. Longev.* **2018**, *2018*, 7280342. [CrossRef]
11. Molehin, O.R.; Adeyanju, A.A.; Adefegha, S.A.; Akomolafe, S.F. Protocatechuic acid mitigates adriamycin-induced reproductive toxicities and hepatocellular damage in rats. *Comp. Clin. Pathol.* **2018**, *27*, 1681–1689. [CrossRef]
12. Jang, S.-E.; Choi, J.-R.; Han, M.J.; Kim, D.-H. The preventive and curative effect of cyanidin-3β-D-glycoside and its metabolite protocatechuic acid against TNBS-induced colitis in mice. *Nat. Prod. Sci.* **2016**, *22*, 282–286. [CrossRef]
13. Bhavani, P.; Subramanian, P.; Kanimozhi, S. Preventive efficacy of vanillic acid on regulation of redox homeostasis, matrix metalloproteinases and cyclin D1 in rats bearing endometrial carcinoma. *Indian J. Clin. Biochem.* **2017**, *32*, 429–436. [CrossRef] [PubMed]
14. Rasheeda, K.; Bharathy, H.; Fathima, N.N. Vanillic acid and syringic acid: Exceptionally robust aromatic moieties for inhibiting in vitro self-assembly of type I collagen. *Int. J. Biol. Macromol.* **2018**, *113*, 952–960. [CrossRef] [PubMed]
15. Khoshnam, S.E.; Farbood, Y.; Moghaddam, H.F.; Sarkaki, A.; Badavi, M.; Khorsandi, L. Vanillic acid attenuates cerebral hyperemia, blood-brain barrier disruption and anxiety-like behaviors in rats following transient bilateral common carotid occlusion and reperfusion. *Metab. Brain Dis.* **2018**, *33*, 785–793. [CrossRef]
16. Tanihara, F.; Hirata, M.; Nhien, N.T.; Hirano, T.; Kunihara, T.; Otoi, T. Effect of ferulic acid supplementation on the developmental competence of porcine embryos during in vitro maturation. *J. Vet. Med Sci.* **2018**, *80*, 1007–1011. [CrossRef]
17. Peresa, D.D.A.; Sarrufb, F.D.; de Oliveirac, C.A.; Velascoa, M.V.R.; Babya, A.R. Ferulic acid photoprotective properties in association with UV filters: Multifunctional sunscreen with improved SPF and UVA-PF. *J. Photochem. Photobiol. B Biol.* **2018**, *185*, 46–49. [CrossRef]
18. Bumrungpert, A.; Lilitchan, S.; Tuntipopipat, S.; Tirawanchai, N.; Komindr, S. Ferulic acid supplementation improves lipid profiles, oxidative stress, and inflammatory status in hyperlipidemic subjects: A randomized, double-blind, placebo-controlled clinical trial. *Nutrients* **2018**, *10*, 713. [CrossRef]
19. Zhang, S.; Wang, P.; Zhao, P.; Wang, D.; Zhang, Y.; Wang, J.; Chen, L.; Guo, W.; Gao, H.; Jiao, Y. Pretreatment of ferulic acid attenuates inflammation and oxidative stress in a rat model of lipopolysaccharide-induced acute respiratory distress syndrome. *Int. J. Immunopathol. Pharmacol.* **2018**, *32*, 394632017750518. [CrossRef]
20. Esposito, D.; Damsud, T.; Wilson, M.; Grace, M.H.; Strauch, R.; Li, X.; Lila, M.A.; Komarnytsky, S. Black currant anthocyanins attenuate weight gain and improve glucose metabolism in diet-induced obese mice with intact, but not disrupted, gut microbiome. *J. Agric. Food Chem.* **2015**, *63*, 6172–6180. [CrossRef]
21. Yang, P.; Yuan, C.; Wang, H.; Han, F.; Liu, Y.; Wang, L.; Liu, Y. Stability of Anthocyanins and Their Degradation Products from Cabernet Sauvignon Red Wine under Gastrointestinal pH and Temperature Conditions. *Molecules* **2018**, *23*, 354. [CrossRef] [PubMed]
22. Cai, H.; Thomasset, S.C.; Berry, D.P.; Garcea, G.; Brown, K.; Stewarda, W.P.; Gescher, A.J. Determination of anthocyanins in the urine of patients with colorectal liver metastases after administration of bilberry extract. *Biomed. Chromatogr.* **2011**, *25*, 660–663. [CrossRef] [PubMed]
23. Talavera, S.; Felgines, C.; Texier, O.; Besson, C.; Lamaison, J.-L.; Remesy, C. Anthocyanins are efficiently absorbed from the stomach in anesthetized rats. *J. Nutr.* **2003**, *133*, 4178–4182. [CrossRef] [PubMed]

24. Moraisa, C.A.; de Rossoa, V.V.; Estadellaa, D.; Pisani, L.P. Anthocyanins as inflammatory modulators and the role of the gut microbiota. *J. Nutr. Biochem.* **2016**, *33*, 1–7. [CrossRef] [PubMed]
25. Jim, F. Some anthocyanins could be efficiently absorbed across the gastrointestinal mucosa: Extensive presystemic metabolism reduces apparent bioavailability. *J. Agric. Food Chem.* **2014**, *62*, 3904–3911.
26. Castañeda-Ovando, A.; de Lourdes Pacheco-Hernández, M.; Páez-Hernández, M.E.; Rodríguez, J.A.; Galán-Vidal, C.A. Chemical studies of anthocyanins: A review. *Food Chem.* **2009**, *113*, 859–871. [CrossRef]
27. Aura, A.-M.; Martin-Lopez, P.; O'Leary, K.A.; Williamson, G.; Oksman-Caldentey, K.M.; Poutanen, K.; Santos-Buelga, C. In vitro metabolism of anthocyanins by human gut microflora. *Eur. J. Nutr.* **2005**, *44*, 133–142. [CrossRef] [PubMed]
28. Hanske, L.; Engst, W.; Loh, G.; Sczesny, S.; Blaut, M.; Braune, A. Contribution of gut bacteria to the metabolism of cyanidin 3-glucoside in human microbiota-associated rats. *Br. J. Nutr.* **2013**, *109*, 1433–1441. [CrossRef]
29. Zhang, X.; Sandhu, A.; Edirisinghe, I.; Burton-Freeman, B. An exploratory study of red raspberry (*Rubus idaeus* L.) (poly)phenols/metabolites in human biological samples. *Food Funct.* **2018**, *9*, 806–818. [CrossRef]
30. Vitaglione, P.; Donnarumma, G.; Napolitano, A.; Galvano, F.; Gallo, A.; Scalfi, L.; Fogliano, V. Protocatechuic acid is the major human metabolite of cyanidin-glucosides. *J. Nutr.* **2007**, *137*, 2043–2048. [CrossRef]
31. Safaeiana, L.; Emamia, R.; Hajhashemia, V.; Haghighatian, Z. Antihypertensive and antioxidant effects of protocatechuic acid in deoxycorticosterone acetate-salt hypertensive rats. *Biomed. Pharmacother.* **2018**, *100*, 147–155. [CrossRef] [PubMed]
32. Lende, A.B.; Kshirsagar, A.D.; Deshpande, A.D.; Muley, M.M.; Patil, R.R.; Bafna, P.A.; Naik, S.R. Anti-inflammatory and analgesic activity of protocatechuic acid in rats and mice. *Inflammopharmacology* **2011**, *19*, 255–263. [CrossRef] [PubMed]
33. Crespo, I.; San-Miguel, B.; Mauriz, J.L.; Ortiz de Urbina, J.; Almar, M.; Tuñón, M.J.; González-Gallego, J. Protective effect of protocatechuic acid on TNBS-induced colitis in mice is associated with modulation of the SphK/S1P signaling pathway. *Nutrients* **2017**, *9*, 288. [CrossRef] [PubMed]
34. Ma, L.; Wang, G.; Chen, Z.; Li, Z.; Yao, J.; Zhao, H.; Wang, S.; Ma, Z.; Chang, H.; Tian, X. Modulating the p66shc signaling pathway with protocatechuic acid protects the intestine from ischemia-reperfusion injury and alleviates secondary liver damage. *Sci. World J.* **2014**, *2014*, 1–11. [CrossRef] [PubMed]
35. Varì, R.; Scazzocchio, B.; Santangelo, C.; Filesi, C.; Galvano, F.; D'Archivio, M.; Masella, R.; Giovannini, C. Protocatechuic acid prevents oxLDL-induced apoptosis by activating JNK/Nrf2 survival signals in macrophages. *Oxid. Med. Cell. Longev.* **2015**, *2015*, 1–11. [CrossRef] [PubMed]
36. Cheng, Y.T.; Lin, J.A.; Jhang, J.J.; Yen, G.C. Protocatechuic acid-mediated DJ-1/PARK7 activation followed by PI3K/mTOR signaling pathway activation as a novel mechanism for protection against ketoprofen-induced oxidative damage in the gastrointestinal mucosa. *Free Radic. Biol. Med.* **2019**, *130*, 35–47. [CrossRef] [PubMed]
37. Amini, A.M.; Spencer, J.P.E.; Yaqoob, P. Effects of pelargonidin-3-O-glucoside and its metabolites on lipopolysaccharide-stimulated cytokine production by THP-1 monocytes and macrophages. *Cytokine* **2018**, *103*, 29–33. [CrossRef]
38. Wang, H.-Y.; Wang, H.; Wang, J.-H.; Wang, Q.; Ma, Q.-F.; Chen, Y.-Y. Protocatechuic acid inhibits inflammatory responses in LPS-stimulated BV2 Microglia via NF-kappaB and MAPKs signaling pathways. *Neurochem. Res.* **2015**, *40*, 1655–1660. [CrossRef]
39. Lin, C.-Y.; Huang, C.-S.; Huang, C.-Y.; Yin, M.-C. Anticoagulatory, antiinflammatory, and antioxidative effects of protocatechuic acid in diabetic mice. *J. Agric. Food Chem.* **2009**, *57*, 6661–6667. [CrossRef]
40. Amini, A.M.; Muzs, K.; Spencer, J.P.; Yaqoob, P. Pelargonidin-3-O-glucoside and its metabolites have modest anti-inflammatory effects in human whole blood cultures. *Nutr. Res.* **2017**, *46*, 88–95. [CrossRef]
41. Wu, S.; Hu, R.; Tan, J.; He, Z.; Liu, M.; Li, Y.; He, X.; Hou, D.-X.; Luo, J.; He, J. Abstract WP534: Cyanidin 3-glucoside and its Metabolites Protect Against Nonalcoholic Fatty Liver Disease: Crosstalk Between Serum Lipids, Inflammatory Cytokines and MAPK/ERK Pathway. *Stroke* **2019**, *50* (Suppl. 1), AWP534. [CrossRef]
42. Amin, F.U.; Shah, S.A.; Kim, M.O. Vanillic acid attenuates Abeta1-42-induced oxidative stress and cognitive impairment in mice. *Sci. Rep.* **2017**, *7*, 40753. [CrossRef] [PubMed]
43. Anbalagan, V.; Raju, K.; Shanmugam, M. Assessment of lipid peroxidation and antioxidant status in vanillic acid treated 7,12-dimethylbenzaanthracene induced hamster buccal pouch carcinogenesis. *J. Clin. Diagn. Res.* **2017**, *11*, BF01–BF04. [PubMed]

44. Vinothiya, K.; Ashokkumar, N. Modulatory effect of vanillic acid on antioxidant status in high fat diet-induced changes in diabetic hypertensive rats. *Biomed. Pharmacother.* **2017**, *87*, 640–652. [CrossRef] [PubMed]
45. Calixto-Campos, C.; Carvalho, T.T.; Hohmann, M.S.; Pinho-Ribeiro, F.A.; Fattori, V.; Manchope, M.F.; Zarpelon, A.C.; Baracat, M.M.; Georgetti, S.R.; Casagrande, R.; et al. Vanillic acid inhibits inflammatory pain by inhibiting neutrophil recruitment, oxidative stress, cytokine production, and NFkB activation in mice. *J. Nat. Prod.* **2015**, *78*, 1799–1808. [CrossRef] [PubMed]
46. Kim, M.-C.; Kim, S.-J.; Kim, D.-S.; Jeon, Y.-D.; Park, S.J.; Lee, H.S.; Um, J.-Y.; Hong, S.-H. Vanillic acid inhibits inflammatory mediators by suppressing NF-kappaB in lipopolysaccharide-stimulated mouse peritoneal macrophages. *Immunopharmacol. Immunotoxicol.* **2011**, *33*, 525–532. [CrossRef] [PubMed]
47. Jeong, H.-J.; Nam, S.-Y.; Kim, H.-Y.; Jin, M.H.; Kim, M.H.; Roh, S.S.; Kim, H.-M. Anti-allergic inflammatory effect of vanillic acid through regulating thymic stromal lymphopoietin secretion from activated mast cells. *Nat. Prod. Res.* **2018**, *32*, 2945–2949. [CrossRef] [PubMed]
48. Ghosh, S.; Chowdhury, S.; Sarkar, P.; Sil, P.C. Ameliorative role of ferulic acid against diabetes associated oxidative stress induced spleen damage. *Food Chem. Toxicol.* **2018**, *118*, 272–286. [CrossRef]
49. He, S.; Guo, Y.; Zhao, J.; Xu, X.; Song, J.; Wang, N.; Liu, Q. Ferulic acid protects against heat stress-induced intestinal epithelial barrier dysfunction in IEC-6 cells via the PI3K/Akt-mediated Nrf2/HO-1 signaling pathway. *Int. J. Hyperth.* **2018**, *35*, 112–121. [CrossRef]
50. Szulc-Kielbik, I.; Kielbik, M.; Klink, M. Ferulic acid but not alpha-lipoic acid effectively protects THP-1-derived macrophages from oxidant and pro-inflammatory response to LPS. *Immunopharmacol. Immunotoxicol.* **2017**, *39*, 330–337. [CrossRef]
51. Das, U.; Manna, K.; Khan, A.; Sinha, M.; Biswas, S.; Sengupta, A.; Chakraborty, A.; Dey, S. Ferulic acid (FA) abrogates gamma-radiation induced oxidative stress and DNA damage by up-regulating nuclear translocation of Nrf2 and activation of NHEJ pathway. *Free Radic. Res.* **2017**, *51*, 47–63. [CrossRef] [PubMed]
52. Liu, J.-L.; He, Y.-L.; Wang, S.; He, Y.; Wang, W.-Y.; Li, Q.-J.; Cao, X.-Y. Ferulic acid inhibits advanced glycation end products (AGEs) formation and mitigates the AGEs-induced inflammatory response in HUVEC cells. *J. Funct. Foods* **2018**, *48*, 19–26. [CrossRef]
53. Zhou, Q.; Gong, X.; Kuang, G.; Jiang, R.; Xie, T.; Tie, H.; Chen, X.; Li, K.; Wan, J.; Wang, B. Ferulic acid protected from kidney ischemia reperfusion injury in mice: Possible mechanism through increasing adenosine generation via HIF-1alpha. *Inflammation* **2018**, *41*, 2068–2078. [CrossRef] [PubMed]
54. Salazar-López, N.J.; Astiazarán-García, H.; González-Aguilar, G.A.; Loarca-Piña, G.; Ezquerra-Brauer, J.M.; Domínguez Avila, J.A.; Robles-Sánchez, M. Ferulic acid on glucose dysregulation, dyslipidemia, and inflammation in diet-induced obese rats: An integrated study. *Nutrients* **2017**, *9*, 675. [CrossRef] [PubMed]
55. Kim, S.-J.; Kim, M.-C.; Um, J.-Y.; Hong, S.-H. The beneficial effect of vanillic acid on ulcerative colitis. *Molecules* **2010**, *15*, 7208–7217. [CrossRef]
56. Nishitani, Y.; Sasaki, E.; Fujisawa, T.; Osawa, R. Genotypic analyses of lactobacilli with a range of tannase activities isolated from human feces and fermented foods. *Syst. Appl. Microbiol.* **2004**, *27*, 109–117. [CrossRef]
57. Szwajgier, D.; Jakubczyk, A. Biotransformation of ferulic acid by *Lactobacillus* acidophilus K1 and selected *Bifidobacterium* strains. *Acta Sci. Pol. Technol. Aliment.* **2010**, *9*, 45–59.
58. Gowd, V.; Bao, T.; Chen, W. Antioxidant potential and phenolic profile of blackberry anthocyanin extract followed by human gut microbiota fermentation. *Food Res. Int.* **2019**, *120*, 523–533. [CrossRef]
59. Keppler, K.; Humpf, H.U. Metabolism of anthocyanins and their phenolic degradation products by the intestinal microflora. *Bioorganic Med. Chem.* **2005**, *13*, 5195–5205. [CrossRef]
60. Wang, D.; Xia, M.; Yan, X.; Li, D.; Wang, L.; Xu, Y.; Jin, T.; Ling, W. Gut microbiota metabolism of anthocyanin promotes reverse cholesterol transport in mice via repressing miRNA-10b. *Circ. Res.* **2012**, *111*, 967–981. [CrossRef]
61. Braga, A.R.C.; Mesquita, L.M.D.S.; Martins, P.L.G.; Habu, S.; De Rosso, V.V.; Habu, S. *Lactobacillus* fermentation of jussara pulp leads to the enzymatic conversion of anthocyanins increasing antioxidant activity. *J. Food Compos. Anal.* **2018**, *69*, 162–170. [CrossRef]
62. Westfall, S.; Lomis, N. Ferulic acid produced by *Lactobacillus* fermentum NCIMB 5221 reduces symptoms of metabolic syndrome in drosophila melanogaster. *J. Microb. Biochem. Technol.* **2016**, *8*, 272–284. [CrossRef]

63. Álvarez-Rodríguez, M.L.; Belloch, C.; Villa, M.; Uruburu, F.; Larriba, G.; Coque, J.-J.R. Degradation of vanillic acid and production of guaiacol by microorganisms isolated from cork samples. *Fems Microbiol. Lett.* **2003**, *220*, 49–55. [CrossRef]
64. Lee, S.; Keirsey, K.I.; Kirkland, R.; Grunewald, Z.I.; Fischer, J.G.; De La Serre, C.B. Blueberry Supplementation Influences the Gut Microbiota, Inflammation, and Insulin Resistance in High-Fat-Diet-Fed Rats. *J. Nutr. Nutr. Dis.* **2018**, *148*, 209–219. [CrossRef] [PubMed]
65. Zhao, S.; Liu, W.; Wang, J.; Shi, J.; Sun, Y.; Wang, W.; Ning, G.; Liu, R.; Hong, J. *Akkermansia* muciniphila improves metabolic profiles by reducing inflammation in chow diet-fed mice. *J. Mol. Endocrinol.* **2016**, *58*, 1–14. [CrossRef] [PubMed]
66. Wang, K.; Wan, Z.; Ou, A.; Liang, X.; Guo, X.; Zhang, Z.; Wu, L.; Xue, X. Monofloral honey from a medical plant, *Prunella vulgaris*, protected against dextran sulfate sodium-induced ulcerative colitis via modulating gut microbial populations in rats. *Food Funct.* **2019**, *10*, 3828–3838. [CrossRef] [PubMed]
67. Wu, S.; Hu, R.; Nakano, H.; Chen, K.; Liu, M.; He, X.; Zhang, H.; He, J.; Hou, D.-X. Modulation of gut microbiota by *Lonicera caerulea* L. Berry polyphenols in a mouse model of fatty liver induced by high fat diet. *Molecules* **2018**, *23*, 2313. [CrossRef] [PubMed]
68. Wang, K.; Jin, X.; Li, Q.; Sawaya, A.C.H.F.; Le Leu, R.K.; Conlon, M.A.; Wu, L.; Hu, F. Propolis from different geographic origins decreases intestinal inflammation and *Bacteroides* spp. populations in a model of DSS-induced colitis. *Mol. Nutr. Food Rese.* **2018**, *62*, e1800080. [CrossRef]
69. Haliru, F.Z.; Saidu, K.; Habibu, R.S.; Ajiboye, T.O.; Uwazie, J.N.; Ibitoye, O.B.; Aliyu, N.O.; Ajiboye, H.O.; Bello, S.A.; Muritala, H.F.; et al. Involvement of oxidative stress in protocatechuic acid-mediated bacterial lethality. *Microbiologyopen* **2017**, *6*, e00472.
70. Zhou, X.; Wu, F. Vanillic acid changed cucumber (*Cucumis sativus* L.) seedling rhizosphere total bacterial, *pseudomonas* and *bacillus* spp. communities. *Sci. Rep.* **2018**, *8*, 4929. [CrossRef]
71. Patzke, H.; Schieber, A. Growth-inhibitory activity of phenolic compounds applied in an emulsifiable concentrate-ferulic acid as a natural pesticide against botrytis cinerea. *Food Res. Int.* **2018**, *113*, 18–23. [CrossRef] [PubMed]
72. Chavarro, J.E.; Toth, T.L.; Sadio, S.M.; Hauser, R. Soy food and isoflavone intake in relation to semen quality parameters among men from an infertility clinic. *Hum. Reprod.* **2008**, *23*, 2584–2590. [CrossRef] [PubMed]
73. Zielinsky, P.; Piccoli, A.L., Jr.; Manica, J.L.; Nicoloso, L.H.; Menezes, H.; Busato, A.; Moraes, M.R.; Silva, J.; Bender, L.; Pizzato, P.; et al. Maternal consumption of polyphenol-rich foods in late pregnancy and fetal ductus arteriosus flow dynamics. *J. Perinatol.* **2010**, *30*, 17–21. [CrossRef] [PubMed]
74. Jacobsen, B.K.; Jaceldo-Siegl, K.; Knutsen, S.F.; Fan, J.; Oda, K.; Fraser, G.E. Soy isoflavone intake and the likelihood of ever becoming a mother: The adventist health study-2. *Int. J. Women's Health* **2014**, *6*, 377–384. [CrossRef] [PubMed]
75. Badary, O.A.; Awad, A.S.; Sherief, M.A.; Hamada, F.M. In vitro and in vivo effects of ferulic acid on gastrointestinal motility: Inhibition of cisplatin-induced delay in gastric emptying in rats. *World J. Gastroenterol.* **2006**, *12*, 5363–5367. [CrossRef] [PubMed]
76. Ferrari, D.; Cimino, F.; Fratantonio, D.; Molonia, M.S.; Bashllari, R.; Busà, R.; Saija, A.; Speciale, A. Cyanidin-3-O-Glucoside modulates the in vitro inflammatory crosstalk between intestinal epithelial and endothelial cells. *Mediat. Inflamm.* **2017**, *2017*, 1–8. [CrossRef] [PubMed]
77. Pereira, S.R.; Pereira, R.; Figueiredo, I.; Freitas, V.; Dinis, T.C.; Almeida, L.M. Comparison of anti-inflammatory activities of an anthocyanin-rich fraction from Portuguese blueberries (*Vaccinium corymbosum* L.) and 5-aminosalicylic acid in a TNBS-induced colitis rat model. *PLoS ONE* **2017**, *12*, e0174116. [CrossRef]
78. Serra, D.; Paixão, J.; Nunes, C.; Dinis, T.C.; Almeida, L.M. Cyanidin-3-glucoside suppresses cytokine-induced inflammatory response in human intestinal cells: Comparison with 5-aminosalicylic acid. *PLoS ONE* **2013**, *8*, e73001. [CrossRef]
79. Jiménez, S.; Gascón, S.; Luquin, A.; Laguna, M.; Ancin-Azpilicueta, C.; Rodríguez-Yoldi, M.J. Rosa canina extracts have antiproliferative and antioxidante effects on caco-2 human colon cancer. *PLoS ONE* **2016**, *11*, e0159136. [CrossRef]
80. Wu, S.; Yano, S.; Chen, J.; Hisanaga, A.; Sakao, K.; He, X.; He, J.; Hou, D.-X. Polyphenols *from Lonicera caerulea* L. berry inhibit LPS-induced inflammation through dual modulation of inflammatory and antioxidant mediators. *J. Agric. Food Chem.* **2017**, *65*, 5133–5141. [CrossRef]

81. Zhang, D.D.; Hannink, M. Distinct cysteine residues in Keap1 are required for Keap1-dependent ubiquitination of Nrf2 and for stabilization of Nrf2 by chemopreventive agents and oxidative stress. *Mol. Cell. Biol.* **2003**, *23*, 8137–8151. [CrossRef] [PubMed]
82. Huang, H.-C.; Nguyen, T.; Pickett, C.B. Phosphorylation of Nrf2 at Ser-40 by protein kinase C regulates antioxidant response element-mediated transcription. *J. Biol. Chem.* **2002**, *277*, 42769–42774. [CrossRef] [PubMed]
83. Zipper, L.M.; Mulcahy, R.T. Inhibition of ERK and p38 MAP kinases inhibits binding of Nrf2 and induction of GCS genes. *Biochem. Biophys. Res. Commun.* **2000**, *278*, 484–492. [CrossRef] [PubMed]
84. Rojo, A.I.; Sagarra, M.R.D.; Cuadrado, A. GSK-3beta down-regulates the transcription factor Nrf2 after oxidant damage: Relevance to exposure of neuronal cells to oxidative stress. *J. Neurochem.* **2008**, *105*, 192–202. [CrossRef] [PubMed]
85. Nakaso, K.; Yano, H.; Fukuhara, Y.; Takeshima, T.; Wada-Isoe, K.; Nakashima, K. PI3K is a key molecule in the Nrf2-mediated regulation of antioxidative proteins by hemin in human neuroblastoma cells. *FEBS Lett.* **2003**, *546*, 181–184. [CrossRef]
86. Varì, R.; D'Archivio, M.; Filesi, C.; Carotenuto, S.; Scazzocchio, B.; Santangelo, C.; Giovannini, C.; Masella, R. Protocatechuic acid induces antioxidant/detoxifying enzyme expression through JNK-mediated Nrf2 activation in murine macrophages. *J. Nutr. Biochem.* **2011**, *22*, 409–417. [CrossRef] [PubMed]
87. Guo, S.; Nighot, M.; Al-Sadi, R.; Alhmoud, T.; Nighot, P.; Ma, T.Y. Lipopolysaccharide regulation of intestinal tight junction permeability is mediated by TLR4 signal transduction pathway activation of FAK and MyD88. *J. Immunol.* **2015**, *195*, 4999–5010. [CrossRef]
88. Im, E.; Riegler, F.M.; Pothoulakis, C.; Rhee, S.H. Elevated lipopolysaccharide in the colon evokes intestinal inflammation, aggravated in immune modulator-impaired mice. *Am. J. Physiol.-Gastrointest. Liver Physiol.* **2012**, *303*, G490–G497. [CrossRef]
89. Cao, M.; Wang, P.; Sun, C.; He, W.; Wang, F. Amelioration of IFN-γ and TNF-α-induced intestinal epithelial barrier dysfunction by berberine via suppression of MLCK-MLC phosphorylation signaling pathway. *PLoS ONE* **2013**, *8*, e61944. [CrossRef]
90. Al-Sadi, R.; Ye, D.; Said, H.M.; Ma, T.Y. Cellular and molecular mechanism of interleukin-1 modulation of Caco-2 intestinal epithelial tight junction barrier. *J. Cell. Mol. Med.* **2011**, *15*, 970–982. [CrossRef]
91. Paris, L.; Tonutti, L.; Vannini, C.; Bazzoni, G. Structural organization of the tight junctions. *Biochim. Biophys. Acta (BBA)/Biomembr.* **2008**, *1778*, 646–659. [CrossRef] [PubMed]
92. Guo, S.; Al-Sadi, R.; Said, H.M.; Ma, T.Y. Lipopolysaccharide causes an increase in intestinal tight junction permeability in vitro and in vivo by inducing enterocyte membrane expression and localization of TLR-4 and CD14. *Am. J. Pathol.* **2013**, *182*, 375–387. [CrossRef] [PubMed]
93. Al-Sadi, R.; Boivin, M.; Ma, T. Mechanism of cytokine modulation of epithelial tight junction barrier. *Front. Biosci.* **2009**, *14*, 2765–2778. [CrossRef] [PubMed]
94. Kurpios-Piec, D.; Grosicka-Maciag, E.; Wozniak, K.; Kowalewski, C.; Kiernozek, E.; Szumi, M.; Rahden-Staron, I. Thiram activates NF-kappaB and enhances ICAM-1 expression in human microvascular endothelial HMEC-1 cells. *Pestic. Biochem. Physiol.* **2015**, *118*, 82–89. [CrossRef] [PubMed]
95. Van de Stolpe, A.; Van Der Saag, P.T. Intercellular adhesion molecule-1. *J. Mol. Med.* **1996**, *74*, 13–33. [CrossRef]
96. Amin, H.P. The vascular and anti-inflammatory activity of cyanidin-3-glucoside and its metabolites in human vascular endothelial cells. Ph.D. Thesis, University of East Anglia, Norwich, UK, 2015.
97. McCarty, M.F.; Iloki Assanga, S.B. Ferulic acid may target MyD88-mediated pro-inflammatory signaling—Implications for the health protection afforded by whole grains, anthocyanins, and coffee. *Med. Hypotheses* **2018**, *118*, 114–120. [CrossRef] [PubMed]
98. Bhattacharya, S.; Ray, R.M.; Johnson, L.R. Cyclin-dependent kinases regulate apoptosis of intestinal epithelial cells. *Apoptosis* **2014**, *19*, 451–466. [CrossRef]
99. Liguori, I.; Russo, G.; Curcio, F.; Bulli, G.; Aran, L.; Della-Morte, D.; Gargiulo, G.; Testa, G.; Cacciatore, F.; Bonaduce, D.; et al. Oxidative stress, aging, and diseases. *Clin. Interv. Aging* **2018**, *13*, 757–772. [CrossRef]
100. Giovannini, C.; Scazzocchio, B.; Matarrese, P.; Varì, R.; D'Archivio, M.; Di Benedetto, R.; Casciani, S.; Dessì, M.R.; Straface, E.; Malorni, W.; et al. Apoptosis induced by oxidized lipids is associated with up-regulation of p66Shc in intestinal Caco-2 cells: Protective effects of phenolic compounds. *J. Nutr. Biochem.* **2008**, *19*, 118–128. [CrossRef]

101. Nair, P.; Lu, M.; Petersen, S.; Ashkenazi, A. Apoptosis initiation through the cell-extrinsic pathway. *Methods Enzymol.* **2014**, *544*, 99–128.
102. Martinez-Caballero, S.; Dejean, L.M.; Jonas, E.A.; Kinnally, K.W. The role of the mitochondrial apoptosis induced channel MAC in cytochrome c release. *J. Bioenerg. Biomembr.* **2005**, *37*, 155–164. [CrossRef] [PubMed]
103. Wang, J.; Li, W. Discovery of novel second mitochondria-derived activator of caspase mimetics as selective inhibitor of apoptosis protein inhibitors. *J. Pharmacol. Exp. Ther.* **2014**, *349*, 319–329. [CrossRef] [PubMed]
104. Grabinger, T.; Bode, K.J.; Demgenski, J.; Seitz, C.; Delgado, M.E.; Kostadinova, F.; Reinhold, C.; Etemadi, N.; Wilhelm, S.; Schweinlin, M.; et al. Inhibitor of apoptosis protein-1 regulates tumor necrosis factor-mediated destruction of intestinal epithelial cells. *Gastroenterology* **2017**, *152*, 867–879. [CrossRef] [PubMed]
105. Kim, W.S.; Lee, K.S.; Kim, J.H.; Kim, C.K.; Lee, G.; Choe, J.; Won, M.H.; Kim, T.H.; Jeoung, D.; Lee, H.; et al. The caspase-8/Bid/cytochrome c axis links signals from death receptors to mitochondrial reactive oxygen species production. *Free Radic. Biol. Med.* **2017**, *112*, 567–577. [CrossRef] [PubMed]
106. Mazewski, C.; Liang, K.; De Mejia, E.G. Inhibitory potential of anthocyanin-rich purple and red corn extracts on human colorectal cancer cell proliferation in vitro. *J. Funct. Foods* **2017**, *34*, 254–265. [CrossRef]
107. Charepalli, V.; Reddivari, L.; Radhakrishnan, S.; Vadde, R.; Agarwal, R.; Vanamala, J.K.P. Anthocyanin-containing purple-fleshed potatoes suppress colon tumorigenesis via elimination of colon cancer stem cells. *J. Nutr. Biochem.* **2015**, *26*, 1641–1649. [CrossRef] [PubMed]
108. Paixão, J.; Dinis, T.C.; Almeida, L.M. Dietary anthocyanins protect endothelial cells against peroxynitrite-induced mitochondrial apoptosis pathway and bax nuclear translocation: An in vitro approach. *Apoptosis* **2011**, *16*, 976–989. [CrossRef]
109. Kim, S.H.; Lee, M.H.; Park, M.; Woo, H.J.; Kim, Y.S.; Tharmalingam, N.; Seo, W.D.; Kim, J.B. Regulatory effects of black rice extract on helicobacter pylori InfectionInduced apoptosis. *Mol. Nutr. Food Res.* **2018**, *62*, 1700586. [CrossRef]
110. Sadar, S.S.; Vyawahare, N.S.; Bodhankar, S.L. Ferulic acid ameliorates TNBS-induced ulcerative colitis through modulation of cytokines, oxidative stress, iNOs, COX-2, and apoptosis in laboratory rats. *Excli J.* **2016**, *15*, 482–499.
111. Khanduja, K.L.; Avti, P.K.; Kumar, S.; Mittal, N.; Sohi, K.K.; Pathak, C.M. Anti-apoptotic activity of caffeic acid, ellagic acid and ferulic acid in normal human peripheral blood mononuclear cells: A Bcl-2 independent mechanism. *Biochim. Biophys. Acta (BBA)-Gen. Subj.* **2006**, *1760*, 283–289. [CrossRef]
112. Moreno-Jiménez, M.R.; López-Barraza, R.; Cervantes-Cardoza, V.; Pérez-Ramírez, I.F.; Reyna-Rojas, J.A.; Gallegos-Infante, J.A.; Rocha-Guzmán, N.E. Mechanisms associated to apoptosis of cancer cells by phenolic extracts from two canned common beans varieties (*Phaseolus vulgaris* L.). *J. Food Biochem.* **2019**, *43*, e12680.

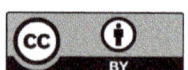

© 2019 by the authors. Licensee MDPI, Basel, Switzerland. This article is an open access article distributed under the terms and conditions of the Creative Commons Attribution (CC BY) license (http://creativecommons.org/licenses/by/4.0/).

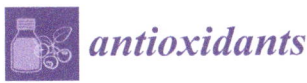

Article

Combined Treatment with Three Natural Antioxidants Enhances Neuroprotection in a SH-SY5Y 3D Culture Model

Pasquale Marrazzo [1], Cristina Angeloni [2],* and Silvana Hrelia [2]

[1] Department for Life Quality Studies, Alma Mater Studiorum, University of Bologna, 47921 Rimini, Italy; pasquale.marrazzo2@unibo.it
[2] School of Pharmacy, University of Camerino, 62032 Camerino, Italy; silvana.hrelia@unibo.it
* Correspondence: cristina.angeloni@unicam.it

Received: 19 August 2019; Accepted: 18 September 2019; Published: 20 September 2019

Abstract: Currently, the majority of cell-based studies on neurodegeneration are carried out on two-dimensional cultured cells that do not represent the cells residing in the complex microenvironment of the brain. Recent evidence has suggested that three-dimensional (3D) *in vitro* microenvironments may better model key features of brain tissues in order to study molecular mechanisms at the base of neurodegeneration. So far, no drugs have been discovered to prevent or halt the progression of neurodegenerative disorders. New therapeutic interventions can come from phytochemicals that have a broad spectrum of biological activities. On this basis, we evaluated the neuroprotective effect of three phytochemicals (sulforaphane, epigallocatechin gallate, and plumbagin) alone or in combination, focusing on their ability to counteract oxidative stress. The combined treatment was found to be more effective than the single treatments. In particular, the combined treatment increased cell viability and reduced glutathione (GSH) levels, upregulated antioxidant enzymes and insulin-degrading enzymes, and downregulated nicotinamide adenine dinucleotide phosphate (NADPH) oxidase 1 and 2 in respect to peroxide-treated cells. Our data suggest that a combination of different phytochemicals could be more effective than a single compound in counteracting neurodegeneration, probably thanks to a pleiotropic mechanism of action.

Keywords: neurodegeneration; SH-SY5Y cell line; 3D cultures; oxidative stress; phytochemicals; antioxidants

1. Introduction

Oxidative stress is strongly involved in the pathogenesis of different neurodegenerative diseases like Alzheimer's disease, Parkinson's disease, and amyotrophic lateral sclerosis [1]. Particularly, an excess of reactive oxygen species (ROS) released by cells promotes oxidative stress, which is a cause of tissue injury and results in dysfunction in the nervous system. So far, no drugs have been discovered to prevent or halt the progression of these widely spread neurological disorders, and the treatments available only manage the symptoms. Therefore, there is an urgent need for new treatments for these diseases, since the World Health Organization (WHO) predicts that by 2040, neurodegenerative diseases will become the second-most prevalent cause of death [2]. New therapeutic approaches can derive from phytochemicals, a huge source of compounds that have been widely investigated in the last years [3]. Sulforaphane (SF) (Figure 1a) is an isothiocyanate derived from *Brassicae* vegetables and has consistent support in the literature for its preventive role against oxidative stress [4], in addition to its well-known role in chemoprevention [5]. Epigallocatechin gallate (EGCG) (Figure 1b), the major catechin found in green tea [6] with diverse medical potential [7] has been demonstrated to promote neuroprotection in numerous studies [8]. Plumbagin (PB) (Figure 1c), a naphthoquinone isolated from the *Plumbaginacae* family, has mainly been studied in respect to its anti-inflammatory [9–11] and antimicrobial activities [12], even though it was also shown to modulate oxidative stress response [13] and precisely target NADPH oxidase 4 (NOX4) [14]. Importantly, the treatment of undifferentiated SH-SY5Y cells with a specific concentration of SF [15], EGCG [16], and PB [17] has been reported to decrease oxidative stress at different levels. On this basis, we hypothesized that a proper combination of such bioactive compounds could possess a higher effect in counteracting oxidative stress-induced neurodegeneration. Within organs, there are various concentration gradients for oxygen as well as for effector molecules, i.e., internal metabolites or exogenous compounds/drugs. Since the human brain cannot be modelled adequately in animals [18], reductionist humanized cellular systems are used and increasingly requested according to the 3Rs (Replacement, Reduction and Refinement) rule.

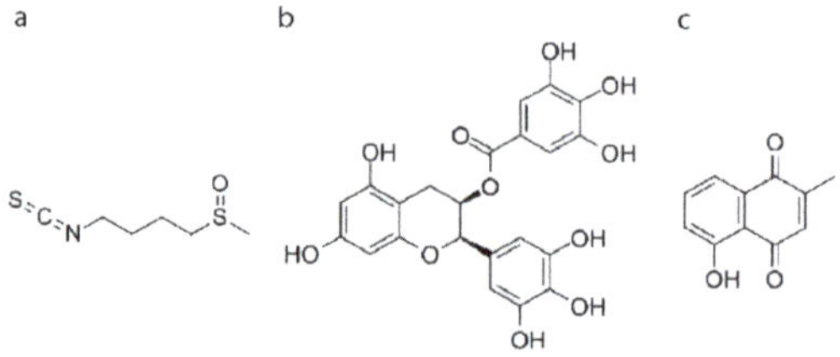

Figure 1. Chemical structures of the natural compounds used in this study. (**a**) Sulforaphane (SF), (**b**) epigallocatechin gallate (EGCG), (**c**) plumbagin (PB).

Currently, the majority of cell-based studies on neurodegeneration have been carried out on cultured cells propagated in two dimensions on plastic surfaces. However, cells cultured in these non-physiological conditions do not represent the cells residing in the complex microenvironment of the brain. With respect to this, recent evidence has suggested that three-dimensional (3D) in vitro microenvironments may better model key features of brain tissues in order to study the molecular mechanisms at the base of neurodegeneration and neurorepair [19,20]. Numerous in vitro approaches have been carried out to mimic human neuronal features, based on neuronal-like cells such as the neuroblastoma line SH-SY5Y. SH-SY5Y is a human cell line that divides quickly and has the ability to differentiate in post-mitotic neurons, thus it is considered a convenient model to study Parkinson's [21] and Alzheimer's diseases [22]. Unlike traditional two-dimensional (2D) cultures, the different availability of oxygen and growth factors in a 3D cell culture should expectantly favor a more in vivo-like morphology and growth of these cells. Indeed, several 3D culture models have been developed with SH-SY5Y cells, in terms of cell aggregates [23], spheroids [24,25], or including different scaffolds [26–28]. To support 3D cultures of SH-SY5Y or neuronal cell lines, collagen has also been used, like collagen hydrogel [29] or porous collagen-based scaffolds [26,30]. To the best of our knowledge, none of the previous models has been used to investigate the ability of natural bioactive molecules to confer resistance to oxidative stress. The aim of this study was to evaluate the neuroprotective effect of a combination of SF, EGCG, and PB in preventing cell damage derived from oxidative stress in a 3D cell culture based on a collagen porous scaffold.

2. Materials and Methods

2.1. Cell Culture and Treatment

The SH-SY5Y human neuroblastoma cell line was obtained from Sigma-Aldrich (cat. n° 94030304) (St. Louis, MO, USA). Cells were expanded in a growth culture medium composed of high glucose Dulbecco's Modified Eagle's medium (DMEM), supplemented with 10% fetal bovine serum (FBS), 2 mM glutamine, 50 U/mL of penicillin, and 50 µg/mL of streptomycin, and cultured at 37 °C with 5% CO_2 as previously reported [31]. Cell differentiation was induced by reducing serum levels of the medium to 1% with 10 µM retinoic acid (RA) for seven days prior to treatments [32]. SF (LKT

Laboratories, Minneapolis, MN, USA), EGCG and PB (Sigma-Aldrich, St. Louis, MO, USA) were dissolved in DMSO, and 10 mM stocks were kept at −20 °C until use. Differentiated SH-SY5Y cells were treated with 1 µM SF, 2.5 µM EGCG, and 0.5 µM PB and SEP (1 µM SF + 2.5 µM EGCG + 0.5 µM PB,) for 24 h or 6 h according to the different experiments. Oxidative stress was induced, as previously reported [33], by exposing cells to 700 µM H_2O_2 in 1% FBS DMEM.

2.2. 3D Model Preparation

To obtain the scaffolds for 3D cultures of SH-SY5Y cells, sterile heterologous native lyophilized collagen type I sponge (BIOPAD™, Angelini Pharma Inc., Gaithersburg, USA) was cut using a sterile scalpel into pieces with squared dimensions able to fit 96-multiwell culture plates. Each piece was divided by subjecting it to a second longitudinal cut, performed in order to present a similar top surface as the cells. The pieces with approximately 1 cm^2 of surface area were inserted into a 24-multiwell plate and constituted the scaffolds for the cell culture. To establish the 3D SH-SY5Y culture, 50 µL of cell suspension in DMEM with 10% FBS was seeded atop of each scaffold. Different cell numbers per scaffold (50×10^3–100×10^3–200×10^3) were seeded to compare cell viability along the culture (1–6 days) and optimize cell seeding for differentiation. To differentiate 3D SH-SY5Y culture, a concentration of 4×10^6 cells/mL equivalent to 200×10^3 cells in 50 uL was used. After 45 min of incubation at 37 °C, 5% CO_2, DMEM with 1% FBS, and 10 µM RA were added to the 3D culture in order to induce cell differentiation. The medium was changed every two days.

2.3. MTT Assay

Before adding 3-(4,5-Dimethylthiazol-2-yl)-2,5-diphenyl-tetrazolium bromide (MTT), 3D cultures were transferred to clean cell culture wells. MTT 0.5 mg/mL was prepared in a cell medium and added to the 3D cultures. To measure the percentage of cells that did not attach to the scaffold, MTT was also added to the wells where cells were initially seeded (Figure S1). The MTT solution was incubated for 2 h at 37 °C, 5% CO_2. After removing the MTT solution, DMSO was added and the absorbance of formazan was measured at 595 nm using a microplate spectrophotometer VICTOR3 V Multilabel plate-reader (PerkinElmer, Wellesley USA). The sum of the two respective absorbance values, the first deriving from the primary wells used during the seeding and the second deriving from the scaffolds, were considered as 100%.

2.4. Prestoblue Assay

A Prestoblue® working solution was prepared in a growth culture medium without phenol red according to the manufacturer's instructions. Briefly, the culture medium was removed from cell culture wells and a Prestoblue working solution was added and incubated at 37 °C, 5% CO_2. After 3 h, the well volumes were collected in a new 96-well plate and the absorbance was read at λ = 570 nm (experimental) and λ = 600 nm (reference wavelength for normalization) using a Victor Multilabel plate-reader (Perkin-Elmer, Wellesley USA).

2.5. Reduced Glutathione (GSH) Level Measurement

A monochlorobimane (MCB) fluorescent probe (Sigma-Aldrich, St. Louis, MO, USA) was used to determine relative intracellular GSH levels as previously reported [34] with some modifications. After 24 h of treatment, the cell culture medium was removed from 3D samples and the scaffolds were transferred to 1.5 mL tubes. The cells were incubated for 15 min in DMEM with 1% FBS containing 50 µM MCB, and for a further 15 min in DMEM with 0.5 mg/mL collagenase I and 50 µM MCB (Sigma-Aldrich). Cells collected by digestion of the scaffold were centrifuged at 250× g. Cells were resuspended in phosphate-buffered saline (PBS) and plated on black 96-well plates. The fluorescence was measured at 355 nm (excitation) and 460 nm (emission) using a Victor Multilabel plate-reader (Perkin-Elmer, Wellesley USA). GSH levels were normalized on the base of the Crystal Violet (CV) assay.

2.6. Crystal Violet Assay

Crystal Violet (CV) staining was performed as follows: Cells were fixed in 50% MeOH-PBS for 3 h at 4 °C. For 15 min at room temperature, a 0.1% (m/v) CV, 5% MeOH staining solution was incubated. The staining solution was removed and the stained cells were washed with distilled water. The plate was left to dry for 5 min under a chemical hood. The bound dye was eluted with MeOH 100% for 30 min at 4 °C. The optical density of each well was measured at 570 nm using a Victor Multilabel plate-reader (Perkin-Elmer, Wellesley USA).

2.7. RNA Extraction and Real-Time PCR

Prior to RNA extraction, cell retrieval was performed by digesting the collagen scaffold in collagenase solution. Collagenase type I (Sigma-Aldrich) was dissolved in DMEM without FBS at a concentration of 0.5 mg/mL. Samples were incubated in collagenase solution for 10 min at 37 °C. Cells suspension was pelleted, and RNA was extracted with an RNeasy® mini kit (Qiagen) following the manufacturer's instruction. A total of 500 ng of RNA was used to obtain cDNA using an iScript™ cDNA Synthesis Kit (BioRad). Real-time PCR was performed using SsoAdvanced Universal SYBR Green Supermix (BioRad), and normalized expression levels were calculated relative to control cells according to the $2-\Delta\Delta CT$ method. Primers were purchased from Sigma-Aldrich. The sequences are listed in Table 1.

Table 1. Primer sequences.

Gene	Sequence	RefSeq Accession n.
RPS18 *	Fw CAGAAGGATGTAAAGGATGG Rv TATTTCTTCTTGGACACACC	NM_022551
MAP2	Fw GAAGATTTACTTACAGCCTCG Rv GGTAAGTTTTAGTTGTCTCTGG	NM_002374
BDNF	Fw CAAAAGTGGAGAACATTTGC Rv AACTCCAGTCAATAGGTCAG	NM_001143811
HMOX1(HO1)	Fw CAACAAAGTGCAAGATTCTG Rv TGCATTCACATGGCATAAAG	NM_002133.2
IDE	Fw CAACCTGAAGTGATTCAGAAC Rv AATATGTGGTTTCACAAGGG	NM_001165946
NOX1	Fw CCGGTCATTCTTTATATCTGTG Rv CAACCTTGGTAATCACAACC	NM_007052
NOX2	Fw AAGATCTACTTCTACTGGCTG Rv AGATGTTGTAGCTGAGGAAG	NM_000397
NQO1	Fw AGTATCCACAATAGCTGACG Rv TTTGTGGGTCTGTAGAAATG	NM_000903
GSR (GR)	Fw GACCTATTCAACGAGCTTTAC Rv CAACCACCTTTTCTTCCTTG	NM_000637
TXNRD1 (TR)	Fw AGACAGTTAAGCATGATTGG Rv AATTGCCCATAAGCATTCTC	NM_001093771

* reference gene.

3. Results

3.1. Development and Characterization of the 3D SH-SY5Y Culture System

To fully assess biocompatibility between the collagen scaffold and SH-SY5Y cells, we evaluated cellular retention to the scaffold and cellular metabolism during 3D culture. The ability of SH-SY5Y cells to attach to the scaffold was evaluated by an MTT viability assay (Figure 2a). This assay was chosen because cells convert MTT to blue formazan that is retained by the cells and, for this reason, it makes it possible to distinguish cells attached to the scaffold from those released from the scaffold (see Figure S1). As reported in Figure 2a, about 95% of the total viable cells were able to attach after the switch from 2D to 3D culture conditions, while only 5% of the cells grew outside of the scaffold.

To check the proliferation of SH-SY5Y cells, we used a Prestoblue assay as it makes it possible to monitor the metabolic activity of the same cell culture over time (Figure 2b). Cells were seeded at different concentrations, and cell viability was evaluated after 1 and 6 days. As expected, cell viability increased with an increasing numbers of cells per scaffold at both time points. Interestingly, the metabolic activity of the 3D culture after 6 days was comparable to that measured after 1 day at all tested seeding densities. Because the scaffold did not allow us to observe the cells under a microscope during growth, to verify that RA-treated SH-SY5Y cells were able to differentiate, we evaluated the mRNA level of the mature neural protein marker MAP2 as well as the secretable neurotrophin BDNF in 3D RA-treated cells (Figure 2c). Interestingly, both markers were upregulated in 3D RA-treated cells in respect to the 3D RA-untreated control, showing their ability to differentiate under 3D culture conditions. Figure S4 reports the macroscopic and microscopic appearance of the 3D SH-SY5Y culture.

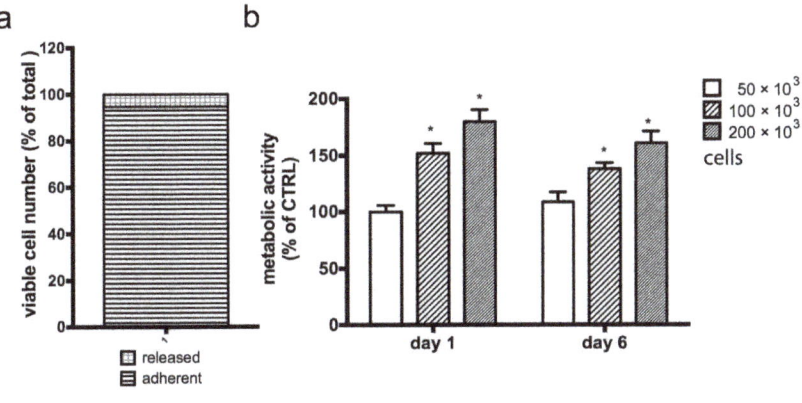

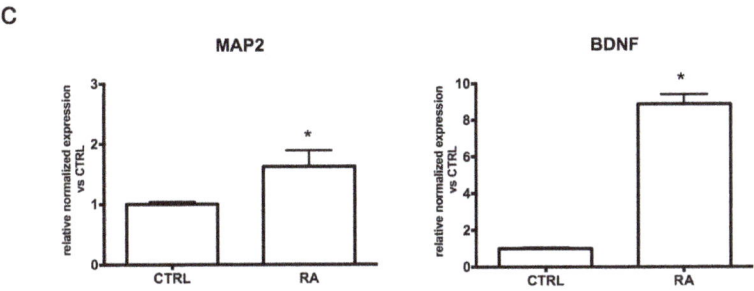

Figure 2. Characterization of the 3D SH-SY5Y model. (**a**) Cellular adhesion to the scaffold was evaluated 24 h after cell seeding by MTT assay as reported in Materials and Methods. Data are expressed as a percentage of total viable cells and represent the mean of three independent experiments. (**b**) Metabolic activity of the 3D model was evaluated after 1 and 6 days from cell seeding by a Prestoblue assay as reported in Materials and Methods. Each bar represents the mean ± SEM of three independent experiments. Data were analyzed with a two-way ANOVA followed by the Fisher's test. * $p < 0.05$. (**c**) Real time-PCR was performed in the 3D culture for neuronal markers. Each bar represents the mean ± SEM of three independent experiments, which were analyzed with an unpaired T-test. * $p < 0.05$.

3.2. SF, EGCG and PB Protect 3D SH-SY5Y Cells from Oxidative-Induced Injury

Before studying the neuroprotective effect of SF, EGCG, and PB, we exposed 3D differentiated SH-SY5Y cells to 1 µM SF, 2.5 µM EGCG, 0.5 µM PB, or to a combination of the three compounds at the same concentrations (SEP) (Figure 3). These concentrations were chosen according to previous reports where these concentrations were not very effective against oxidative stress [15–17]. Our results showed that all the tested concentrations—1 µM SF, 2.5 µM EGCG, and 0.5 µM PB—were not toxic.

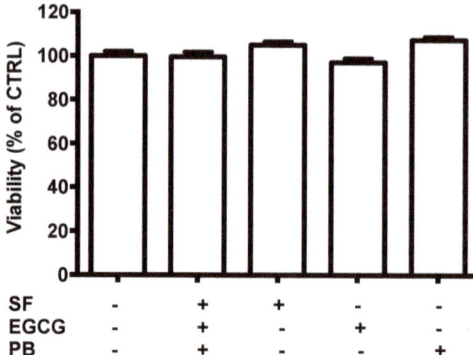

Figure 3. Potential cytotoxicity of sulforaphane (SF), epigallocatechin gallate (EGCG), and plumbagin (PB) on SH-SY5Y cells. Cells were treated with 1 µM SF, 2.5, µM EGCG, and 0.5 µM PB, and after 24 h, viability was evaluated by a Prestoblue assay as reported in Materials and Methods. Results are expressed as a percentage of untreated cells. Each bar represents the mean ± SEM of three independent experiments, which were analyzed with a one-way ANOVA followed by the Fisher's test.

We then investigated the potential protective effect of the single treatments or a combination of them against H_2O_2-induced oxidative stress (Figure 4). As expected, incubation with 700 µM H_2O_2 for 2 h induced a significant reduction of cell viability compared to the control cells (Figure S2). Only 0.5 µM PB, 1 µM SF, and the co-treatment (1 µM SF, 2.5 µM EGCG, and 0.5 µM PB) were able to protect the cells against H_2O_2-induced damage. Of note, SEP co-treatment was the most effective treatment as it significantly increased cell viability compared to the other treatments.

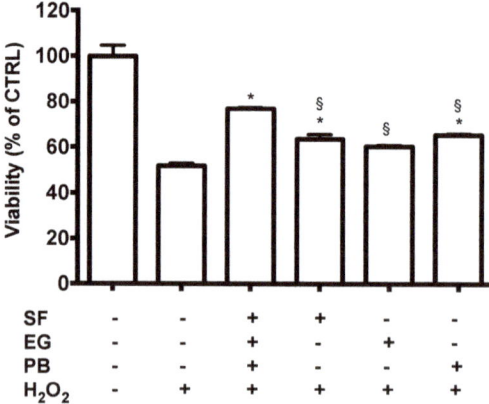

Figure 4. Neuroprotective activity of SF, EGCG, and PB compounds against H_2O_2-induced damage. Cells were treated with 1 µM SF, 2.5 µM EGCG, and 0.5 µM PB, and after 24 h, were exposed to 700 µM H_2O_2 to induce oxidative stress. Cell viability in 3D cultures was measured by a Prestoblue assay as reported in Materials and Methods. Data are expressed as a percentage of untreated cells. Each bar represents mean ± SEM of three independent experiments. Data were analyzed with a one-way ANOVA followed by the Fisher's test. * $p < 0.05$ vs. H_2O_2 treated cells; § $p < 0.05$ vs. sulforaphane, epigallocatechin gallate, and plumbagin (SEP) co-treatment.

3.3. SEP Co-Treatment Enhances Antioxidant Defenses

As our results showed a higher neuroprotective activity of SEP co-treatment (1 µM SF, 2.5 µM EGCG, and 0.5 µM PB) compared to the single treatments of 1 µM SF, 2.5, µM EGCG, or 0.5 µM PB, we investigated the ability of SEP co-treatment to modulate the cellular redox state by evaluating GSH levels with an MCB assay. The effect of the different treatments after 24 h on GSH levels is reported in Figure 5. All the treatments were able to significantly increase GSH levels in respect to control cells. In agreement with the viability data, we observed the most effective increase of GSH levels after SEP co-treatment (1 µM SF, 2.5 µM EGCG, and 0.5 µM PB) in comparison to the single treatment of 1 µM SF, 2.5 µM EGCG, or 0.5 µM PB.

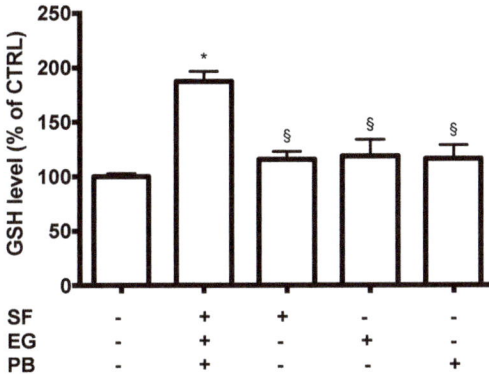

Figure 5. Antioxidant activity of SF, EGCG, and PB compounds on SH-SY5Y cells. Cells were treated with 1 µM SF, 2.5 µM EGCG, and 0.5 µM PB, and after 24 h GSH levels were evaluated with an monochlorobimane (MCB) assay as reported in Materials and Methods. Data are expressed as a percentage of untreated cells (CTRL). Each bar represents mean ± SEM of three independent experiments. Data were analyzed with a one-way ANOVA followed by the Fisher's test. * $p < 0.05$ vs. untreated cells; § $p < 0.05$ vs. SEP co-treatment.

3.4. SEP Co-Treatment Modulates Genes Involved in Oxidative Stress Control

As the previous data showed that SEP co-treatment was significantly more effective compared to the single treatments, we decided to study its ability to modulate cellular antioxidant status. Real-time PCR analysis was employed to investigate the ability of SEP co-treatment to modulate the mRNA level of different antioxidant enzymes. The cDNA was obtained from 3D SH-SY5Y cultures that were co-treated (1 µM SF, 2.5 µM EGCG, and 0.5 µM PB) for 6 h. The 3D cultures were then exposed to 700 µM H_2O_2 for 1 h prior to lysis (Figure 6). Importantly, SEP co-treatment induced a significant and marked upregulation of heme oxygenase 1 (HO1), NADPH: quinone oxidoreductase 1 (NQO1), glutathione reductase (GR), and thioredoxin reductase (TR) in 3D cultures although with different levels of upregulation (Figure 6). Moreover, SEP co-treatment in the presence of oxidative stress induced a significant upregulation of all tested genes in respect to H_2O_2-treated cells.

NADPH oxidase (NOX) enzymes have been shown to be a major source of ROS in the brain and to be involved in several neurological diseases [35]. On this basis, we studied the modulatory effect of SEP co-treatment on NOX1 and NOX2 expression using real-time PCR analysis (Figure 7). In the absence of oxidative stress, SEP co-treatment had a strong effect on these enzymes as it significantly reduced NOX1 and NOX2 expression compared to untreated cells. In the presence of oxidative stress (700 µM H_2O_2), SEP co-treatment significantly reduced NOX1 and NOX2 expression compared to H_2O_2-treated cells. Of note, SEP co-treatment before peroxide exposure maintained NOX1 levels at a value comparable to control cells.

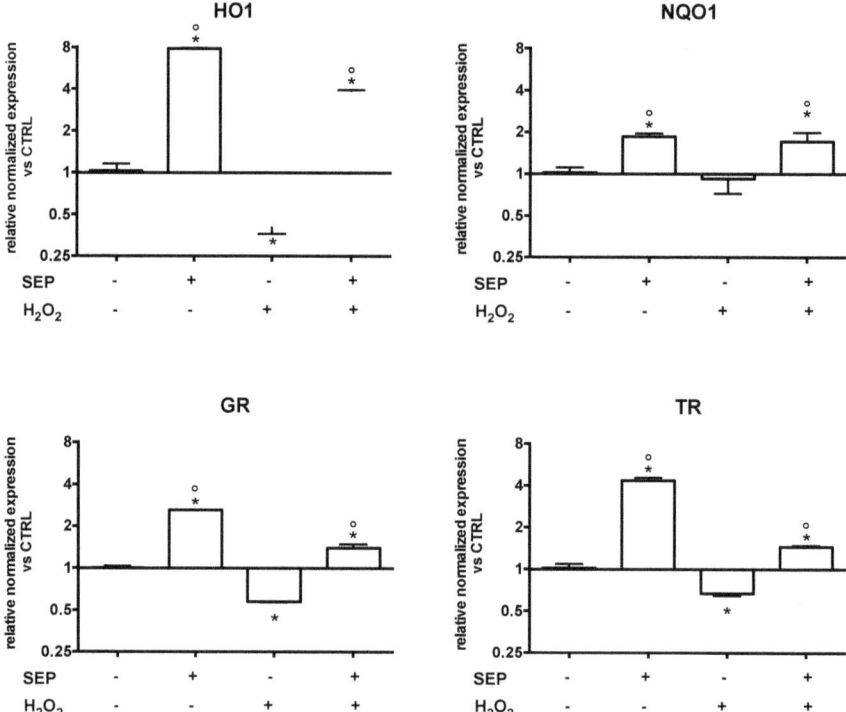

Figure 6. Effect of SEP co-treatment on antioxidant enzyme expression. Cells were co-treated with 1 µM SF, 2.5 µM EGCG, and 0.5 µM PB for 6 h. Oxidative stress was induced with 700 µM H_2O_2 for 1 h prior to lysis. Real time-PCR was performed to detect heme oxygenase 1 (HO1), NADPH: quinone oxidoreductase 1 (NQO1), glutathione reductase (GR), and thioredoxin reductase (TR) mRNA levels. Data are expressed as relative abundance compared to untreated cells. Each bar represents mean ± SEM of three independent experiments. Data were analyzed with a one-way ANOVA followed by the Fisher's test. * $p < 0.05$ vs. untreated cells, ° $p < 0.05$ vs. H_2O_2.

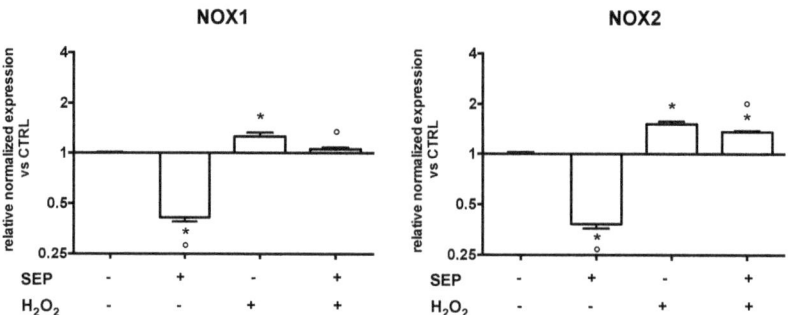

Figure 7. Effect of SEP co-treatment on NADPH oxidase 1 (NOX1) and NADPH oxidase 2 (NOX2). Cells were co-treated with 1 µM SF, 2.5 µM EGCG, and 0.5 µM PB for 6 h. Oxidative stress was induced with 700 µM H_2O_2 for 1 h prior to lysis. Real time-PCR was performed to detect NOX1 and NOX2 mRNA levels. Data are expressed as relative abundance compared to untreated cells. Each bar represents mean ± SEM of three independent experiments. Data were analyzed using a one-way ANOVA followed by the Fisher's test. * $p < 0.05$ vs. untreated cells, ° $p < 0.05$ vs. H_2O_2.

3.5. SEP Co-Treatment is able to Modulate Insulin-Degrading Enzyme (IDE) Gene Expression

To investigate if SEP co-treatment had other neuroprotective activities besides the antioxidant one, we studied its effect on insulin-degrading enzyme (IDE) expression. IDE plays a significant role in Aβ degradation [36], which is one of the main hallmarks of Alzheimer's disease. Moreover, recent studies have demonstrated that increasing Aβ degradation as opposed to inhibiting synthesis is a more effective strategy for preventing Aβ build-up [37]. In our 3D SH-SY5Y cultures, IDE mRNA levels were downregulated by oxidative stress, but, interestingly, SEP co-treatment (1 μM SF, 2.5 μM EGCG, and 0.5 μM PB) was able to upregulate its expression at levels comparable to untreated cells (Figure 8).

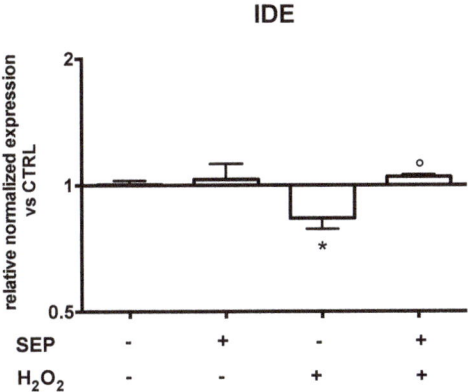

Figure 8. Effect of SEP co-treatment on insulin-degrading enzyme (IDE). Cells were co-treated with 1 μM SF, 2.5 μM EGCG, and 0.5 μM PB for 6 h. Oxidative stress was induced with 700 μM H_2O_2 for 1 h prior to lysis. Real time-PCR was performed to detect IDE mRNA levels. Data are expressed as relative abundance compared to untreated cells. Each bar represents mean ± SEM of three independent experiments. Data were analyzed with a one-way ANOVA followed by the Fisher's test. * $p < 0.05$ vs. untreated cells, ° $p < 0.05$ vs. H_2O_2.

4. Discussion

The prevalence of neurodegenerative disorders is growing [2,38] in parallel to the urgency to find new compounds for the treatment of such diseases, in which oxidative stress is a common hallmark and has been suggested to play a causative role [39,40]. Unfortunately, the screening of drug leads and natural compounds to counteract neurodegeneration using 2D cell cultures often results in the unsuccessful translation of data to clinics. Neurons are strongly influenced by their immediate extracellular environment, and there is a great need to develop new culture systems that more faithfully reproduce the complexity of this milieu in vivo. Human 3D cell culture models are a good alternative to animal models [41,42]. In contrast to 2D cell cultures, 3D cell cultures do not overlook the physical interactions existing between cell–cell and cell–matrix and have a higher resemblance to the in vivo phenotype. Ideal scaffolds for neuronal tissue or disease modelling should exhibit suitable 3D architecture for in vitro manipulation, should facilitate cell adhesion while promoting neurites outgrowth, and have high biocompatibility [43]. Collagen type I is highly used as scaffold because of its abundance and ubiquity in most of the hard and soft tissues in the human body [44]. Porous collagen sponges have been used to grow various cell types in vitro [45] and collagen derived scaffolds have been widely used in neural tissue engineering for drug delivery [46]. Furthermore, the extracellular matrix (ECM) in nerves is mainly composed of type I collagen [47] and is a commonly used material in nerve tissue engineering [47] and for peripheral nerve regeneration [48]. ECM geometry and composition are well known to influence cell morphology and gene expression. It has been shown that SH-SY5Y cells extended longer neurites in 3D collagen I hydrogel cultures than in 2D cultures [26]. On this basis, we used equine native collagen, commercially available for clinical application, as scaffold to support 3D cultures of differentiated SH-SY5Y cells.

Our aim was to study the neuroprotective activity of a combination of SF, EGCG, and PB in counteracting peroxide-induced damage in 3D cultures of differentiated SH-SY5Y cells.

Taking into account previous studies showing the protective effects of these compounds against oxidative stress [49,50], we decided to treat SH-SY5Y cells with specific concentrations of SF, EGCG, and PB to better mimic concentrations that could be measured in plasma after oral intake of the three compounds [51]. We selected a porous instead of a hydrogel scaffold because it easily permits the removal of apoptotic blebs and dead cells by washing during medium exchange. The used collagenous scaffold was found to be highly biocompatible since it supported the adhesion and proliferation of SH-SY5Y cells in the 3D environment.

Our data demonstrated that SEP co-treatment was significantly more effective against oxidative stress than the single treatments of PB, EGCG, or SF, suggesting a synergistic protective mechanism of the co-treatment. In particular, SEP was more effective in limiting cell injury induced by H_2O_2 exposure. These data were also demonstrated in our 2D cell model, and we confirmed the superior efficacy in enhancing GSH levels by SEP co-treatment compared the single treatments both in 2D and 3D models (Figure S3). Although different reports have discussed the neuroprotective effect of PB, EGCG, and SF against brain-induced toxicity [52–54], there is no documented work on the effect of their combination. Our results are in agreement with other papers demonstrating the synergistic protective effect of different combinations of natural compounds against neurodegeneration [55–57]. In general, the superior protection of co-treatments compared to the single treatments could be probably ascribed to the concurrent modulation of different molecular targets involved in the pathogenesis and progression of these multi-factorial diseases.

To better elucidate the mechanisms behind SEP protection against H_2O_2 in SH-SY5Y cells, we investigated the effect of the co-treatment on the expression of different antioxidant enzymes: heme oxygenase 1 (HO1), NADPH: quinone oxidoreductase 1 (NQO1), glutathione reductase (GR) and thioredoxin reductase (TR).

The enzyme HO1 converts heme to three end products, namely biliverdin, CO, and ferrous ion [58], then biliverdin reductase activity produces the antioxidant bilirubin. NQO1 is a highly inducible detoxifying flavoenzyme. It catalyzes the reduction of quinones generating stable hydroquinones and possesses superoxide scavenging activity [59]. GR is responsible for maintaining a storage amount of reduced glutathione [60]. The thioredoxin (Trx) system, composed of Trx, TR, and NADPH as a cofactor, is a cellular defense system that is ubiquitously involved in converting ROS to nontoxic metabolites [61]. In such a system, the Trx in reduced status can be oxidized into oxidized Trx during the degradation of H_2O_2 and then reduced by TR [62].

SF is known to upregulate antioxidant defense through the induction of HO1, NQO1, and GR in SH-SY5Y cells [15,63], while GR, TR, and NQO1 have been observed to be upregulated in cortical neurons [64]. EGCG induced HO1 expression in rat-cultured neurons [65] and increased protein levels in treated rats following focal cerebral ischemia [66]. PB treatment led to increased levels of HO1, NQO1, and TR in SH-SY5Y cells [17]. Interestingly, our data showed that SEP co-treatment, in the absence of oxidative stress, strongly upregulated these enzymes compared to control cells (the same results were also obtained in the 2D model (Figure S3)), and, in the presence of oxidative stress, it was able to significantly increase the expression of these enzymes compared to H_2O_2 exposed cells. In agreement with our data that showed the enhanced effect of a combination of different compounds compared to treatment with the single compounds, in a previous work, we observed that a combination of EGCG and SF counteracts in vitro oxidative stress and delays stemness loss of amniotic fluid stem cells [67]. Moreover, a combination of berberine with resveratrol had enhanced hypolipidemic effects in high fat diet-induced mice and was able to decrease the lipid accumulation in adipocytes to a level significantly lower than that of the treatment with the single compounds [68].

Recently, it has been suggested that inhibition of the generation, rather than the scavenging, of ROS may be a more successful strategy to counteract oxidative stress-induced neurodegeneration [69]. ROS can be produced by many enzymes in the cells such as mitochondria respiratory complexes, NADPH oxidase, nitric oxide synthase, cytochrome 450, cyclooxygenase, lipoxygenase, and xanthine oxidase [14,70]. Interestingly, all these enzymes except NADPH oxidase produce ROS as a byproduct, while NOX enzymes generate ROS as a principal aim [71–73]. Moreover, different studies have shown the involvement of NADPH oxidase family members in brain injury and neurodegenerative disorders (reviewed in [69]). Our data demonstrated that SEP co-treatment was effective in reducing NOX1 and NOX2 expression compared to control cells and was also able to counteract the increase of NOX1 and NOX2 expression induced by H_2O_2. This means that SEP not only potentiates the antioxidant defense system upregulating fundamental enzymes, but also reduces the intracellular production of ROS.

The last aim of this paper was to investigate if SEP could modulate other hallmarks of neurodegeneration in addition to its ability to counteract oxidative stress. We decided to focus our attention on IDE, the main protease responsible for amyloid β clearance [74–76]. A reduction of IDE activity in the brain with age and during the early stages of Alzheimer's disease (AD) has been observed [74], suggesting that IDE downregulation may be among the triggers of AD. Of note, SEP counteracted the strong downregulation of IDE induced by oxidative stress, maintaining IDE expression at a level comparable to control cells, suggesting a potential role of SEP in counteracting AD.

In conclusion, we highlighted that an appropriate synergistic combination of natural antioxidants such as SF, EGCG, and PB can help to rescue neuronal cells from oxidative stress cell death. The protective effect of the co-treatment was observed in a novel 3D model of SH-SY5Y cells that we developed. In agreement with other authors [77–79], we suggest that a 3D culture system better mimics cell–cell interactions and cell–ECM interactions compared to the traditional 2D monolayer. In particular, our 3D model would be useful for future investigations of the neuroprotective activity of natural compounds [80]. In the present study, we observed the protective effect of an "acute" co-treatment with SF, EGCG, and PB but, taking into account the nature of neurodegeneration, a subchronic/chronic administration should be even more effective. For this reason, future studies will have to be carried out to investigate the effect of chronic SEP treatment against oxidative stress in neurodegeneration. The present findings underscore the importance of a combinatorial approach for effective treatments against oxidative damage in neurodegeneration. Moreover, 3D SH-SY5Y cell culture systems appear to be the ideal environment for in vitro assays regarding the effects of phytochemicals on cell viability.

Supplementary Materials: The following are available online at http://www.mdpi.com/2076-3921/8/10/420/s1. Figure S1: Visual explanation of MTT assay as used in this study, Figure S2: Cell viability of SH-SY5Y incubated with H_2O_2, Figure S3: Results obtained with SEP co-treatement in SH-SY5Y 2D model. Figure S4: Images of SH-SY5Y 3D model.

Author Contributions: Conceptualization, P.M. and C.A.; methodology, P.M. and C.A.; data curation, P.M. and C.A.; writing—original draft preparation, P.M.; writing—review and editing, C.A. and S.H.; funding acquisition, S.H.

Funding: This work was supported by MIUR-PRIN 2015 (N. 20152HKF3Z) to S.H.

Conflicts of Interest: The authors declare that there is no conflict of interest regarding the publication of this paper.

Abbreviations

2D	Two-dimensional
3D	Three-dimensional
BDNF	Brain-derived neurotrophic factor
DCFH-DA	2,7-dichlorodihydrofluorescein diacetate
DMEM	Dulbecco's Modified Eagle's medium
DMSO	Dimethyl sulfoxide
ECM	Extra cellular matrix
EGCG	Epigallocatechin gallate
GR	Glutathione reductase

GSH	Reduced glutathione
H_2O_2	Hydrogen peroxide
HO1	Heme oxygenase 1
IDE	Insulin-degrading enzyme
MAP2	Microtubule-associated protein 2
MCB	Monochlorobimane
MTT	3-(4,5-dimethylthiazol-2-yl)-2,5-diphenyl-tetrazolium bromide)
NOX1	NADPH oxidase 1
NOX2	NADPH oxidase 2
NQO1	NAD(P)H: quinone oxidoreductase 1
PB	Plumbagin
PBS	Phosphate buffered saline
PCR	Polymerase chain reaction
RA	All-trans retinoic acid
ROS	Reactive oxygen species
RPS18	Ribosomal protein S18
SEP	Sulforaphane, Epigallocatechin gallate, Plumbagin
SF	Sulforaphane
TR	Thioredoxin reductase 1

References

1. Barnham, K.J.; Masters, C.L.; Bush, A.I. Neurodegenerative diseases and oxidative stress. *Nat. Rev. Drug Discov.* **2004**, *3*, 205–214. [CrossRef]
2. Gammon, K. Neurodegenerative disease: Brain windfall. *Nature* **2014**, *515*, 299–300. [CrossRef] [PubMed]
3. Tarozzi, A.; Angeloni, C.; Malaguti, M.; Morroni, F.; Hrelia, S.; Hrelia, P. Sulforaphane as a Potential Protective Phytochemical against Neurodegenerative Diseases. *Oxid. Med. Cell. Longev.* **2013**, *2013*, 415078. [CrossRef] [PubMed]
4. Angeloni, C.; Malaguti, M.; Hrelia, S. Antiglycative activity of sulforaphane: A new avenue to counteract neurodegeneration? *Neural Regen. Res.* **2015**, *10*, 1750. [CrossRef] [PubMed]
5. Lenzi, M.; Fimognari, C.; Hrelia, P. Sulforaphane as a Promising Molecule for Fighting Cancer. In *Advances in Nutrition and Cancer*; Cancer Treatment and Research; Springer: Berlin/Heidelberg, Germany, 2014; Volume 159, pp. 207–223.
6. Bordoni, A.; Hrelia, S.; Angeloni, C.; Giordano, E.; Guarnieri, C.; Caldarera, C.M.; Biagi, P.L. Green tea protection of hypoxia/reoxygenation injury in cultured cardiac cells. *J. Nutr. Biochem.* **2002**, *13*, 103–111. [CrossRef]
7. Singh, B.N.; Shankar, S.; Srivastava, R.K. Green tea catechin, epigallocatechin-3-gallate (EGCG): Mechanisms, perspectives and clinical applications. *Biochem. Pharmacol.* **2011**, *82*, 1807–1821. [CrossRef] [PubMed]
8. Singh, N.A.; Mandal, A.K.A.; Khan, Z.A. Potential neuroprotective properties of epigallocatechin-3-gallate (EGCG). *Nutr. J.* **2016**, *15*, 60. [CrossRef]
9. Chen, X.-J.; Zhang, J.-G.; Wu, L. Plumbagin inhibits neuronal apoptosis, intimal hyperplasia and also suppresses TNF-α/NF-κB pathway induced inflammation and matrix metalloproteinase-2/9 expression in rat cerebral ischemia. *Saudi J. Biol. Sci.* **2017**, *25*, 1033–1039. [CrossRef]
10. Yuan, J.-H.; Pan, F.; Chen, J.; Chen, C.-E.; Xie, D.-P.; Jiang, X.-Z.; Guo, S.-J.; Zhou, J. Neuroprotection by plumbagin involves BDNF-TrkB-PI3K/Akt and ERK1/2/JNK pathways in isoflurane-induced neonatal rats. *J. Pharm. Pharmacol.* **2017**, *69*, 896–906. [CrossRef]
11. Luo, P.; Wong, Y.F.; Ge, L.; Zhang, Z.F.; Liu, Y.; Liu, L.; Zhou, H. Anti-inflammatory and analgesic effect of plumbagin through inhibition of nuclear factor-κB activation. *J. Pharmacol. Exp. Ther.* **2010**, *335*, 735–742. [CrossRef]
12. Padhye, S.; Dandawate, P.; Yusufi, M.; Ahmad, A.; Sarkar, F.H. Perspectives on medicinal properties of plumbagin and its analogs. *Med. Res. Rev.* **2012**, *32*, 1131–1158. [CrossRef] [PubMed]
13. Arruri, V.; Komirishetty, P.; Areti, A.; Dungavath, S.K.N.; Kumar, A. Nrf2 and NF-κB modulation by Plumbagin attenuates functional, behavioural and biochemical deficits in rat model of neuropathic pain. *Pharmacol. Rep.* **2017**, *69*, 625–632. [CrossRef] [PubMed]

14. Maraldi, T. Natural compounds as modulators of NADPH oxidases. *Oxid. Med. Cell. Longev.* **2013**, *2013*, 271602. [CrossRef] [PubMed]
15. Tarozzi, A.; Morroni, F.; Merlicco, A.; Hrelia, S.; Angeloni, C.; Cantelli-Forti, G.; Hrelia, P. Sulforaphane as an inducer of glutathione prevents oxidative stress-induced cell death in a dopaminergic-like neuroblastoma cell line. *J. Neurochem.* **2009**, *111*, 1161–1171. [CrossRef] [PubMed]
16. Jeong, J.H.; Kim, H.J.; Lee, T.J.; Kim, M.K.; Park, E.S.; Choi, B.S. Epigallocatechin 3-gallate attenuates neuronal damage induced by 3-hydroxykynurenine. *Toxicology* **2004**, *195*, 53–60. [CrossRef] [PubMed]
17. Son, T.G.; Camandola, S.; Arumugam, T.V.; Cutler, R.G.; Telljohann, R.S.; Mughal, M.R.; Moore, T.A.; Luo, W.; Yu, Q.-S.; Johnson, D.A.; et al. Plumbagin, a novel Nrf2/ARE activator, protects against cerebral ischemia. *J. Neurochem.* **2010**, *112*, 1316–1326. [CrossRef] [PubMed]
18. Holmes, A.M.; Charlton, A.; Derby, B.; Ewart, L.; Scott, A.; Shu, W. Rising to the challenge: Applying biofabrication approaches for better drug and chemical product development. *Biofabrication* **2017**, *9*, 033001. [CrossRef] [PubMed]
19. Papadimitriou, C.; Celikkaya, H.; Cosacak, M.I.; Mashkaryan, V.; Bray, L.; Bhattarai, P.; Brandt, K.; Hollak, H.; Chen, X.; He, S.; et al. 3D Culture Method for Alzheimer's Disease Modeling Reveals Interleukin-4 Rescues Aβ42-Induced Loss of Human Neural Stem Cell Plasticity. *Dev. Cell* **2018**, *46*, 85–101. [CrossRef]
20. Zhang, D.; Pekkanen-Mattila, M.; Shahsavani, M.; Falk, A.; Teixeira, A.I.; Herland, A. A 3D Alzheimer's disease culture model and the induction of P21-activated kinase mediated sensing in iPSC derived neurons. *Biomaterials* **2014**, *35*, 1420–1428. [CrossRef]
21. Xicoy, H.; Wieringa, B.; Martens, G.J.M. The SH-SY5Y cell line in Parkinson's disease research: A systematic review. *Mol. Neurodegener.* **2017**, *12*, 10. [CrossRef]
22. Lázaro, D.F.; Angeliki, M.; Pavlou, S.; Outeiro, T.F. Cellular models as tools for the study of the role of alpha-synuclein in Parkinson's disease. *Exp. Neurol.* **2017**, *298*, 162–171. [CrossRef] [PubMed]
23. Morabito, C.; Steimberg, N.; Mazzoleni, G.; Guarnieri, S.; Fanò-Illic, G.; Mariggiò, M.A.; Mariggi, M.A. RCCS Bioreactor-Based Modelled Microgravity Induces Significant Changes on In Vitro 3D Neuroglial Cell Cultures. *BioMed Res. Int.* **2015**, *2015*, 754283. [CrossRef] [PubMed]
24. Seidel, D.; Krinke, D.; Jahnke, H.G.; Hirche, A.; Kloß, D.; Mack, T.G.A.; Striggow, F.; Robitzki, A. Induced Tauopathy in a Novel 3D-Culture Model Mediates Neurodegenerative Processes: A Real-Time Study on Biochips. *PLoS ONE* **2012**, *7*, e49150. [CrossRef] [PubMed]
25. De Simone, U.; Roccio, M.; Gribaldo, L.; Spinillo, A.; Caloni, F.; Coccini, T. Human 3D Cultures as Models for Evaluating Magnetic Nanoparticle CNS Cytotoxicity after Short-and Repeated Long-Term Exposure. *Int. J. Mol. Sci.* **2018**, *19*, 1993. [CrossRef] [PubMed]
26. Li, G.N.; Livi, L.L.; Gourd, C.M.; Deweerd, E.S.; Hoffman-Kim, D. Genomic and Morphological Changes of Neuroblastoma Cells in Response to Three-Dimensional Matrices. *Tissue Eng.* **2007**, *13*, 1035–1047. [CrossRef] [PubMed]
27. Innala, M.; Riebe, I.; Kuzmenko, V.; Sundberg, J.; Gatenholm, P.; Hanse, E.; Johannesson, S. 3D Culturing and differentiation of SH-SY5Y neuroblastoma cells on bacterial nanocellulose scaffolds. *Artif. Cells Nanomed. Biotechnol.* **2014**, *42*, 302–308. [CrossRef] [PubMed]
28. Tunesi, M.; Fusco, F.; Fiordaliso, F.; Corbelli, A.; Biella, G.; Raimondi, M.T. Optimization of a 3D Dynamic Culturing System for In Vitro Modeling of Frontotemporal Neurodegeneration-Relevant Pathologic Features. *Front. Aging Neurosci.* **2016**, *8*, 146. [CrossRef] [PubMed]
29. Desai, A.; Kisaalita, W.S.; Keith, C.; Wu, Z.-Z. Human neuroblastoma (SH-SY5Y) cell culture and differentiation in 3-D collagen hydrogels for cell-based biosensing. *Biosens. Bioelectron.* **2006**, *21*, 1483–1492. [CrossRef] [PubMed]
30. Lv, D.; Yu, S.-C.; Ping, Y.-F.; Wu, H.; Zhao, X.; Zhang, H.; Cui, Y.; Chen, B.; Zhang, X.; Dai, J.; et al. A three-dimensional collagen scaffold cell culture system for screening anti-glioma therapeutics. *Oncotarget* **2016**, *7*, 56904–56914. [CrossRef] [PubMed]
31. Angeloni, C.; Teti, G.; Barbalace, M.C.; Malaguti, M.; Falconi, M.; Hrelia, S. 17β-Estradiol enhances sulforaphane cardioprotection against oxidative stress. *J. Nutr. Biochem.* **2017**, *42*, 26–36. [CrossRef] [PubMed]
32. Lopes, F.M.; Schroder, R.; da Frota Junior, M.L.C.; Zanotto-Filho, A.; Muller, C.B.; Pires, A.S.; Meurer, R.T.; Colpo, G.D.; Gelain, D.P.; Kapczinski, F.; et al. Comparison between proliferative and neuron-like SH-SY5Y cells as an in vitro model for Parkinson disease studies. *Brain Res.* **2010**, *1337*, 85–94. [CrossRef] [PubMed]

33. Giusti, L.; Angeloni, C.; Barbalace, M.; Lacerenza, S.; Ciregia, F.; Ronci, M.; Urbani, A.; Manera, C.; Digiacomo, M.; Macchia, M.; et al. A Proteomic Approach to Uncover Neuroprotective Mechanisms of Oleocanthal against Oxidative Stress. *Int. J. Mol. Sci.* **2018**, *19*, 2329. [CrossRef] [PubMed]
34. Angeloni, C.; Malaguti, M.; Rizzo, B.; Barbalace, M.C.; Fabbri, D.; Hrelia, S. Neuroprotective Effect of Sulforaphane against Methylglyoxal Cytotoxicity. *Chem. Res. Toxicol.* **2015**, *28*, 1234–1245. [CrossRef] [PubMed]
35. Angeloni, C.; Prata, C.; Vieceli Dalla Sega, F.; Piperno, R.; Hrelia, S. Traumatic Brain Injury and NADPH Oxidase: A Deep Relationship. *Oxid. Med. Cell. Longev.* **2015**, *2015*, 370312. [CrossRef] [PubMed]
36. Kurochkin, I.V.; Guarnera, E.; Berezovsky, I.N. Insulin-Degrading Enzyme in the Fight against Alzheimer's Disease. *Trends Pharmacol. Sci.* **2018**, *39*, 49–58. [CrossRef] [PubMed]
37. Sikanyika, N.L.; Parkington, H.C.; Smith, A.I.; Kuruppu, S. Powering Amyloid Beta Degrading Enzymes: A Possible Therapy for Alzheimer's Disease. *Neurochem. Res.* **2019**, *44*, 1289–1296. [CrossRef] [PubMed]
38. Heemels, M.-T. Neurodegenerative diseases. *Nature* **2016**, *539*, 179. [CrossRef] [PubMed]
39. Chen, X.; Guo, C.; Kong, J. Oxidative stress in neurodegenerative diseases. *Neural Regen. Res.* **2012**, *7*, 376–385. [CrossRef] [PubMed]
40. Uttara, B.; Singh, A.V.; Zamboni, P.; Mahajan, R.T. Oxidative stress and neurodegenerative diseases: A review of upstream and downstream antioxidant therapeutic options. *Curr. Neuropharmacol.* **2009**, *7*, 65–74. [CrossRef]
41. Mazzoleni, G.; Di Lorenzo, D.; Steimberg, N. Modelling tissues in 3D: The next future of pharmaco-toxicology and food research? *Genes Nutr.* **2009**, *4*, 13–22. [CrossRef]
42. Marrazzo, P.; Maccari, S.; Taddei, A.; Bevan, L.; Telford, J.; Soriani, M.; Pezzicoli, A. 3D Reconstruction of the Human Airway Mucosa In Vitro as an Experimental Model to Study NTHi Infections. *PLoS ONE* **2016**, *11*, e0153985. [CrossRef] [PubMed]
43. Brännvall, K.; Bergman, K.; Wallenquist, U.; Svahn, S.; Bowden, T.; Hilborn, J.; Forsberg-Nilsson, K. Enhanced neuronal differentiation in a three-dimensional collagen-hyaluronan matrix. *J. Neurosci. Res.* **2007**, *85*, 2138–2146. [CrossRef] [PubMed]
44. Dong, C.; Lv, Y. Application of Collagen Scaffold in Tissue Engineering: Recent Advances and New Perspectives. *Polymers* **2016**, *8*, 42. [CrossRef] [PubMed]
45. Glowacki, J.; Mizuno, S. Collagen scaffolds for tissue engineering. *Biopolymers* **2008**, *89*, 338–344. [CrossRef] [PubMed]
46. Willerth, S.M.; Sakiyama-Elbert, S.E. Approaches to neural tissue engineering using scaffolds for drug delivery. *Adv. Drug Deliv. Rev.* **2007**, *59*, 325–338. [CrossRef] [PubMed]
47. Gao, X.; Wang, Y.; Chen, J.; Peng, J. The role of peripheral nerve ECM components in the tissue engineering nerve construction. *Rev. Neurosci.* **2013**, *24*, 443–453. [CrossRef]
48. Gonzalez-Perez, F.; Udina, E.; Navarro, X. Extracellular Matrix Components in Peripheral Nerve Regeneration. *Int. Rev. Neurobiol.* **2013**, *108*, 257–275. [CrossRef]
49. Kelsey, N.A.; Wilkins, H.M.; Linseman, D.A. Nutraceutical antioxidants as novel neuroprotective agents. *Molecules* **2010**, *15*, 7792–7814. [CrossRef] [PubMed]
50. Tilak, J.C.; Adhikari, S.; Devasagayam, T.P.A. Antioxidant properties of *Plumbago zeylanica*, an Indian medicinal plant and its active ingredient, plumbagin. *Redox Rep.* **2004**, *9*, 219–227. [CrossRef]
51. Vashist, A.; Kaushik, A.; Vashist, A.; Bala, J.; Nikkhah-Moshaie, R.; Sagar, V.; Nair, M. Nanogels as potential drug nanocarriers for CNS drug delivery. *Drug Discov. Today* **2018**, *23*, 1436–1443. [CrossRef]
52. Wang, K.-H.; Li, B.-Z. Plumbagin protects against hydrogen peroxide-induced neurotoxicity by modulating NF-κB and Nrf-2. *Arch. Med. Sci.* **2018**, *14*, 1112–1118. [CrossRef]
53. Wang, S.; Zhang, Z.; Zhao, S. Plumbagin inhibits amyloid-β-induced neurotoxicity. *Neuroreport* **2018**, *29*, 1269–1274. [CrossRef] [PubMed]
54. Sun, Y.; Yang, T.; Leak, R.K.; Chen, J.; Zhang, F. Preventive and Protective Roles of Dietary Nrf2 Activators Against Central Nervous System Diseases. *CNS Neurol. Disord. Drug Targets* **2017**, *16*, 326–338. [CrossRef] [PubMed]
55. Khan, M.B.; Hoda, M.N.; Ishrat, T.; Ahmad, S.; Moshahid Khan, M.; Ahmad, A.; Yusuf, S.; Islam, F. Neuroprotective efficacy of Nardostachys jatamansi and crocetin in conjunction with selenium in cognitive impairment. *Neurol. Sci.* **2012**, *33*, 1011–1020. [CrossRef] [PubMed]

56. Zaky, A.; Bassiouny, A.; Farghaly, M.; El-Sabaa, B.M. A Combination of Resveratrol and Curcumin is Effective Against Aluminum Chloride-Induced Neuroinflammation in Rats. *J. Alzheimer's Dis.* **2017**, *60*, S221–S235. [CrossRef] [PubMed]
57. Dhitavat, S.; Ortiz, D.; Rogers, E.; Rivera, E.; Shea, T.B. Folate, vitamin E, and acetyl-l-carnitine provide synergistic protection against oxidative stress resulting from exposure of human neuroblastoma cells to amyloid-beta. *Brain Res.* **2005**, *1061*, 114–117. [CrossRef]
58. Cheng, Y.; Rong, J. Therapeutic Potential of Heme Oxygenase-1/carbon Monoxide System Against Ischemia-Reperfusion Injury. *Curr. Pharm. Des.* **2017**, *23*. [CrossRef]
59. Ross, D.; Siegel, D. Functions of NQO1 in Cellular Protection and CoQ10 Metabolism and its Potential Role as a Redox Sensitive Molecular Switch. *Front. Physiol.* **2017**, *8*, 595. [CrossRef]
60. Couto, N.; Wood, J.; Barber, J. The role of glutathione reductase and related enzymes on cellular redox homoeostasis network. *Free Radic. Biol. Med.* **2016**, *95*, 27–42. [CrossRef]
61. Lu, J.; Holmgren, A. The thioredoxin antioxidant system. *Free Radic. Biol. Med.* **2014**, *66*, 75–87. [CrossRef]
62. Li, J.; Li, W.; Jiang, Z.G.; Ghanbari, H. Oxidative stress and neurodegenerative disorders. *Int. J. Mol. Sci.* **2013**, *14*, 24438–24475. [CrossRef] [PubMed]
63. De Oliveira, M.R.; Brasil, F.B.; Fürstenau, C.R. Sulforaphane Attenuated the Pro-Inflammatory State Induced by Hydrogen Peroxide in SH-SY5Y Cells Through the Nrf2/HO-1 Signaling Pathway. *Neurotox. Res.* **2018**, *34*, 241–249. [CrossRef]
64. Vauzour, D.; Buonfiglio, M.; Corona, G.; Chirafisi, J.; Vafeiadou, K.; Angeloni, C.; Hrelia, S.; Hrelia, P.; Spencer, J.P.E. Sulforaphane protects cortical neurons against 5-S-cysteinyl-dopamine-induced toxicity through the activation of ERK1/2, Nrf-2 and the upregulation of detoxification enzymes. *Mol. Nutr. Food Res.* **2010**, *54*, 532–542. [CrossRef] [PubMed]
65. Romeo, L.; Intrieri, M.; D'Agata, V.; Mangano, N.G.; Oriani, G.; Ontario, M.L.; Scapagnini, G. The major green tea polyphenol, (-)-epigallocatechin-3-gallate, induces heme oxygenase in rat neurons and acts as an effective neuroprotective agent against oxidative stress. *J. Am. Coll. Nutr.* **2009**, *28*, S492–S499. [CrossRef] [PubMed]
66. Han, J.; Wang, M.; Jing, X.; Shi, H.; Ren, M.; Lou, H. (−)-Epigallocatechin Gallate Protects Against Cerebral Ischemia-Induced Oxidative Stress via Nrf2/ARE Signaling. *Neurochem. Res.* **2014**, *39*, 1292–1299. [CrossRef] [PubMed]
67. Marrazzo, P.; Angeloni, C.; Freschi, M.; Lorenzini, A.; Prata, C.; Maraldi, T.; Hrelia, S. Combination of epigallocatechin gallate and sulforaphane counteracts in vitro oxidative stress and delays stemness loss of amniotic fluid stem cells. *Oxid. Med. Cell. Longev.* **2018**, *2018*, 5263985. [CrossRef] [PubMed]
68. Zhu, X.; Yang, J.; Zhu, W.; Yin, X.; Yang, B.; Wei, Y.; Guo, X. Combination of Berberine with Resveratrol Improves the Lipid-Lowering Efficacy. *Int. J. Mol. Sci.* **2018**, *19*, 3903. [CrossRef] [PubMed]
69. Ma, M.W.; Wang, J.; Zhang, Q.; Wang, R.; Dhandapani, K.M.; Vadlamudi, R.K.; Brann, D.W. NADPH oxidase in brain injury and neurodegenerative disorders. *Mol. Neurodegener.* **2017**, *12*, 7. [CrossRef] [PubMed]
70. Shyu, K.-G.; Chang, C.-C.; Yeh, Y.-C.; Sheu, J.-R.; Chou, D.-S. Mechanisms of Ascorbyl Radical Formation in Human Platelet-Rich Plasma. *Biomed Res. Int.* **2014**, *2014*, 614506. [CrossRef]
71. Coso, S.; Harrison, I.; Harrison, C.B.; Vinh, A.; Sobey, C.G.; Drummond, G.R.; Williams, E.D.; Selemidis, S. NADPH Oxidases as Regulators of Tumor Angiogenesis: Current and Emerging Concepts. *Antioxid. Redox Signal.* **2012**, *16*, 1229–1247. [CrossRef]
72. Selemidis, S.; Sobey, C.G.; Wingler, K.; Schmidt, H.H.H.W.; Drummond, G.R. NADPH oxidases in the vasculature: Molecular features, roles in disease and pharmacological inhibition. *Pharmacol. Ther.* **2008**, *120*, 254–291. [CrossRef] [PubMed]
73. Armitage, M.E.; Wingler, K.; Schmidt, H.H.H.W.; La, M. Translating the oxidative stress hypothesis into the clinic: NOX versus NOS. *J. Mol. Med.* **2009**, *87*, 1071–1076. [CrossRef] [PubMed]
74. Stargardt, A.; Gillis, J.; Kamphuis, W.; Wiemhoefer, A.; Kooijman, L.; Raspe, M.; Benckhuijsen, W.; Drijfhout, J.W.; Reits, E. Reduced amyloid-β degradation in early Alzheimer's disease but not in the APPswePS1dE9 and 3xTg-AD mouse models. *Aging Cell* **2013**, *12*, 499–507. [CrossRef] [PubMed]
75. Portelius, E.; Mattsson, N.; Pannee, J.; Zetterberg, H.; Gisslén, M.; Vanderstichele, H.; Gkanatsiou, E.; Crespi, G.A.N.; Parker, M.W.; Miles, L.A.; et al. Ex vivo 18O-labeling mass spectrometry identifies a peripheral amyloid β clearance pathway. *Mol. Neurodegener.* **2017**, *12*, 18. [CrossRef] [PubMed]

76. Farris, W.; Mansourian, S.; Chang, Y.; Lindsley, L.; Eckman, E.A.; Frosch, M.P.; Eckman, C.B.; Tanzi, R.E.; Selkoe, D.J.; Guenette, S. Insulin-degrading enzyme regulates the levels of insulin, amyloid beta-protein, and the beta-amyloid precursor protein intracellular domain in vivo. *Proc. Natl. Acad. Sci. USA* **2003**, *100*, 4162–4167. [CrossRef] [PubMed]
77. Langhans, S.A. Three-Dimensional in Vitro Cell Culture Models in Drug Discovery and Drug Repositioning. *Front. Pharmacol.* **2018**, *9*, 6. [CrossRef]
78. Fang, Y.; Eglen, R.M. Three-Dimensional Cell Cultures in Drug Discovery and Development. *SLAS Discov. Adv. Life Sci. R D* **2017**, *22*, 456–472. [CrossRef]
79. Ko, K.R.; Frampton, J.P. Developments in 3D neural cell culture models: The future of neurotherapeutics testing? *Expert Rev. Neurother.* **2016**, *16*, 739–741. [CrossRef]
80. Maraldi, T.; Prata, C.; Marrazzo, P.; Hrelia, S.; Angeloni, C. Natural compounds as a strategy to optimize "in vitro" expansion of stem cells. *Rejuvenation Res.* **2019**. [CrossRef]

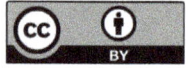

© 2019 by the authors. Licensee MDPI, Basel, Switzerland. This article is an open access article distributed under the terms and conditions of the Creative Commons Attribution (CC BY) license (http://creativecommons.org/licenses/by/4.0/).

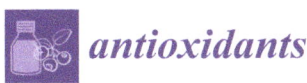

Review

Hormetic and Mitochondria-Related Mechanisms of Antioxidant Action of Phytochemicals

Rafael Franco [1,2,*], Gemma Navarro [2,3] and Eva Martínez-Pinilla [4,5,6,*]

1. Chemistry School, University of Barcelona, 08028 Barcelona, Spain
2. Centro de Investigación Biomédica en Red Enfermedades Neurodegenerativas (CiberNed), Instituto de Salud Carlos III, 28031 Madrid, Spain
3. Department of Biochemistry and Physiology, Faculty of Pharmacy and Food Sciences, University of Barcelona, 02028 Barcelona, Spain
4. Departamento de Morfología y Biología Celular, Facultad de Medicina, Universidad de Oviedo, 33006 Oviedo, Spain
5. Instituto de Neurociencias del Principado de Asturias (INEUROPA), 33003 Oviedo, Spain
6. Instituto de Investigación Sanitaria del Principado de Asturias (ISPA), 33011 Oviedo, Spain
* Correspondence: rfranco@ub.edu (R.F.); martinezpinillaeva@gmail.com (E.M.-P.); Tel.: +34-934-021-208 (R.F.); +34-985-102-774 (E.M.-P.)

Received: 23 July 2019; Accepted: 28 August 2019; Published: 4 September 2019

Abstract: Antioxidant action to afford a health benefit or increased well-being may not be directly exerted by quick reduction-oxidation (REDOX) reactions between the antioxidant and the pro-oxidant molecules in a living being. Furthermore, not all flavonoids or polyphenols derived from plants are beneficial. This paper aims at discussing the variety of mechanisms underlying the so-called "antioxidant" action. Apart from antioxidant direct mechanisms, indirect ones consisting of fueling and boosting innate detox routes should be considered. One of them, hormesis, involves upregulating enzymes that are needed in innate detox pathways and/or regulating the transcription of the so-called vitagenes. Moreover, there is evidence that some plant-derived compounds may have a direct role in events taking place in mitochondria, which is an organelle prone to oxidative stress if electron transport is faulty. Insights into the potential of molecules able to enter into the electron transport chain would require the determination of their reduction potential. Additionally, it is advisable to know both the oxidized and the reduced structures for each antioxidant candidate. These mechanisms and their related technical developments should help nutraceutical industry to select candidates that are efficacious in physiological conditions to prevent diseases or increase human health.

Keywords: CNS; fava beans; glucose; fructose; oxidative stress; vitagenes

1. Chemical Basis of Antioxidant Action

Any reduction-oxidation (REDOX) reaction follows well-established chemical laws. Almost any substance can be oxidized or reduced and this depends on a second reagent. In fact, a REDOX reaction requires two semi-reactions and two molecules: one that is oxidized (the reductant) and another that is reduced (the oxidant). Accordingly, any antioxidant molecule is a reductant able to reduce an oxidized reagent. The chemical laws guiding REDOX processes are valid in vivo and in vitro (i.e., in a test tube). As commented in a previous paper, the canonical function of antioxidants in the food industry is to increase the useful life of processed foods. In the case of animal-derived products, antioxidants are added to avoid/delay rotting (i.e., their action is to prevent putrefaction of dead matter) [1].

Nowadays, "antioxidants" is a word also used to refer to substances that provide benefit to humans due to REDOX-related capabilities. Importantly, it is often assumed that these capabilities are directly exerted on a given tissue or a given oxidative stressor. However, antioxidants may indirectly exert their beneficial effect. This paper aims at highlighting the hormetic and mitochondria-related mechanisms of antioxidants action that can be changed by the phytochemical use.

2. Are Antioxidants Needed for Human Life?

The use of phytochemicals dates back to ancestral times. Paleontological and anthropological evidence demonstrates that Neanderthals, who until quite recently were regarded predominantly as meat-eaters, included plants in their diet. Valuous studies aimed at identifying entrapped material in calcified dental plaque show, quite surprisingly, that a Neanderthal group of hominids who inhabited El Sidrón cave (Asturias, Spain) 49,000 years ago, did not consume foods of animal origin but moved in the direction of a more "healthy" vegetable/plant-based diet, including mushrooms, pine nuts, and moss [2,3]. Apparently, our ancestors already noticed that some plants helped, not only calorically, but also in terms of well-being. More prevalent in higher primates, this "self-medication" is not exclusive to them but it is widespread within the animal kingdom [4–6].

A newborn does not need any plant derived antioxidant for living. If the child takes milk from the mother it may be hypothesized that mother's milk already had its own antioxidants some of which could derive from ingested plants. But the use of formula milks and the lack of increased health problems in children raised with artificial milk prove that antioxidants are not required for a child's healthy life. Commercially available infant milk contains plant derived products but few (or none) that are considered as "antioxidants". On the one hand, they contain sugars and fatty acids/lipids, which are oxidants, in other words very reduced molecules that are oxidized in infant's cells. On the other hand, they contain vitamins and no added antioxidant apart from, eventually, one acting as preservative. As we have previously argued, vitamins may have in vitro antioxidant action, but none in the basis of chemical rules, so they do not act as in vivo antioxidants [1]. According to Mayo Clinic the daily requirement of vitamin A for adult men is 900 µg (i.e., very low to have any overall direct antioxidant effect).

Fruits are among the first plant-derived foods introduced in child's nutrition. Indeed, fruit has antioxidants but is the antioxidant content the reason for such early introduction of fruits in human diet? The answer is, likely not. Another relevant question is whether sugars (from fruits) can be the only sugar energy source in humans. Despite glucose and fructose in human nutrition derive from vegetables, the answer is that human metabolism has evolved to use glucose instead of fructose as main energy source.

But are glucose or fructose antioxidants? From a chemical point of view, glucose is a reducing sugar whereas fructose is a non-reducing sugar. This nomenclature goes back to the first reactions using biological compounds that were designed to identify sugars in a mixture or in blood. Reduction is a relative term since it depends on the properties of a second component that may be reduced or oxidized. The classical technique to measure the reducing potential was to observe whether Cu^{2+} could be reduced to Cu^+ in basic conditions of pH. In mild circumstances, this technique results in glucose being a reducing sugar (an aldose) and fructose (a ketose) being a non-reducing sugar. But if conditions are forced, fructose, due to ketose-aldose tautomerism may lead to the Cu^{2+}/Cu^+ reduction (i.e., fructose could react as a reducing sugar). Very importantly, these in vitro assays are of little usefulness in physiological conditions. In fact, may a reducing sugar (glucose) or a non-reducing sugar (fructose) be in vivo antioxidants? None of two sugars acts as antioxidants in humans [7–9], both are oxidized to obtain energy and, in the case of glucose, to (also) obtain reducing power to be used in innate antioxidant mechanisms. In summary, the non-reducing sugar, fructose, and the reducing sugar, glucose, are not in vivo-acting antioxidants, but the latter is required to provide the molecules needed by innate antioxidant human systems (see [1] for further details).

3. When Does Antioxidant Intake Become Beneficial in Human Life?

Some evidence suggests that a high fructose dietary intake, in the form of cultivated fruits or sweeteners (sucrose or high fructose corn syrup), is related to the development of a variety of metabolic diseases [10,11]. Fructose absorbed in the gut is completely converted into triose-phosphate by fructokinase, aldolase B and triokinase, in the sequential steps of a metabolic pathway which is not controlled through feedback inhibition (ADP or citrate) [12]. Resulting metabolites may be oxidized, and converted into glucose and lactate to be released into the bloodstream, or converted into hepatic glycogen or triacylglycerol in liver cells by de novo lipogenesis, in an insulin-independent process. All together leads to increases in plasma triglycerides, insulin resistance, or high blood pressure [10,13,14]. Although the data about the adverse metabolic effects of fructose in humans are controversial [14], rodents fed with a high-fructose diet show fatty liver, impaired insulin sensitivity, or dyslipidemia [13,15–17], also affecting (negatively) the antioxidant status [8,9]. Similar results were reported in *Macaca fascicularis* and rhesus monkeys exposed to high fructose over a long period of time [18,19] (Table 1).

Table 1. Sources, mechanism of action and effects of dietary phytochemicals.

Phytochemicals	Sources	Mechanism of Action	Effects	References
Fructose	Cultivated fruits or sweeteners	Increases in plasma triglycerides, insulin resistance, high blood pressure, etc.	Fatty liver, insulin resistance, dyslipidemia, etc.	[8,9,12–20]
Coenzyme Q10	Oranges, spinach, broccoli, soybeans, nuts, sesame seeds, etc.	Correct function of the electron chain transport in mitochondria	Improvement in orthostatic hypotension, renal alterations in type II diabetes	[21–24]
Lipoic acid	Potatoes, spinach, broccoli, carrots, tomatoes, rice bran, etc.	Correct function of different enzymatic systems	To combat oxidative stress (by mechanisms not known)	[25]
Vicine and convicine	Fava beans	"Hormetic" maintenance of high levels of glucose-6-phosphate dehydrogenase	Maintenance hemoglobin in a functional state and the innate antioxidant mechanism of red blood cells	[26–30]

Current human dietary habits are inherited from our ancient hominid specimens and are similar to that of wild monkeys and apes. How is it possible that dietary habits may cause chronic illnesses and health problems, mainly in Western societies? One answer comes from tackling the changes in food staples and food-processing procedures. In fact, some studies suggest that many harvested fruits and vegetables eaten by humans differ from the wild versions in regards to fatty acid level, macronutrients and phytochemical composition or fiber content. It is even possible that the use of food additives and supplements have detrimental effects. Let us take "designed fruits" as an example. These fruits are optimized by seed selection and cross-fertilization to have succulent pulps with dew or no seeds, thus becoming more attractive for the consumers. Surely, the most important difference lies on sweetness and, consequently, on the sugar content. Whereas wild fruits are rich in hexoses, as glucose and fructose, cultivated fruits have been genetically modified to be higher in sucrose, a glucose and fructose disaccharide for which our metabolism is not properly adapted [4,5]. In the seminal work of Schwitzer et al., (2008) we can find an exhaustive comparison between wild and cultivated fruits and vegetables in terms of nutrients and energy content. For example, the major sugars in harvested figs are 0.40% sucrose, 25.5% glucose and 23.40% fructose, in contrast to the pattern of the wild variety *Ficus insipida* that shows a 0.4% of sucrose, a 0.6% of glucose and a 0.3% of fructose [20]. In this sense, other studies have also identified lower monosaccharides/disaccharides ratios in modified fruits and vegetables [31–33]. Compelling evidence in recent years, has shown that, apart from the fructose content, the processing operations of commercial forms of fruit and vegetable food products influence the levels of a myriad of dietary phytochemicals [34]. In addition, additive and/or synergistic role of some flavonols present in culinary plants has been demonstrated and among them, myricetin, fisetin, quercetin, catechin and curcumin seem to inhibit fructose gut transport by glucose transporter 2 (GLUT2) and 5 (GLUT5), as shown in *Xenopus laevis* oocytes and in human intestinal Caco-2 cells [35,36].

When this nutritional information is added to physiological burden due to wear and/or malfunction occurring in aging or disease, humans need help. According to our view, the need of "so-called" antioxidants begins upon aging (i.e., when innate antioxidant mechanisms start to have some dysfunctions and alter well-being). Then, the search for interventions to keep healthiness is of vital importance and, in this sense, "antioxidants" have a huge potential. However, in our opinion, to take optimal profit of antioxidant-related interventions, more knowledge on mechanisms is needed.

4. Direct Mechanisms of Plant Antioxidant/Nutraceutical Action

A REDOX reaction may immediately take place when a reductant and an antioxidant meet. The kinetics coordinate is very important as there are some rules to fulfil to delay antioxidant actions. The naked eye is able to see quick oxidation when fruits, for instance bananas and apples, are peeled off. Instantaneously some component(s) of the fruit (reductant(s)), reacts with atmospheric oxygen (oxidant) and the process is visible by the appearance of a brown color. As the process is relatively quick, similar reactions take place when a human eats bananas or apples but locally (i.e., along the gastrointestinal tract). It is very unlikely that reductants remain intact until reaching a given tissue and reacting with "the undesirable" oxidant. In summary, ready-to-use reduction potential likely occurs locally [1]; in the case of food, thus potential is limited to the proximal structures of the gastrointestinal tract: esophagus and stomach (Figure 1).

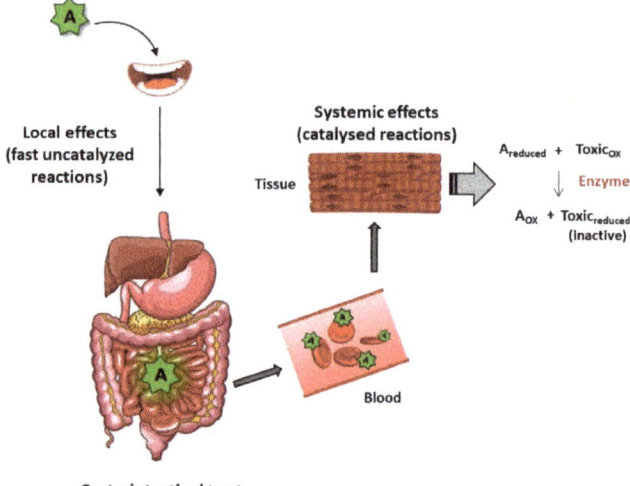

Figure 1. Scheme of direct antioxidant mechanisms including local effects by fast uncatalyzed reactions and systemic effects due to catalyzed reactions. A—antioxidant, A_{ox}—oxidized antioxidant, $A_{reduced}$—reduced antioxidant, $Toxic_{ox}$—oxidized toxic, $Toxic_{reduced}$—reduced toxic (non-toxic in reduced form).

Surely, REDOX reactions may be "delayed" if time of reaction is the limiting factor. The most common way to increase reaction rate in living organisms is by the action of bio-catalysts (i.e., of enzymes). In such cases, the reductant present in a plant-derived product may be considered as a drug orally taken which reaches the blood, is distributed and acts in the targeted tissue by, among other, activating a receptor or inhibiting an enzyme. In the case of a reductant able to act like a drug, it would reach the targeted tissue and react with a specific (undesirable) oxidant. In summary, this mechanism requires a reductant that travels to the target tissue(s) to meet a specific oxidant and a specific enzyme able to catalyze the REDOX reaction (Figure 1). Somewhat expected, such reductant has not yet been described (to our knowledge). A reductant acting by this mechanism would be a nutraceutical—"a type of food substance that helps to maintain health and prevent illness"—according with the Encyclopedia Britannica. Antioxidants research is a relatively young field and the tendency is to group molecules:

polyphenols, flavonoids, etc. However, each molecule is different and it is likely that there are "good" and "bad" polyphenols. Identifying the "good" ones and demonstrating that there is a specific mechanism able to inactivate a noxious oxidant in a given tissue is an attractive possibility, even a necessity. In one of the most recent studies, toxicity of polyphenols or polyphenol-rich plant extracts has been addressed by quantitating and comparing the effects on survival in hepatic (HepG2), fibroblast (3T3), epithelial (A549 and Caco-2), and endothelial (HMEC-1) human cell lines. As a conclusion a list of the five most toxic and the five least toxic polyphenol-rich compounds was provided [37]. As pure molecules, naringin was the less toxic and kaempferol the most toxic. Accordingly, in the data sheet of kaempferol from Cayman chemical company indicates "acute toxicity and germ cell mutagenicity" (in humans); in addition, the product is "H301: toxic if swallowed" and "H341: suspect of causing genetic defects" [38]. It is important to highlight that any nutraceutical must be tested for genotoxicity to get approval to be released into the market.

From both human health and industrial point of views, another relevant aspect should not be forgotten which is bioavailability and the possibility that per-oral consumed molecules are transformed upon in vivo metabolism or gut fermentation/biotransformation [39]. On the one hand, bioaccessibility of the administered compound and its metabolites may vary depending on the "galenic" formulation of the phytochemical-containing product. One example is provided by comparing creams with microencapsulated phenolic acids and flavanols [40]; another is to find the best vehicle to increase the bioavailability of curcumin incorporated to bread [41]. On the other hand, total antioxidant capacity, measured for instance in blood, may be a convenient tool to quickly decide whether to continue or not the research and development of a substance or of an extract [42]. Nevertheless, caution is needed as total antioxidant capacity is not reflecting the whole potential of substances indirectly reinforcing antioxidant mechanisms.

5. Hormetic and Replenishment Mechanisms of Indirect Antioxidant/Nutraceutical Action

Faulty oxidation in cells results in oxidative stress, which is harmful [43]. For instance, the electron transport and oxidative phosphorylation events taking place in the mitochondria are self-regulated; if cells have all the required components and the mitochondria are healthy no undesired REDOX-related effect is expected to occur. Oxidative stress appears as a threat to cell/organism survival when a component is reduced or the mitochondria do not properly work.

A well-known indirect antioxidant strategy is to provide components (or precursors) of REDOX-related routes. One option is to supply molecules that participate in events whose dysfunction leads to oxidative stress. A second option is providing molecules that participate in innate mechanisms of detoxification. A few examples of those strategies are provided below.

A very successful way to use plant antioxidants is by increasing the concentration of endogenous substances that participate in REDOX mechanisms. A complete list of antioxidant supplements and its "galenic" formulations is out of the scope of the present paper; therefore, we will provide some examples of antioxidants derived from plants that are quite fruitful. For instance, supplement of coenzyme Q10, ubiquinol (ubiquinone in oxidized form), may replenish the compound if there is a shortage due to aging, disease or, eventually, malnutrition. The coenzyme Q10, essential for electron chain transport in mitochondria, can be found in a variety of vegetable sources: oranges, spinach, broccoli, soybeans, nuts, sesame seeds, etc. A recent report has confirmed shortage of coenzyme Q10 in centenarians and a correlation with increased oxidative stress [21]. Other benefits of supplementation with ubiquinol/ubiquinone include improvement in orthostatic hypotension [22], and prevention of renal alterations in a model of type II diabetes [23]. Interestingly, a recent double-blind placebo-controlled clinical trial has shown that ubiquinol is better than ubiquinone to increase the total levels of coenzyme Q10 [24] (Table 1).

Lipoic (or thioctic) acid is another endogenous component that may lead to oxidative stress if cell concentrations decay. It is found in a variety of plant-derived products: potatoes, spinach, broccoli, carrots, tomatoes, rice bran, etc. In mammalians, lipoic acid participates in at least five different enzymatic systems. For example, two of the enzymes of the Kreb's cycle, which occurs in mitochondria to produce reducing power in the form of reducing nicotine adenine dinucleotide (NADH) and reduced flavin-adenine dinucleotide (FADH$_2$), need lipoic acid. Benefits of lipoic acid supplementation are less evident than those attributed to coenzyme Q10 but it is thought that they may be helpful to combat oxidative stress (by mechanisms not yet deciphered). A systematic review and meta-analysis indicates that these benefits include improvement of biomarkers of diabetes and of inflammation [25] (Table 1).

Whereas supplements of lipoic acid in diets are obtained from plant-derived products, coenzyme Q10 used in the food or cosmetic industry is synthetic or produced by microbes in fermenters. The latter leads to a low yield and is relatively expensive. Plant-derived raw materials or products are cost-effective alternatives. Production of coenzyme Q10 from plants may be a relatively cheap but environment-friendly approach that is explored by the supplement's industry [44].

Probably, one of the main antioxidant mechanisms exerted by plant components gets unnoticed. It is indirect and counterintuitive and consists of boosting the innate mechanism of defense against oxidative stress. Such "hormetic" mechanisms have been likely shaped by Evolution. They are well characterized, for instance, in the case of ionizing radiation (radioactivity), in the sense that limited exposure is beneficial while high exposure is detrimental [45]. In fact, there is a background of radioactivity, mainly due to ^{40}K, that is not detrimental to species that have evolved to coexist with such environmental conditions. A significant example of hormetic mechanism in humans was serendipitously discovered as patients of glucose-6-phosphate dehydrogenase (G6PDH) deficiency presented clinical symptoms after intake of antimalaria drug (primaquine) or of fava beans. In fact, in some rural zones the disease was known as favism. When the enzyme is missing the reduced nicotine adenine dinucleotide phosphate (NADPH) required to maintain a functional hemoglobin is not produced, erythrocytes die and hemolysis occurs. In healthy people, intake of fava beans maintains high the levels of G6PDH and, hence, the innate antioxidant mechanism of red blood cells is efficient in keeping significant amounts of reduced glutathione and/or rapidly converting oxidized glutathione into reduced glutathione [26–30] (Figure 2). As mentioned, this mechanism is triggered by the pro-oxidant action of a drug (primaquine) or of a phytochemical (vicine or convicine in fava beans) [29,30] (Table 1). In summary, a pro-oxidant compound wakes-up an antioxidant defense mechanism that is innate in humans. The nutraceutical industry may take advantage of such pro-oxidants to be used at low doses and/or intermittently (a chronic high-dose supplementation is not advisable and would go against the hormetic principle).

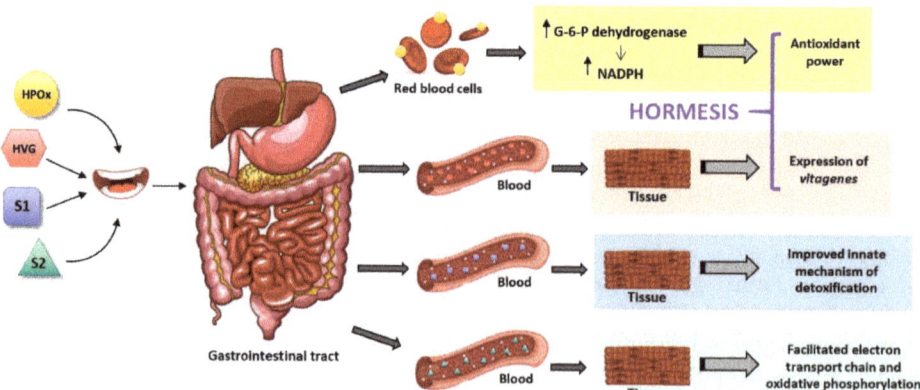

Figure 2. Scheme of indirect antioxidant mechanisms including hormetic actions exerted by pro-oxidants or vitagene expression regulators, and the use of supplements that improves innate mechanisms of detoxification or facilitates mitochondrial function. HPOX—hormetic pro-oxidant, HVG—vitagene-enhancing hormetic compound, S1—supplement type 1, S2—supplement type 2.

Contrary to what one might think, hormesis is less strange than it seems. Physical training is also an hormetic-like mechanism because sedentary life may lead to oxidative stress due to malfunctioning of cell metabolic events. The oxidative stress in any exercise will be higher in a non-trained individual. Therefore, training in the case of athletes is not only needed to have good scores but to minimize oxidative stress. Trained individuals have all the machinery ready for the exercise and, consequently, oxidative events take place very efficiently and with minimal production of undesired compounds. Furthermore, studies in exercise-trained rats show that diet affects muscle expression of G6PDH [46]. Finally, it has been considered that caloric restriction is an hormetic antiaging mechanism that may increase life span [47], and that antioxidant phytochemicals may be neuroprotective by hormetic processes that involve the engagement of "vitagenes" [48] (Figure 2). The word was coined to highlight those genes that are involved in repair and maintenance processes; Rattan SI (1998) wrote that: the "complex network of the so-called longevity assurance processes is composed of several genes, which may be called vitagenes" [49]. Genes that encode some heat-shock proteins are considered as vitagenes because temperature is one of the most employed hormetic factors. Heat shock produces upregulation of heat-shock proteins, chaperones that preserve the tridimensional structure of proteins and help newly synthesized proteins to be properly folded [49,50].

Another example is the protective role of superoxide radicals on hydrogen peroxide stress [51]. Whereas the excess of superoxide radicals is detrimental for cells, the occasional presence of low levels of these species are beneficial not only for cells but for the whole animal. Rattan SI, already in 1998, demonstrated that mild heat shock retards ageing of human fibroblasts and concluded that "These hormesis-like effects of stress-induced defense processes can be useful to elucidate the role of maintenance and repair mechanisms in ageing" [50]. A similar procedure has recently shown that neuronal survival is enhanced. Mild stress applied to primary cultures of cortical neurons decreases the chance of deposition of lipofuscin granules and of pathological aggregates (neurofibrillary tangles or senile plaques) [52]. Mild oxidative stress achieved in worms by downregulating the electron transport chain, affords protection against age-related proteostasis collapse and restores the heat-shock response [53]. At moderate doses, green tea polyphenols reduce the pathological signs in an experimental rodent model of colitis, while unwanted side-effects appear at high doses [54].

Glycation is a very well-known phenomenon but difficult to address from a technological point of view. Part of the reason is the structural diversity of sugars coupled to proteins and/or lipids. The simplest example is, perhaps, the so-called advanced glycation endproducts (AGEs) constituted by a sugar and a protein that are formed in the absence of any catalyst. Formation occurs in any condition but it is enriched when sugar blood levels rise (e.g., in diabetes). They are supposedly involved in a variety of diseases from hypertension to neurodegeneration; however, some evidence indicates that AGEs may be protective. For example, ischemic preconditioning is a mechanism of protecting heart from occlusive cardiovascular disease. Murry et al. (1986) showed that cardioprotection can be achieved by short cycles of ischemia-reperfusion [55]. It seems that AGEs formation in these circumstances is part of the protection mechanism (see [56,57]). Hence, it is suggested that moderate stress by AGEs may potentiate innate defense mechanisms in various illnesses [57]. Therefore, protein glycation may be beneficial or detrimental, thus constituting a hormetic response that may be, likely, modulated by plant-derived products. Indeed, this is an attractive field of research.

It has been shown in an invertebrate animal model, *Caenorhabditis elegans*, that variation in hormetic effects is genetically determined [58]. Translated to humans, these findings confirm that hormesis is constituted by mechanisms that have been optimized upon evolution. The challenge is to identify plant-derived products able to restore the efficacy of those mechanisms of protection when they become disfuntional by ageing or by disease. A recent report, has shown that ampelopsin, rosmarinic acid and amorfrutin-A are "hormetins" in human skin fibroblasts undergoing senescence. They protect against telomere length reduction and accumulation of 8-OH-deoxyguanosine, an oxidative DNA damage product, while they upregulate heat-shock protein Hsp70 [59].

6. Mitochondria-Related Mechanisms of Plant Antioxidant/Nutraceutical Action

It is well known that polyphenols and other bioactive compounds derived from plants may act on mitochondria. As an example, isoflavones, trans-resveratrol and resveratrol analogues, activate peroxisome proliferator—activated receptor γ (PPARγ) coactivator-1β (PGC-1β) leading to increase the levels of medium-chain acyl-CoA dehydrogenase, a mitochondrial enzyme that participates in lipid metabolism, in a transgenic model of PGC-1β overexpression [60]. The mode of action of these phytochemicals is unclear as PPARγ is a nuclear receptor and the upregulated enzyme is mitochondrial. Daidzein and genistein, two widely-studied phytoflavonoids, protect cerebellum granule neurons from apoptosis by interacting with the mitochondria. In conditions of induced apoptosis, the two compounds "prevented the impairment of glucose oxidation and mitochondrial coupling, reduced cytochrome C release, and prevented both impairment of the adenine nucleotide translocator and opening of the mitochondrial permeability transition pore" [61]. The underlying molecular mechanisms of these effects are not known and the relevant question is whether some pathway or another REDOX reactions are involved. The finding, by Atlante and co-workers (2010), that superoxide compounds decreased the level of reactive oxygen species in conditions of apoptosis is not a proof that anti-apoptotic action is due to any intrinsic antioxidant power of daidzein and genistein.

Plants have chloroplasts and mitochondria both of which are involved in REDOX reactions. Therefore, some of components of these plant organelles, which upon oral intake reach significant levels in blood, may arrive to the mitochondria of mammalian cells and participate in electron transport, or in oxidative phosphorylation or both. Refilling the metabolites in mitochondria by plant-derived products may result in preventing oxidative stress (Figure 2). Conceptually, this antioxidant indirect mechanism is similar to providing supplements to increase the concentration of mammalian cell molecules, the difference is that plant-specific components may directly participate in mammalian mitochondrial REDOX pathways. There is evidence of such possibility. On the one hand, there are reasons to believe that plant-specific mitochondrial components could readily act as mediators of the electron transport events in mammalian cells. On the other hand, it has been shown that polyphenols may act in the mitochondrial machinery independently of reactive oxygen species scavenging; the authors of this study also indicate that "certain polyphenols affect mitochondrial electron transport chain and ATP synthesis" [62]. Thermogenesis and mitochondrial biogenesis are other processes regulated by polyphenols, at least in vitro [63]. However, and despite suggestive data [62,64], it is unlikely that plant polyphenols may act as real anti-cancer compounds by releasing cytochrome C and unrolling apoptosis in tumor cells.

Hints on the direct engagement of endogenous compounds in electron transport chain are many-fold, but two properties are required: (i) the compound reaches the mitochondria, and (ii) the compound has a reduction potential ($\varepsilon^{o'}$) between that of the global semi-reaction—soxygen to water and NAD$^+$ to NADH; standard reduction potentials in cellular conditions of pH and ion composition ($\varepsilon^{o'}$) are, respectively, 0.81 and -0.32 Volts. As a reference the $\varepsilon^{o'}$ of ubiquinone to ubiquinol semi-reaction is 0.05 Volts. Since an exhaustive review is not yet possible due to the need of more reports on the subject, a couple of examples will be given. The first is related to quercetin, one of the most studied plant antioxidant. Quercetin is a flavonoid included in human diet because it is present, among other vegetable products, in apples, oranges, lemons, onions, tomatoes and broccoli. Red wine, St John's wort (*Hypericum perforatum*), or *Ginkgo biloba* are also sources of this compound which, in addition, is sold as a dietary supplement. A very recent study using astrocytes deficient in methyl-CpG-binding protein 2 transcription factor showed that quercetin rescued the reduced activity of mitochondrial respiratory chain complex-II and complex-III [65]. Another recent study demonstrated benefits for mitochondrial function of kolaviron, a biflavonoid found in the seeds of *Garcinia kola* [66]. Kolaviron is able to reverse mitochondrial electron transport chain dysfunction after brain ischemia/reperfusion injury. In this sense, authors conclude that "kolaviron ... is a promising candidate for drug development against stroke" [67]. What remains to be established are the details of the mode of action of kolaviron, for instance, which is the targeted mitochondrial complex: I, II, III or IV.

7. Conclusions

Plant antioxidant action for the benefit of human health/well-being may occur by a variety of mechanisms. As in the case of therapeutic drugs, industry has to address the mode of action of "antioxidants". Direct mechanisms include quick REDOX reactions occurring locally but, also, the action of a given compound that after blood-mediated distribution into a target tissue participates in an enzyme-catalyzed REDOX reaction.

Indirect mechanisms, more difficult to measure but with significant potential to help in development of the industry of plant supplements and nutraceuticals, include actions such as boosting innate mechanisms of detoxification. Hormetic processes, also indirect, should be considered since plant derivatives may provide pro-oxidants able to upregulate the expression of enzymes of innate detox pathways or, alternatively, regulators of the expression of vitagenes (as defined in [48]).

Finally, it is likely that molecules present in chloroplast and mitochondria of plant cells (and therefore in plant extracts) may reach the mitochondria of mammalian cells to make electron transport and oxidative phosphorylation more efficient. One of the causes of oxidative stress is malfunctioning of mitochondria due to a disease and/or to aging.

Nutraceutical industry, focusing more on mechanisms, could select the best candidates from the myriad of plant-derived molecules that can be divided as more beneficious or as detrimental (or less beneficious). Furthermore, the industry must consider that, often, in vitro measured antioxidant power does not correlate with antioxidant action at the physiological level.

Author Contributions: R.F., G.N. and E.M.-P. scanned the literature, retrieved and processed papers referenced in the review. R.F. compiled all the information and wrote the first version of the manuscript. G.N. and E.M.-P. critically read the manuscript, prepared a second version and the tables/figures in all versions of the paper. All authors edited the manuscript and revised the final submitted version.

Funding: This research received no external funding.

Acknowledgments: In Memoriam: Adela Mazo, a brilliant chemistry student, a master of REDOX chemistry and stunning as colleague. In Memoriam: Jesús (Suso) Pintor who produced stunning papers and was as good as scientist as a person (we miss you Suso). We acknowledge the inspiring work of Vince Gilligan and his team, especially for this quote: "I simply respect Chemistry. Chemistry must be respected"—Walter White. Anything good or bad occurring in life has a common factor: Chemistry.

Conflicts of Interest: The authors declare no conflict of interest.

References

1. Franco, R.; Martínez-Pinilla, E. Chemical rules on the assessment of antioxidant potential in food and food additives aimed at reducing oxidative stress and neurodegeneration. *Food Chem.* **2017**, *235*, 318–323. [CrossRef] [PubMed]
2. Hardy, K.; Buckley, S.; Collins, M.J.; Estalrrich, A.; Brothwell, D.; Copeland, L.; García-Tabernero, A.; García-Vargas, S.; de la Rasilla, M.; Lalueza-Fox, C.; et al. Neanderthal medics? Evidence for food, cooking, and medicinal plants entrapped in dental calculus. *Naturwissenschaften* **2012**, *99*, 617–626. [CrossRef] [PubMed]
3. Weyrich, L.S.; Duchene, S.; Soubrier, J.; Arriola, L.; Llamas, B.; Breen, J.; Morris, A.G.; Alt, K.W.; Caramelli, D.; Dresely, V.; et al. Neanderthal behaviour, diet, and disease inferred from ancient DNA in dental calculus. *Nature* **2017**, *544*, 357–361. [CrossRef]
4. Milton, K. Nutritional characteristics of wild primate foods: Do the diets of our closest living relatives have lessons for us? *Nutrition* **1999**, *15*, 488–498. [CrossRef]
5. Milton, K. Back to basics: Why foods of wild primates have relevance for modern human health. *Nutrition* **2000**, *16*, 480–483. [CrossRef]
6. Cordain, L.; Eaton, S.B.; Sebastian, A.; Mann, N.; Lindeberg, S.; Watkins, B.A.; O'Keefe, J.H.; Brand-Miller, J. Origins and evolution of the Western diet: Health implications for the 21st century. *Am. J. Clin. Nutr.* **2005**, *81*, 341–354. [CrossRef]

7. García-Arroyo, F.E.; Gonzaga, G.; Muñoz-Jiménez, I.; Osorio-Alonso, H.; Iroz, A.; Vecchio, M.; Tapia, E.; Roncal-Jiménez, C.A.; Johnson, R.J.; Sánchez-Lozada, L.G. Antioxidant supplements as a novel mean for blocking recurrent heat stress-induced kidney damage following rehydration with fructose-containing beverages. *Free Radic. Biol. Med.* **2019**, *141*, 182–191. [CrossRef]
8. Girard, A.; Madani, S.; Boukortt, F.; Cherkaoui-Malki, M.; Belleville, J.; Prost, J. Fructose-enriched diet modifies antioxidant status and lipid metabolism in spontaneously hypertensive rats. *Nutrition* **2006**, *22*, 758–766. [CrossRef]
9. Song, M.; Schuschke, D.A.; Zhou, Z.; Chen, T.; Pierce, W.M.; Wang, R.; Johnson, W.T.; McClain, C.J. High fructose feeding induces copper deficiency in Sprague-Dawley rats: A novel mechanism for obesity related fatty liver. *J. Hepatol.* **2012**, *56*, 433–440. [CrossRef]
10. Tappy, L.; Lê, K.A.; Tran, C.; Paquot, N. Fructose and metabolic diseases: New findings, new questions. *Nutrition* **2010**, *26*, 1044–1049. [CrossRef]
11. Bray, G.A. Energy and Fructose From Beverages Sweetened With Sugar or High-Fructose Corn Syrup Pose a Health Risk for Some People. *Adv. Nutr.* **2013**, *4*, 220–225. [CrossRef] [PubMed]
12. Feinman, R.D.; Fine, E.J. Fructose in perspective. *Nutr. Metab.* **2013**, *10*, 45. [CrossRef] [PubMed]
13. Jensen, T.; Abdelmalek, M.F.; Sullivan, S.; Nadeau, K.J.; Green, M.; Roncal, C.; Nakagawa, T.; Kuwabara, M.; Sato, Y.; Kang, D.-H.; et al. Fructose and sugar: A major mediator of non-alcoholic fatty liver disease. *J. Hepatol.* **2018**, *68*, 1063–1075. [CrossRef] [PubMed]
14. Van Buul, V.J.; Tappy, L.; Brouns, F.J.P.H. Misconceptions about fructose-containing sugars and their role in the obesity epidemic. *Nutr. Res. Rev.* **2014**, *27*, 119–130. [CrossRef] [PubMed]
15. Nakagawa, T.; Hu, H.; Zharikov, S.; Tuttle, K.R.; Short, R.A.; Glushakova, O.; Ouyang, X.; Feig, D.I.; Block, E.R.; Herrera-Acosta, J.; et al. A causal role for uric acid in fructose-induced metabolic syndrome. *Am. J. Physiol. Physiol.* **2006**, *290*, F625–F631. [CrossRef] [PubMed]
16. Sánchez-Lozada, L.G.; Mu, W.; Roncal, C.; Sautin, Y.Y.; Abdelmalek, M.; Reungjui, S.; Le, M.; Nakagawa, T.; Lan, H.Y.; Yu, X.; et al. Comparison of free fructose and glucose to sucrose in the ability to cause fatty liver. *Eur. J. Nutr.* **2010**, *49*, 1–9. [CrossRef] [PubMed]
17. Castro, M.C.; Massa, M.L.; Arbeláez, L.G.; Schinella, G.; Gagliardino, J.J.; Francini, F. Fructose-induced inflammation, insulin resistance and oxidative stress: A liver pathological triad effectively disrupted by lipoic acid. *Life Sci.* **2015**, *137*, 1–6. [CrossRef] [PubMed]
18. Cydylo, M.A.; Davis, A.T.; Kavanagh, K. Fatty liver promotes fibrosis in monkeys consuming high fructose. *Obesity* **2017**, *25*, 290–293. [CrossRef] [PubMed]
19. Bremer, A.A.; Stanhope, K.L.; Graham, J.L.; Cummings, B.P.; Wang, W.; Saville, B.R.; Havel, P.J. Fructose-fed rhesus monkeys: A nonhuman primate model of insulin resistance, metabolic syndrome, and type 2 diabetes. *Clin. Transl. Sci.* **2011**, *4*, 243–252. [CrossRef]
20. Schwitzer, C.; Polowinsky, S.Y.; Solman, C. Fruits as foods-common misconceptions about frugivory. In *Zoo Animal Nutrition IV*; Clauss, M., Fidgett, A., Janssens, J., Hatt, J.-M., Huisman, T., Hummel, J., Nijboer, J., Plowman, A., Eds.; Filander Verlag: Fürth, Germany, 2008; pp. 131–168.
21. Nagase, M.; Yamamoto, Y.; Matsumoto, N.; Arai, Y.; Hirose, N. Increased oxidative stress and coenzyme Q10 deficiency in centenarians. *J. Clin. Biochem. Nutr.* **2018**, *63*, 129–136. [CrossRef]
22. Rembold, C.M. Coenzyme Q10 Supplementation in Orthostatic Hypotension and Multiple-System Atrophy: A Report on 7 Cases. *Am. J. Med.* **2018**, *131*, 444–446. [CrossRef] [PubMed]
23. Sourris, K.C.; Harcourt, B.E.; Tang, P.H.; Morley, A.L.; Huynh, K.; Penfold, S.A.; Coughlan, M.T.; Cooper, M.E.; Nguyen, T.-V.; Ritchie, R.H.; et al. Ubiquinone (coenzyme Q10) prevents renal mitochondrial dysfunction in an experimental model of type 2 diabetes. *Free Radic. Biol. Med.* **2012**, *52*, 716–723. [CrossRef] [PubMed]
24. Zhang, Y.; Liu, J.; Chen, X.-Q.; Oliver Chen, C.-Y. Ubiquinol is superior to ubiquinone to enhance Coenzyme Q10 status in older men. *Food Funct.* **2018**, *9*, 5653–5659. [CrossRef] [PubMed]
25. Rahimlou, M.; Asadi, M.; Banaei Jahromi, N.; Mansoori, A. Alpha-lipoic acid (ALA) supplementation effect on glycemic and inflammatory biomarkers: A Systematic Review and meta-analysis. *Clin. Nutr. ESPEN* **2019**, *32*, 16–28. [CrossRef] [PubMed]
26. Van Zwieten, R.; Verhoeven, A.J.; Roos, D. Inborn defects in the antioxidant systems of human red blood cells. *Free Radic. Biol. Med.* **2014**, *67*, 377–386. [CrossRef] [PubMed]
27. Luzzatto, L.; Nannelli, C.; Notaro, R. Glucose-6-Phosphate Dehydrogenase Deficiency. *Hematol. Oncol. Clin. North Am.* **2016**, *30*, 373–393. [CrossRef] [PubMed]

28. Ho, H.; Cheng, M.; Chiu, D.T. Glucose-6-phosphate dehydrogenase—from oxidative stress to cellular functions and degenerative diseases. *Redox Rep.* **2007**, *12*, 109–118. [CrossRef]
29. Baker, M.A.; Bosia, A.; Pescarmona, G.; Turrini, F.; Arese, P. Mechanism of Action of Divicine in a Cell-free System and in Glucose-6-phosphate Dehydrogenase-deficient Red Cells. *Toxicol. Pathol.* **1984**, *12*, 331–336. [CrossRef]
30. Vural, N.; Sardas, S. Biological activities of broad bean (*Vicia faba* L.) extracts cultivated in South Anatolia in favism sensitive subjects. *Toxicology* **1984**, *31*, 175–179. [CrossRef]
31. Mikulic-Petkovsek, M.; Schmitzer, V.; Slatnar, A.; Stampar, F.; Veberic, R. Composition of Sugars, Organic Acids, and Total Phenolics in 25 Wild or Cultivated Berry Species. *J. Food Sci.* **2012**, *77*, C1064–C1070. [CrossRef]
32. Simsek, S.; Ozcan, M.M.; Al Juhaimi, F.; ElBabiker, E.; Ghafoor, K. Amino Acid and Sugar Contents of Wild and Cultivated Carob (*Ceratonia siliqua*) Pods Collected in Different Harvest Periods. *Chem. Nat. Compd.* **2017**, *53*, 1008–1009. [CrossRef]
33. Ma, B.; Chen, J.; Zheng, H.; Fang, T.; Ogutu, C.; Li, S.; Han, Y.; Wu, B. Comparative assessment of sugar and malic acid composition in cultivated and wild apples. *Food Chem.* **2015**, *172*, 86–91. [CrossRef] [PubMed]
34. Tiwari, U.; Cummins, E. Factors influencing levels of phytochemicals in selected fruit and vegetables during pre- and post-harvest food processing operations. *Food Res. Int.* **2013**, *50*, 497–506. [CrossRef]
35. Kwon, O.; Eck, P.; Chen, S.; Corpe, C.P.; Lee, J.-H.; Kruhlak, M.; Levine, M. Inhibition of the intestinal glucose transporter GLUT2 by flavonoids. *FASEB J.* **2007**, *21*, 366–377. [CrossRef] [PubMed]
36. Lee, Y.; Lim, Y.; Kwon, O. Selected Phytochemicals and Culinary Plant Extracts Inhibit Fructose Uptake in Caco-2 Cells. *Molecules* **2015**, *20*, 17393–17404. [CrossRef] [PubMed]
37. Boncler, M.; Golanski, J.; Lukasiak, M.; Redzynia, M.; Dastych, J.; Watala, C. A new approach for the assessment of the toxicity of polyphenol-rich compounds with the use of high content screening analysis. *PLoS ONE* **2017**, *12*, e0180022. [CrossRef] [PubMed]
38. Cayman Chemical Co. Kaempferol Data Sheet. Available online: https://www.caymanchem.com/product/11852 (accessed on 26 August 2019).
39. Fogliano, V.; Corollaro, M.L.; Vitaglione, P.; Napolitano, A.; Ferracane, R.; Travaglia, F.; Arlorio, M.; Costabile, A.; Klinder, A.; Gibson, G. In vitro bioaccessibility and gut biotransformation of polyphenols present in the water-insoluble cocoa fraction. *Mol. Nutr. Food Res.* **2011**, *55*, S44–S55. [CrossRef] [PubMed]
40. Vitaglione, P.; Barone Lumaga, R.; Ferracane, R.; Sellitto, S.; Morelló, J.R.; Reguant Miranda, J.; Shimoni, E.; Fogliano, V. Human bioavailability of flavanols and phenolic acids from cocoa-nut creams enriched with free or microencapsulated cocoa polyphenols. *Br. J. Nutr.* **2013**, *109*, 1832–1843. [CrossRef]
41. Vitaglione, P.; Barone Lumaga, R.; Ferracane, R.; Radetsky, I.; Mennella, I.; Schettino, R.; Koder, S.; Shimoni, E.; Fogliano, V. Curcumin Bioavailability from Enriched Bread: The Effect of Microencapsulated Ingredients. *J. Agric. Food Chem.* **2012**, *60*, 3357–3366. [CrossRef]
42. Pellegrini, N.; Vitaglione, P.; Granato, D.; Fogliano, V. Twenty-five years of total antioxidant capacity measurement of foods and biological fluids: Merits and limitations. *J. Sci. Food Agric.* **2019**. [CrossRef]
43. Pham-Huy, L.A.; He, H.; Pham-Huy, C. Free radicals, antioxidants in disease and health. *Int. J. Biomed. Sci.* **2008**, *4*, 89–96. [PubMed]
44. Parmar, S.S.; Jaiwal, A.; Dhankher, O.P.; Jaiwal, P.K. Coenzyme Q10 production in plants: Current status and future prospects. *Crit. Rev. Biotechnol.* **2015**, *35*, 152–164. [CrossRef] [PubMed]
45. Calabrese, E.J. The threshold vs LNT showdown: Dose rate findings exposed flaws in the LNT model part 1. The Russell-Muller debate. *Environ. Res.* **2017**, *154*, 435–451. [CrossRef] [PubMed]
46. Morifuji, M.; Sakai, K.; Sanbongi, C.; Sugiura, K. Dietary whey protein downregulates fatty acid synthesis in the liver, but upregulates it in skeletal muscle of exercise-trained rats. *Nutrition* **2005**, *21*, 1052–1058. [CrossRef] [PubMed]
47. Masoro, E.J. Hormesis and the Antiaging Action of Dietary Restriction. *Exp. Gerontol.* **1998**, *33*, 61–66. [CrossRef]
48. Calabrese, V.; Cornelius, C.; Dinkova-Kostova, A.T.; Iavicoli, I.; Di Paola, R.; Koverech, A.; Cuzzocrea, S.; Rizzarelli, E.; Calabrese, E.J. Cellular stress responses, hormetic phytochemicals and vitagenes in aging and longevity. *Biochim. Biophys. Acta* **2012**, *1822*, 753–783. [CrossRef] [PubMed]
49. Rattan, S.I.S. The Nature of Gerontogenes and Vitagenes: Antiaging Effects of Repeated Heat Shock on Human Fibroblasts. *Ann. N. Y. Acad. Sci.* **1998**, *854*, 54–60. [CrossRef]

50. Rattan, S.I. Repeated mild heat shock delays ageing in cultured human skin fibroblasts. *Biochem. Mol. Biol. Int.* **1998**, *45*, 753–759. [CrossRef] [PubMed]
51. Thorpe, G.W.; Reodica, M.; Davies, M.J.; Heeren, G.; Jarolim, S.; Pillay, B.; Breitenbach, M.; Higgins, V.J.; Dawes, I.W. Superoxide radicals have a protective role during H_2O_2 stress. *Mol. Biol. Cell* **2013**, *24*, 2876–2884. [CrossRef]
52. Mane, N.R.; Gajare, K.A.; Deshmukh, A.A. Mild heat stress induces hormetic effects in protecting the primary culture of mouse prefrontal cerebrocortical neurons from neuropathological alterations. *IBRO Rep.* **2018**, *5*, 110–115. [CrossRef] [PubMed]
53. Labbadia, J.; Brielmann, R.M.; Neto, M.F.; Lin, Y.-F.; Haynes, C.M.; Morimoto, R.I. Mitochondrial Stress Restores the Heat Shock Response and Prevents Proteostasis Collapse during Aging. *Cell Rep.* **2017**, *21*, 1481–1494. [CrossRef] [PubMed]
54. Murakami, A. Dose-dependent functionality and toxicity of green tea polyphenols in experimental rodents. *Arch. Biochem. Biophys.* **2014**, *557*, 3–10. [CrossRef] [PubMed]
55. Murry, C.E.; Jennings, R.B.; Reimer, K.A. Preconditioning with ischemia: a delay of lethal cell injury in ischemic myocardium. *Circulation* **1986**, *74*, 1124–1136. [CrossRef] [PubMed]
56. Bartling, B.; Friedrich, I.; Silber, R.E.; Simm, A. Ischemic preconditioning is not cardioprotective in senescent human myocardium. *Ann. Thorac. Surg.* **2003**, *76*, 105–111. [CrossRef]
57. Simm, A.; Müller, B.; Nass, N.; Hofmann, B.; Bushnaq, H.; Silber, R.E.; Bartling, B. Protein glycation—Between tissue aging and protection. *Exp. Gerontol.* **2015**, *68*, 71–75. [CrossRef] [PubMed]
58. Rodriguez, M.; Snoek, L.B.; Riksen, J.A.G.; Bevers, R.P.; Kammenga, J.E. Genetic variation for stress-response hormesis in *C. elegans* lifespan. *Exp. Gerontol.* **2012**, *47*, 581–587. [CrossRef] [PubMed]
59. Sodagam, L.; Lewinska, A.; Kwasniewicz, E.; Kokhanovska, S.; Wnuk, M.; Siems, K.; Rattan, S.I.S. Phytochemicals Rosmarinic Acid, Ampelopsin, and Amorfrutin-A Can Modulate Age-Related Phenotype of Serially Passaged Human Skin Fibroblasts in vitro. *Front. Genet.* **2019**, *10*, 81. [CrossRef]
60. Uchitomi, R.; Nakai, S.; Matsuda, R.; Onishi, T.; Miura, S.; Hatazawa, Y.; Kamei, Y. Genistein, daidzein, and resveratrols stimulate PGC-1β-mediated gene expression. *Biochem. Biophys. Rep.* **2019**, *17*, 51–55. [CrossRef]
61. Atlante, A.; Bobba, A.; Paventi, G.; Pizzuto, R.; Passarella, S. Genistein and daidzein prevent low potassium-dependent apoptosis of cerebellar granule cells. *Biochem. Pharmacol.* **2010**, *79*, 758–767. [CrossRef]
62. Sandoval-Acuña, C.; Ferreira, J.; Speisky, H. Polyphenols and mitochondria: An update on their increasingly emerging ROS-scavenging independent actions. *Arch. Biochem. Biophys.* **2014**, *559*, 75–90. [CrossRef]
63. Wood dos Santos, T.; Cristina Pereira, Q.; Teixeira, L.; Gambero, A.; A. Villena, J.; Lima Ribeiro, M. Effects of Polyphenols on Thermogenesis and Mitochondrial Biogenesis. *Int. J. Mol. Sci.* **2018**, *19*, 2757. [CrossRef] [PubMed]
64. Mouria, M.; Gukovskaya, A.S.; Jung, Y.; Buechler, P.; Hines, O.J.; Reber, H.A.; Pandol, S.J. Food-derived polyphenols inhibit pancreatic cancer growth through mitochondrial cytochrome C release and apoptosis. *Int. J. Cancer* **2002**, *98*, 761–769. [CrossRef] [PubMed]
65. Dave, A.; Shukla, F.; Wala, H.; Pillai, P. Mitochondrial Electron Transport Chain Complex Dysfunction in MeCP2 Knock-Down Astrocytes: Protective Effects of Quercetin Hydrate. *J. Mol. Neurosci.* **2019**, *67*, 16–27. [CrossRef] [PubMed]
66. Farombi, E.O.; Adedara, I.A.; Ajayi, B.O.; Ayepola, O.R.; Egbeme, E.E. Kolaviron, a Natural Antioxidant and Anti-Inflammatory Phytochemical Prevents Dextran Sulphate Sodium-Induced Colitis in Rats. *Basic Clin. Pharmacol. Toxicol.* **2013**, *113*, 49–55. [CrossRef] [PubMed]
67. Ojo, O.B.; Amoo, Z.A.; Saliu, I.O.; Olaleye, M.T.; Farombi, E.O.; Akinmoladun, A.C. Neurotherapeutic potential of kolaviron on neurotransmitter dysregulation, excitotoxicity, mitochondrial electron transport chain dysfunction and redox imbalance in 2-VO brain ischemia/reperfusion injury. *Biomed. Pharmacother.* **2019**, *111*, 859–872. [CrossRef] [PubMed]

© 2019 by the authors. Licensee MDPI, Basel, Switzerland. This article is an open access article distributed under the terms and conditions of the Creative Commons Attribution (CC BY) license (http://creativecommons.org/licenses/by/4.0/).

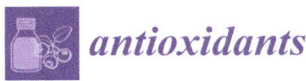

Article

The Skin-Whitening Effects of Ectoine via the Suppression of α-MSH-Stimulated Melanogenesis and the Activation of Antioxidant Nrf2 Pathways in UVA-Irradiated Keratinocytes

You-Cheng Hseu [1,2,3,4], Xuan-Zao Chen [1], Yugandhar Vudhya Gowrisankar [1], Hung-Rong Yen [3,4,5,6], Jing-Yuan Chuang [7] and Hsin-Ling Yang [8,*]

[1] Department of Cosmeceutics, College of Biopharmaceutical and Food Sciences, China Medical University, Taichung 40402, Taiwan; ychseu@mail.cmu.edu.tw (Y.-C.H.); x28753281@gmail.com (X.-Z.C.); dr.vgyugandhar@mail.cmu.edu.tw (Y.V.G.)
[2] Department of Health and Nutrition Biotechnology, Asia University, Taichung 41354, Taiwan
[3] Chinese Medicine Research Center, China Medical University, Taichung 40402, Taiwan; hungrongyen@gmail.com
[4] Research Center of Chinese Herbal Medicine, China Medical University, Taichung 40402, Taiwan
[5] Department of Medical Research, China Medical University Hospital, Taichung 40402, Taiwan
[6] School of Chinese Medicine, China Medical University, Taichung 40402, Taiwan
[7] Department of Medical Laboratory Science and Biotechnology, China Medical University, Taichung 40402, Taiwan; jychuang@mail.cmu.edu.tw
[8] Institute of Nutrition, College of Biopharmaceutical and Food Sciences, China Medical University, 91 Hsueh-Shih Road, Taichung 40402, Taiwan
* Correspondence: hlyang@mail.cmu.edu.tw

Received: 23 December 2019; Accepted: 8 January 2020; Published: 10 January 2020

Abstract: Ultraviolet A (UVA)-irradiation induced reactive oxygen species (ROS) production mediates excessive melanogenesis in skin cells leading to pigmentation. We demonstrated the depigmenting and anti-melanogenic effects of Ectoine, a natural bacterial osmolyte, in UVA-irradiated human (HaCaT) keratinocytes, and the underlying molecular mechanisms were elucidated. HaCaT cells were pre-treated with low concentrations of Ectoine (0.5–1.5 µM) and assayed for various depigmenting and anti-melanogenic parameters. This pre-treatment significantly downregulated ROS generation, α-melanocyte-stimulating hormone (α-MSH) production, and proopiomelanocortin (POMC) expression in UVA-irradiated HaCaT cells. Also, antioxidant heme oxygenase-1 (HO-1), NAD(P)H dehydrogenase [quinone 1] (NQO-1), and γ-glutamate-cysteine ligase catalytic subunit (γ-GCLC) protein expressions were mediated via the nuclear translocation of nuclear factor erythroid 2-related factor 2 (Nrf2) whose knockdown indeed impaired this effect signifying the importance of the Nrf2 pathway. Ectoine was mediating the activation of Nrf2 via the p38, protein kinase B (also known as AKT), protein kinase C (PKC), and casein kinase II protein kinase (CKII) pathways. The conditioned medium obtained from the Ectoine pre-treated and UVA-irradiated HaCaT cells downregulated the tyrosinase, tyrosinase-related protein-1 and -2 (TRP-1/-2), cyclic AMP (c-AMP) protein kinase, c-AMP response element-binding protein (CREB), and microphthalmia-associated transcription factor (MITF) expressions leading to melanoma B16F10 cells having inhibited melanin synthesis. Interestingly, this anti-melanogenic effect in α-MSH-stimulated B16F10 cells was observable only at 50–400 µM concentrations of Ectoine, signifying the key role played by Ectoine (0.5–1 µM)-treated keratinocytes in skin whitening effects. We concluded that Ectoine could be used as an effective topical natural cosmetic agent with depigmenting and anti-melanogenic efficacy.

Keywords: Ectoine; keratinocytes; melanogenesis; tyrosinase; α-MSH; Nrf2

1. Introduction

Exposing human skin to UVA radiation triggers ROS generation and also over-producing melanin in the skin cells. The uncontrolled production of ROS could lead to melanoma conditions as well. Most skin whitening agents are targeting and trying to minimize the melanogenesis process through the inhibition of α-MSH and tyrosinase productions [1]. Most skin-tone lightening creams are composed of hydroquinone [2] or hydrocortisone [3], that are known to decrease the formation of melanin, but are also associated with severe side effects. For example, acne, flaky and itchy skin, blue and black discoloration of the skin, ochronosis, burning and stinging, skin irritation, and even inflammation. However, skin whitening agents from the natural sources, for example, Kojic acid (a fungal derivative obtained from *Penicillium* and *Aspergillus* species) is also reported to cause 'contact dermatitis' in individuals who have sensitive skin. In these individuals, more than 1% of kojic acid could cause severe hypersensitive side effects [4,5]. Therefore, only a few naturally derived skin whitening products (oleosin, licorice extract, ascorbic acid, soy protein, and N-acetyl glucosamine, etc.) are currently being used in the cosmetic industry [6]. However, the skincare products that are principally targeting the depigmenting properties have at times failed to focus on counteracting the deleterious effects posed by the UVA irradiation-induced ROS production mediated excess melanogenesis in skin cells.

Ectoine is a 'natural extremolyte' produced from several species of microorganisms under stressful conditions [7,8]. This compound was first isolated from the *Ectothiorhodospira* species of bacteria that are living in the Egyptian desert. The cascade of *ect* operon genes (*ect*A, *ect*B, *ect*C, or *ect*D) are involved in the production of this compound. Ectoine is chemically designated as 1,4,5,6-tetrahydro-2-methyl-4-pyrimidinecarboxylic acid [9]. As a moisture binder, Ectoine helps in, restructuring of the skin cell membrane [10], protection from UV damage and pollution [11,12], moisturizing the skin [13], delaying the premature skin aging [14], etc. In addition to the skin protective roles, Ectoine has been shown to be useful in the treatment of atopic dermatitis [15], Alzheimer's [16], as well as the inhibition of HIV replication [17], radio and chemotherapy [18], and liver cirrhosis [19]. Ectoine is speculated to exhibit its depigmenting and skin whitening properties without causing undesirable side effects [20]. Contrastingly, the molecular mechanisms elicited by Ectoine are not known. Therefore, the objective of this study was to delineate the Ectoine mediated depigmenting and anti-melanogenic mechanisms elicited in UVA-irradiated human (HaCaT) keratinocytes as the cellular model system. The effect of Ectoine induced secretions of skin-protecting agents from the HaCaT cells to the culture medium (conditioned medium) was also tested using a typical melanoma cell (B16F10) line as well.

2. Materials and Methods

2.1. Reagents and Antibodies

Ectoine (Product no: 81619, purity ≥ 95%) was purchased from Sigma-Aldrich (Taufkichen, Germany). Fetal bovine serum (FBS), penicillin/streptomycin, Dulbecco's modified Eagle's medium (DMEM) and L-glutamine were bought from Invitrogen/Gibco BRL (Carlsbad, CA, USA). L-DOPA, melanin, 3-4,5-dimethyl-2-yl-2,5-diphenyl tetrazolium bromide (MTT), and α-MSH were procured from Sigma Chemical Co (St. Louis, MO, USA). N-acetylcysteine (NAC) and 2′,7′-dichlorofluorescein-diacetate ($DCFH_2$-DA) were procured from Sigma-Aldrich (St. Louis, MO, USA). All pharmacological inhibitors required for JNK (SP600125), ERK1/2 (PD98059), p38 (SB203580), PKC (GF109203X), and CKII were obtained from Calbiochem (La Jolla, CA, USA) PI3K/AKT inhibitor (LY294002) was obtained from Sigma-Aldrich (St. Louis, MO, USA). All antibodies for POMC, CREB, β-actin, tyrosinase, Nrf2, p-CREB, NQO-1, PKC, Kelch-like ECH-associated protein-1 (Keap-1), and TRP-1, TRP-2 were obtained from Santa Cruz Biotechnology Inc. (Heidelberg, Germany). Antibodies against γ-GCLC and HO-1 were procured from Gene Tex Inc. (San Antonio, TX, USA). We obtained antibodies against c-AMP protein kinase and CKII from Abcam (Cambridge, MA, USA). Histones, MITF, p-p38, p38, p-AKT, and AKT were obtained from Cell Signal Technology (Beverly, MA, USA).

Enhanced chemiluminescence (ECL) detection reagents were obtained from Millipore, (Billerica, MA, USA). All other reagents (at HPLC grade) were either purchased from Sigma-Aldrich or Merck & Co., Inc. (Darmstadt, Germany).

2.2. Cell Culture

We obtained immortalized human skin keratinocyte HaCaT and murine melanoma B16F10 cells from both Cell Line Services (CLS, Eppelheim, Germany) and American Type Culture Collection (ATCC, VA, USA). The cells were cultured in DMEM supplemented with 10% heat-activated FBS, 1% streptomycin/penicillin, and 2 mM L-glutamine in a humidified incubator supplemented with 5% CO_2 at 37 °C.

2.3. Cell Treatments and UVA-Irradiation

Before UVA irradiation, the cells were pre-treated with Ectoine (0.5–1.5 µM for 24 h) or vehicle (PBS). Post incubation, PBS washed cells were exposed to 3 J/cm^2 UVA radiations (for 27 min, λ_{max}, 365 nm, no detectable emissions below 320 nm) using the UV CROSS-LINKER CL-508 (UVItec, Cambridge, UK) [21].

2.4. Cell Viability Assay

HaCaT cells (5×10^4 cells/well) were seeded in a 24-well plate containing DMEM and supplemented with 10% FBS and varying concentrations of Ectoine (0.5–1.5 µM, 24 h). Then it was irradiated in the absence or presence of UVA (3 J/cm^2). B16F10 cells (5×10^4 cells/well) were seeded in a 24-well plate containing DMEM and supplemented with 10% FBS and varying concentrations of Ectoine (100–400 µM, 72 h). The cells were washed with PBS and an MTT cell viability assay was conducted [21].

2.5. Intracellular ROS Assay

HaCaT cells were seeded at a density of 1.5×10^5 in 8-well Lab Teck chamber containing DMEM supplemented with 10% FBS and were grown to 80% confluence. These cells were first treated with 1.5 µM Ectoine, followed by exposure to 3 J/cm^2 UVA irradiation for the prescribed amount of time. Cells were washed with PBS and $DCFH_2$-DA method was used to determine the intracellular ROS production using the Olympus Software solution software for each condition [21].

2.6. Melanin Quantification

In a 6-well plate, murine melanoma B16F10 cells were seeded at a density of 2.5×10^5 cells/well. They were pre-treated with 100, 200, and 400 µM of Ectoine for 2 h in the absence or presence of α-MSH (1 µM). The protocol used for the quantification of melanin followed a previously described method [21]. We measured melanin content with the ELISA microplate reader with an absorbance wavelength of 470 nm.

2.7. Western Blot

HaCaT (1×10^6 cells/10 cm dish) or B16F10 (1×10^6 cells/10 cm dish) cells were pre-treated with varying concentrations of Ectoine (0.5, 1, and 1.5 µM) or α-MSH (1 µM) followed by irradiation in the absence or presence of UVA for the prescribed amount of time. PBS washed cells were harvested, the protein content (nuclear and cytosolic) was isolated after treatment. Then, the cells were subjected to the Western blot method used previously for the determination of expressions of various nuclear and cytosolic proteins [21].

2.8. RNA Extraction and RT-PCR

Ectoine pre-treated (1.5 µM, 24 h) HaCaT cells were subjected to the TRIzol reagent (Invitrogen, Carlsbad) for the isolation of total RNA from these cells. 1 µg of total RNA and the reagents supplied by the SuperScript-III One-Step RT-PCR platinum *Taq* kit (Invitrogen, Carlsbad) were used in the PCR experiment with the Bio-Rad iCycler PCR instrument (Bio-Rad, Hercules, CA, United States). The forward and reverse primers for Nrf2 used were: F: 5′-AAACCAGTGGATCTGCCAAC-3′, R-5′-GCAATGAAGACTGGGCTCTC-3′. The forward and reverse primers for GAPDH used were: F: 5′-GCATCCTGGGCTACACTGA-3′, R: 5′-CCACCACCCTGTTGCTGTA-3′. At the end of the experiment, PCR product was analyzed using 1% agarose gel. Then, it was visualized with ethidium bromide staining. As an internal control, we used GAPDH [22].

2.9. Immunofluorescence Assay

HaCaT cells were cultured at a density of 1×10^4 cells/well in DMEM supplement with 10% FBS in an 8-well Lab Tek chamber (Thermo Fisher Scientific, Waltham, MA, USA). We pretreated the cells with 1.5 µM Ectoine for the indicated time followed by irradiation in the absence or presence of UVA. The cells were subjected to an immunofluorescence assay, which uses a method previously described [21].

2.10. siRNA Transfection

For siRNA transfection, HaCaT cells were plated in a 6-well plate and were grown till it has reached a confluence of 40–60% at the time of transfection. The remaining protocol was followed according to a method that was explained before [21].

2.11. Statistical Analysis

We used the mean ± standard deviation (mean ± SD) for all the results used in this study. All data were analyzed with an analysis of variance (ANOVA), followed by Dunnett's test for pair-wise comparisons and presented as mean ± SD of three or more independent experiments. Statistical significance was set at * $p < 0.05$; ** $p < 0.01$; *** $p < 0.001$ when compared with untreated control cells, and # $p < 0.05$; ## $p < 0.01$; ### $p < 0.001$ when compared with the UVA-exposed HaCaT cells or α-MSH treated B16F10 cells.

3. Results

3.1. Ectoine Inhibited UVA-Induced ROS Generation in HaCaT Cells

First, we tested for the cytotoxic effects of Ectoine (Figure 1A) on UVA-irradiated HaCaT cells. Our MTT data indicated that when compared to the untreated control cells, Ectoine pre-treated (0.5–1.5 µM) and 3 J/cm^2 UVA exposed HaCaT cells were unable to show a significant decrease in cell viability (Figure 1B). Further, Ectoine pretreatment attenuated the UVA (3 J/cm^2)-induced cell death in a dose-dependent manner (Figure 1B). In addition to our fluorescence data, which indicated that, when compared to the control cells, 3 J/cm^2 UVA irradiation and Ectoine alone treatments (1.5 µM) significantly upregulated ROS levels by 5- and 2-fold, respectively. However, in the case of Ectoine pretreatment ROS levels were significantly downregulated and we can infer that Ectoine has an antioxidant effect against UVA irradiation. This also induces basal levels of ROS in HaCaT cells (Figure 1C,D).

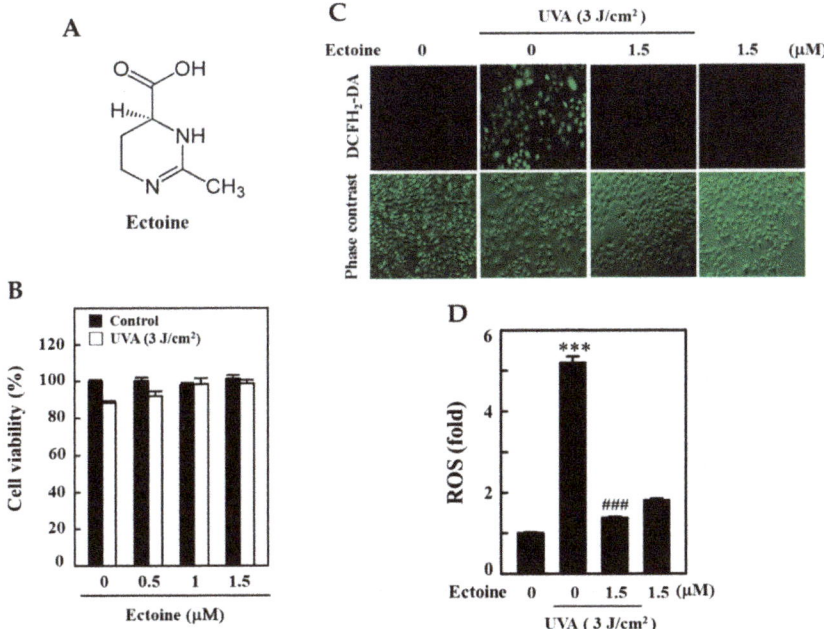

Figure 1. Ectoine inhibits UVA-induced ROS production in human keratinocyte (HaCaT) cells. (**A**) Ectoine's chemical structure. (**B**) To determine cell viability, an MTT assay was used. Cells were treated with Ectoine (0.5, 1, and 1.5 µM) for 24 h. Then, they were irradiated with 3 J/cm² or without UVA. (**C,D**) Cells were pre-treated with Ectoine (0 or 1.5 µM) for 24 h and then irradiated with 3 J/cm² or without UVA. For each condition, we used the percentage of the fluorescence intensity of the DCF-stained cells as determined by Olympus Softimage. Statistical significance was assigned as *** $p < 0.001$ compared to the untreated control cells and ### $p < 0.001$ compared to the UVA-exposed HaCaT cells.

3.2. Ectoine Suppressed POMC and α-MSH Expressions in UVA-Irradiated HaCaT Cells

UVA exposed keratinocytes were stimulated for their ROS-p53 mediated POMC and also a small peptide hormone α-MSH that is derived from POMC [23]. Therefore, we determined the alterations in expression patterns of α-MSH, POMC, and other associated proteins in Ectoine pre-treated HaCaT cells and then exposed them to UVA (3 J/cm²). Western blot data indicated that UVA-induced upregulation of α-MSH and POMC expressions were downregulated by Ectoine pretreatment; whereas, Ectoine treatment without UVA irradiation has completely inhibited the α-MSH and POMC expressions of non-irradiated HaCaT cells (Figure 2A). Later, we tested the effect of 'conditioned-medium' (10 mL/100 mm plate), obtained from the Ectoine pre-treated and UVA irradiated HaCaT cells, on the melanogenesis of B16F10 melanoma cells. Figure 2B shows this conditioned medium downregulated the tyrosinase, TRP-1, TRP-2, c-AMP protein kinase, p-CREB, CREB, and MITF levels in B16F10 cells.

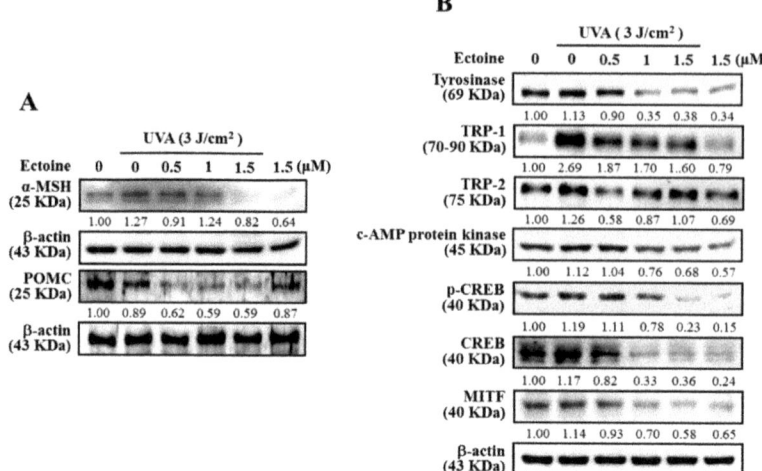

Figure 2. Ectoine suppresses UVA-induced POMC and α-MSH expression in HaCaT cells. (**A**) Western blotting showed us protein levels of α-MSH and POMC. Cells were pre-treated with Ectoine (0–1.5 µM) for 24 h and then irradiated or not with 3 J/cm² UVA. (**B**) Effect of HaCaT conditioned medium on B16F10 cells melanin synthesis. HaCaT cells were pre-treated with vehicle (PBS) or Ectoine (0.5–1.5 µM) for 24 h. Subsequently, these cells were exposed or non-exposed to the 3 J/cm² UVA-irradiation. After 1–24 h, the conditioned medium (10 mL/100 mm dish) was collected and tested on B16F10 cells for the expression of various proteins through western blot method. Lanes 1 and 2 were indicating the experimental conditions of conditioned medium obtained from vehicle (PBS) pre-treated and UVA non exposed (lane #1) and exposed (lane #2). Whereas, lanes 3–5, and 6 were indicating the experimental conditions of conditioned medium obtained from Ectoine pre-treated (0.5–1.5 µM) and UVA exposed, and non-exposed, respectively. Western blot analysis measured the protein levels of tyrosinase, TRP-1, TRP-2 (for 24 h), c-AMP protein kinase (for 1 h), p-CREB, CREB (for 2 h), and MITF (for 4 h).

3.3. Ectoine Downregulated Melanin and Tyrosinase Expression in α-MSH-Stimulated B16F10 Cells

B16F10 melanoma cells were first subjected to the higher concentrations of Ectoine and the effect of cytotoxicity was determined using MTT assay. Figure 3A shows that Ectoine had no significant impact on the viability of B16F10 cells at higher concentrations (100–400 µM for 72 h). However, cell viability was not effected at 24 and 48 h of Ectoine treatment (data not shown). Therefore, these concentrations were used to determine the effect of Ectoine on α-MSH-stimulated melanogenesis in B16F10 cells. Melanin quantification data showed that, compared to the control cells, treatment with α-MSH (1 µM) alone significantly upregulated the melanin levels by more than 25%. However, compared to α-MSH alone treatment, cells exposed to increasing concentrations of Ectoine (100–400 µM at 72 h) dose-dependently and significantly downregulated the percentage of melanin content with maximum downregulation of only 85% (or −15% than untreated control) was observed at 400 µM of Ectoine pretreatment (Figure 3B). Moreover, our Western blot data also showed that α-MSH stimulated tyrosinase (24 h) and p-CREB (2 h) expressions were significantly downregulated with increasing concentrations of Ectoine pretreatments in these melanoma cells (Figure 3C).

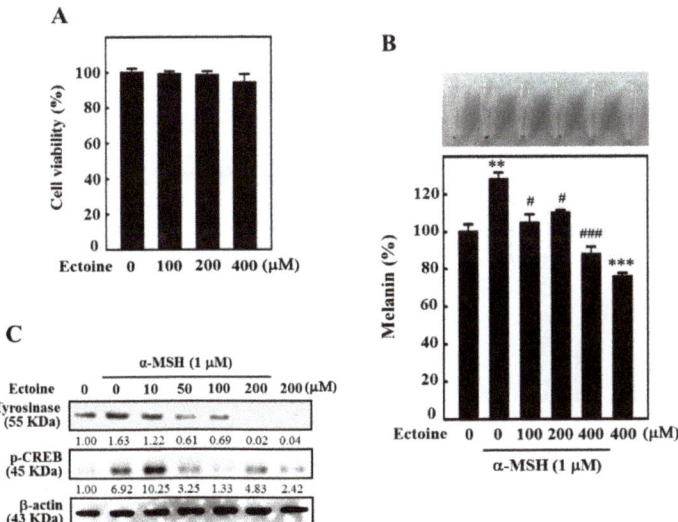

Figure 3. Ectoine downregulated the melanogenesis in α-MSH-stimulated B16F10 cells. (**A**) High concentrations of Ectoine (100–400 μM, 72 h) affect the cell viability of B16F10 as determined by an MTT assay. (**B**) Cells were pre-treated with Ectoine (0–400 μM, 1 h) followed by stimulation without or with 1 μM α-MSH for 72 h. The percentage of melanin content was quantified from total cell lysates. (**C**) Cells were pre-treated with Ectoine (0–200 μM for 1 h) and then treated with or without α-MSH (1 μM) for 24 or 2 h. Western blot analysis measured the expressions of tyrosinase and p-CREB proteins. Statistical significance was assigned as ** $p < 0.01$; *** $p < 0.001$ compared to the untreated control cells and # $p < 0.05$, ### $p < 0.001$ compared to the α-MSH treated B16F10 cells.

3.4. Ectoine Facilitated Nrf2 Nuclear Translocation in HaCaT Cells

Nrf2-Keap-1 is an important cytoprotective pathway that protects the skin cells from ROS and electrophile insult caused by UVA exposure. Nrf2 and Keap1 maintain a stoichiometric ratio in the cytoplasm. In a cytoprotective pathway, Nrf2 dissociates from Keap-1 and, for the expression of various antioxidant genes, translocate to the cellular nucleus. Therefore, the ratio of Nrf2/Keap-1 is a key factor. Here, our Western blot data indicated a shift in the ratio of Nrf2/Keap-1 that was towards more Nrf2 expression with the increasing concentrations of Ectoine, signifying that Ectoine favors the nuclear translocation of Nrf2 in HaCaT cells (Figure 4A,B). Also, the expression of Nrf2 mRNA levels was shown to be significantly elevated in the 1.5 μM Ectoine pre-treated cells (Figure 4C). This was also consistent with our fluorescence image data (Figure 4D).

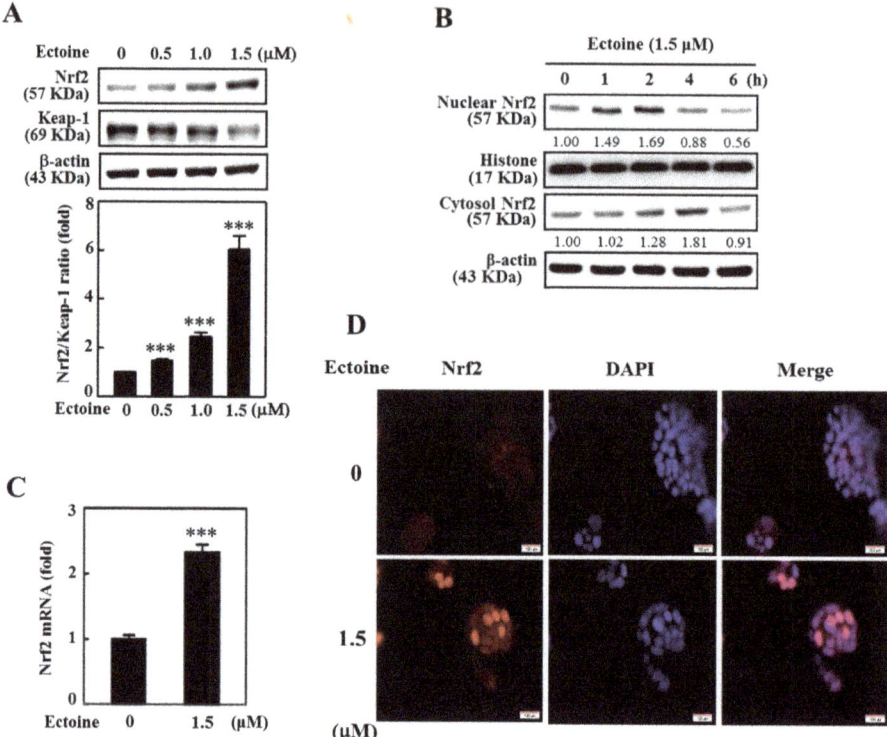

Figure 4. Ectoine upregulated the nuclear translocation of antioxidant marker Nrf2 in HaCaT cells. (**A**) Effect of Ectoine on protein expressions of Nrf2 and Keap-1 in HaCaT cells. Western blot method measured the expressions of Nrf2 and Keap-1 in cells treated with Ectoine (0–1.5 µM) for 2 h (**B**) Effect of time on the Ectoine mediated nuclear and cytosolic expressions of Nrf2. Cells were exposed to 1.5 µM Ectoine for different time points and Western blot method measured the expressions of nuclear and cytosolic Nrf2. (**C**) Cells were pre-treated with Ectoine (1.5 µM, 1 h) followed by the isolation of total mRNA from HaCaT cells. 1 µg of total mRNA was used to measure the expression of the Nrf2 gene through the RT-PCR method. As an internal control, GAPDH was used. (**D**) Immunofluorescence staining of HaCaT cells. Cells were treated with 1.5 µM of Ectoine for 2 h and the nuclear localization of Nrf2 were visualized by immunofluorescence method. Cells were stained with DAPI (1 µg/mL) for 5 min and examined by fluorescence microscopy (scale bar 100 µM). Statistical significance was assigned as *** $p < 0.001$ compared to the untreated control cells.

3.5. Ectoine Upregulated the Expression of HO-1, NQO-1, and γ-GCLC Proteins in HaCaT Cells

To determine the effect of time on Ectoine mediated nuclear translocation of Nrf2 and the subsequent downstream expression of HO-1, NQO-1, and γ-GCLC proteins, HaCaT cells were exposed to 1.5 µM Ectoine and the cellular proteins were harvested 0.5, 1, 2, 4, 8, or 12 h after the Ectoine treatment. Western blot data indicated that, except for the γ-GCLC protein, 1.5 µM Ectoine caused the maximum expression of HO-1, Nrf2, and NQO-1 proteins at the 4 h time point. γ-GCLC was shown at 8 h time point (Figure 5A). Data obtained from the time-curve lead us to test the effect of Ectoine concentration on the expression of antioxidant proteins at 4 h time point. Figure 5B shows that all three antioxidant proteins exhibited maximum expression at 1.5 µM of Ectoine concentration. Later, the effects of Ectoine pre-treatment were tested on the expression of Nrf2 and Keap-1 ratio in the UVA-irradiated HaCaT cells. Western data analysis indicated that pre-treatment with 1.5 µM of

Ectoine exhibited an increase in the ratio of Nrf2/Keap-1 in UVA-irradiated HaCaT cells (Figure 5C). We also saw consistent data with the increased expression of NQO-1, HO-1, and γ-GCLC proteins in Ectoine pre-treated HaCaT cells that were irradiated with 3 J/cm^2 UVA (Figure 5D). This data infers that Ectoine pre-treatment plays a protective role in UVA-irradiated HaCaT cells.

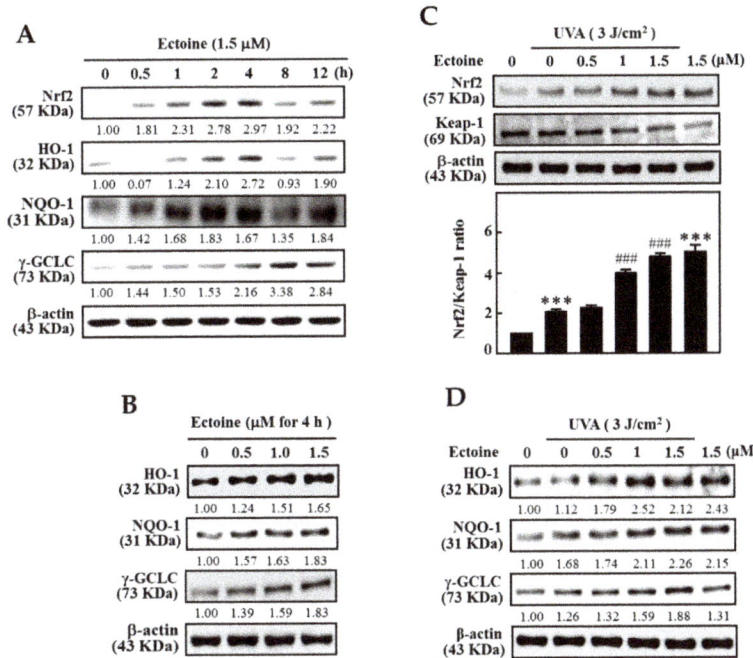

Figure 5. Ectoine mediated differential expressions of antioxidant genes in UVA irradiated HaCaT cells. (**A,B**) Western blot method was used to determine the effects of time (0–12 h) and Ectoine concentrations (0–1.5 µM) on the expressions of Nrf2 and antioxidant genes (HO-1, NQO-1, and γ-GCLC) in HaCaT cells. (**C,D**) Effect of Ectoine pretreatment effect on the Nrf2/Keap-1 ratio of HaCaT cells irradiated with UVA. Cells were pre-treated with Ectoine (0–1.5 µM for 24 h), and then irradiated in the absence or presence of 3 J/cm^2 UVA. The ratio of Nrf2/Keap-1 (**C**) and antioxidant gene (HO-1, NQO-1, and γ-GCLC) expressions (**D**) were determined by Western blotting. Statistical significance was assigned as *** $p < 0.001$ compared to the untreated cells and ### $p < 0.001$ compared to the UVA exposed HaCaT cells.

3.6. Various Signaling Pathways Were Involved in the Activation of Nrf2 in Ectoine Treated HaCaT Cells

We determined the signaling pathways involved in the Ectoine mediated nuclear translocation of Nrf2. HaCaT cells were pre-treated with pharmacological inhibitors of PI3K/AKT, ERK, p38, JNK, PKC, ROS, and CKII signaling pathways, followed by 1.5 µM Ectoine. Western blot data of nuclear Nrf2 showed that p38 MAPK, PI3K/AKT, PKC, and CKII pathways were involved in this mechanism (Figure 6A). From the obtained information, we also determined the effect of Ectoine pre-treatment on the role played by these pathways in the expression of antioxidant proteins. Figure 6B shows that pharmacological inhibition of MAPK, p38, PI3K/AKT, CKII, and PKC pathways down-regulated the expression of NQO-1, HO-1, and γ-GCLC antioxidant proteins in HaCaT cells. Moreover, the time taken for the phosphorylation of AKT, p38, and the expression of PKC and CKII while exposed to Ectoine indicates that, except for the p-AKT, the phosphorylation of p38 and the expressions of PKC and CKII took place at the later time points only (after 30 min) (Figure 6C). In the case of AKT, phosphorylation was observed from the 15 min time point that has reached a peak at 30 min (Figure 6C). These cumulative results suggested that p38, AKT, PKC, and CKII signaling pathways activated the Ectoine mediated nuclear translocation of Nrf2 leading to the expression of antioxidant proteins.

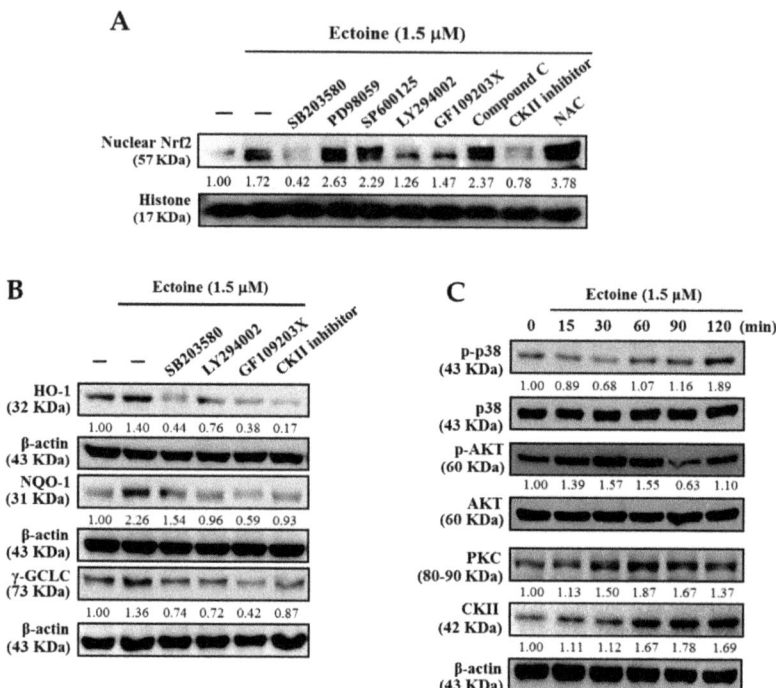

Figure 6. Ectoine mediated the activation of nuclear Nrf2 through p38, AKT, PKC, and CKII signaling pathways in HaCaT cells. (**A**) Cells were pre-treated with p38 inhibitor (SB203580, 20 µM), ERK inhibitor (PD98059, 30 µM), JNK inhibitor (SP600125, 25 µM), PI3K/AKT inhibitor (LY294002, 30 µM), PKC inhibitor (GF109203X, 2.5 µM), AMPK inhibitor (compound C, 10 µM), Casein kinase II inhibitor (CKII, 20 µM), or antioxidant NAC (1 mM) for 30 min, followed by exposure to Ectoine (1.5 µM) for 2 h. Western blot was performed to analyze the nuclear Nrf2 expression against histone proteins as internal control (**B**) HO-1, NQO-1, and γ-GCLC protein levels were evaluated using immunoblot analysis. Cells were pre-treated with inhibitors for p38 (SB203580, 20 µM), PI3K/AKT (LY294002, 30 µM), PKC (GF109203X, 2.5 µM), and CKII (20 µM) for 30 min followed by exposure to Ectoine (1.5 µM) for 4–8 h. (**C**) Ectoine activated the p38, AKT, PKC, and CKII signaling pathways. Cells were pre-treated with Ectoine (1.5 µM) for 0–120 min, and the protein expressions of p-p38, p38, p-AKT, AKT, PKC, and CKII were measured by immunoblot analysis.

3.7. Ectoine Mediated Anti-Melanogenic Effect was Suppressed due to the Knockdown of Nrf2

The role of Nrf2 in Ectoine mediated anti-melanogenesis was determined by silencing the Nrf2 in HaCaT cells. Data from the Western blot indicated that Nrf2 knockdown cells exposed to 1.5 µM Ectoine showed minimum expression of NQO-1, HO-1, and γ-GCLC antioxidant proteins (Figure 7A). Later, we tested the effect of Nrf2 knockdown on the expression of α-MSH levels in UVA irradiated (3 J/cm^2) HaCaT cells. Western blot results indicated that to control the siRNA transfected cells, UVA-irradiation was significant in the upregulation of the expression of α-MSH levels in cells unexposed to Ectoine (Figure 7B). However, 1.5 µM Ectoine has suppressed this effect. For the other case, cells transfected with siNrf2 showed a decrease in the expression of α-MSH levels in both untreated and treated cells (Figure 7B). Similar to α-MSH data, our fluorescence data also indicated that UVA irradiation significantly upregulated the ROS production in Ectoine untreated control siRNA cells (Figure 7C,D). However, this effect was significantly suppressed when the cells exposed to 1.5 µM Ectoine. On the other hand, Nrf2 transfected and UVA-irradiated HaCaT cells showed an approximately 8-fold increase in ROS levels compared to the Nrf2 transfected cells that were not irradiated with UVA but exposed to Ectoine treatment (Figure 7C,D). All this data signifies the Ectoine mediated protective role played by Nrf2 in the minimization of melanin production in UVA-irradiated HaCaT cells.

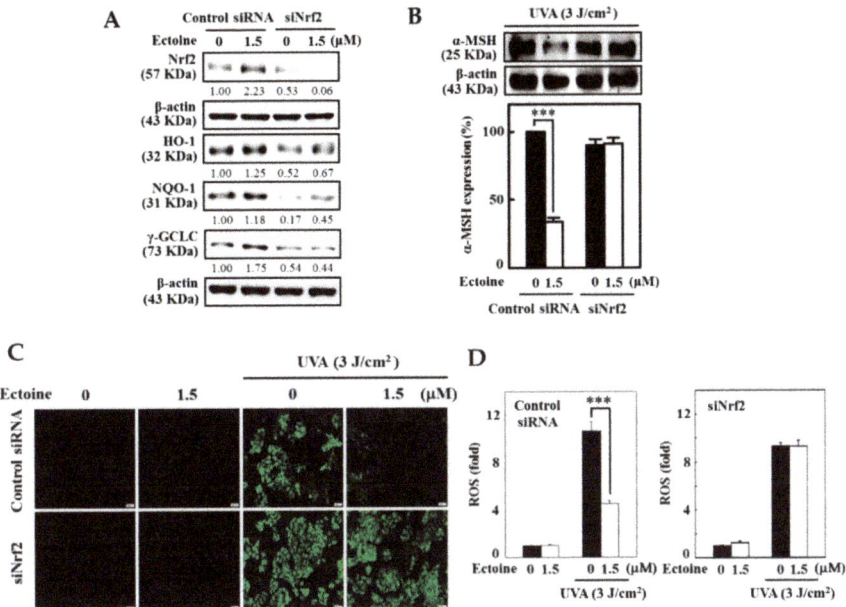

Figure 7. Nrf2 knockdown attenuated the protective effects of Ectoine in UVA-irradiated HaCaT cells. Cells were transfected with siRNA that is specific to either Nrf2 or a non-silencing control. (A) Transfected cells were pre-treated with Ectoine (0 or 1.5 µM for 2 or 12 h) and the expression of Nrf2 (for 2 h), or HO-1, NQO-1, and γ-GCLC (for 12 h) proteins in both control and siNrf2 were measured by Western blot analysis. (B) The effect of Nrf2 knockdown on the expression of α-MSH levels in UVA irradiated HaCaT cells were determined. Transfected cells were pre-treated with or without Ectoine (1.5 µM for 24 h) and then irradiated with 3 J/cm^2 UVA. The Western blot method measured the percentage of α-MSH levels (C,D) The effect of Nrf2 knockdown on the UVA radiation-induced ROS levels in transfected cells were measured by DCF fluorescence microscopy. Statistical significance was assigned as *** $p < 0.001$ compared to the untreated cells.

4. Discussion

Various skin-whitening agents are in use in the cosmetic industry. Many of these agents are from the chemical origin and are suffering from the limitations of causing various side effects including the cancers [24–26]. Therefore, the identification of safe and natural skin-whitening agents represent the need of the hour. Ectoine (Figure 1A) has been known to be used as an active ingredient in face creams and other cosmetic agents. This acts as a skin moisturizing agent and also considered to delay the premature skin-aging as well [27]. Almost all known skin-whitening agents target the downregulation of tyrosinase enzyme activity in UV-irradiated cells that decreases the melanogenesis in skin cells. Yao et al. demonstrated the whitening properties of biosynthesized Ectoine and suggested that it is a putative whitening agent. In their study, they tested the high concentration (500 µM) of Ectoine for its whitening effect on mouse melanoma (B16F0) and human melanoma (A2058) cell lines and concluded that Ectoine is a safe and potential agent for the cosmetic and clinical application [20]. However, in this study, we further tested the beneficial effects of low concentrations of Ectoine (0.5–1.5 μM) on UVA-irradiated HaCaT cells and the underlying molecular mechanisms were deciphered. In our study, it was shown that Ectoine, through the Nrf2/ARE pathway, has not only induced the expression of antioxidant gene expression but also downregulated the α-MSH levels in UVA-irradiated HaCaT cells via the suppression of POMC. A decrease in the α-MSH levels was correlated with downregulation of tyrosinase enzyme activity leading to the decrease in the melanin production. From our knowledge, this is first the report that was evidenced by the mechanism elicited by Ectoine in UVA-irradiated HaCaT cells. This study delineated the molecular mechanisms exhibited by Ectoine in HaCaT cells as the cellular model system.

We first determined the sub-lethal concentrations of Ectoine as well as the effect of UVA radiation on the viability of HaCaT cells. Our MTT data indicated that low concentrations of Ectoine (0.5–1.5 μM) had no significant effect on the viability of HaCaT cells (Figure 1B). Ectoine pre-treatment increased the viability of 3 J/cm^2 UVA-irradiated HaCaT cells (Figure 1B). Based on these observations, we continued our further experiments using 1.5 μM of Ectoine pre-treatment and UVA irradiation at 3 J/cm^2 dosage.

UVA irradiation-induced ROS production in skin keratinocytes is a well-known fact [28]. Therefore, we also tested for any beneficial effects from Ectoine pre-treatment in the UVA-radiation induced ROS production in HaCaT cells. Our DCF-fluorescence intensity data indicated that pre-treatment with 1.5 μM of Ectoine significantly downregulated the UVA-radiation induced ROS production in keratinocytes. It was also observable that 1.5 μM of Ectoine could cause a basal level increase in the ROS levels in HaCaT cells that were shown to be statistically significant (Figure 1D,E).

Rousseau et al. reported that POMC, is secreted by human epidermal keratinocytes and melanocytes and has stimulated the melanogenesis [29]. By keeping this in view, we too tested the effect of UVA irradiation and Ectoine pre-treatments on the melanogenesis associated proteins in HaCaT cells. Our Western blot data indicated the dose-dependent downregulation of the expression of α-MSH and POMC proteins in UVA-irradiated HaCaT cells was caused by the pretreatment by Ectoine. Conversely, Ectoine pre-treatment has a differential effect on the expression pattern of melanogenesis associated proteins. Notably, almost all tested proteins (Tyrosinase, TRP-1, TRP-2, c-AMP protein kinase, CREB, and MITF) showed decreased expressions with increasing concentrations of Ectoine pre-treatment in UVA-irradiated HaCaT cells (Figure 2A,B). This data signifies the fact that Ectoine possesses anti-melanogenic properties in UVA-irradiated HaCaT cells.

The anti-melanogenic efficacy of Ectoine was further tested in B16F10 cells, a well-known melanoma cell line used in melanogenesis studies [30]. One of the notable observations in our study was that, in contrast to the HaCaT cells, high concentrations of Ectoine (100–400 μM) were necessary to suppress the melanin synthesis in α-MSH-stimulated B16F10 cells (Figure 3B). Our Western blot data indicated that Ectoine dose-dependently downregulated the expression of tyrosinase and p-CREB proteins in α-MSH-stimulated B16F10 cells, leading to the aforesaid effect (Figure 3C). Therefore, we also tested if these high concentrations of Ectoine could affect the viability of B16F10 cells. Our MTT results indicated that high concentrations of Ectoine (100–400 μM) had no effect on the viability of B16F10 cells (Figure 3A). These results signify that keratinocytes play a key role in Ectoine mediated anti-melanogenesis and depigmenting effects.

The role of transcription factor Nrf2 in skin cells metabolism was well documented [31]. Therefore, we further tested the mechanisms played by Nrf2/Keap-1 pathway in Ectoine mediated effects in keratinocytes. Figure 4A shows that Ectoine dose-dependently and significantly increased the Nrf2/Keap-1 ratio with a maximum effect was observed at 1.5 μM Ectoine concentration. It was also observed that 1.5 μM Ectoine favored the nuclear translocation of Nrf2 protein with the maximum expression of Nrf2 from the nuclear protein fraction observed at the 2 h time point (Figure 4B). Data obtained from the immunofluorescence staining of HaCaT cells has also supported this effect (Figure 4D).

In human melanocytes and keratinocytes, Marrot et al. and others have explained the importance of Nrf2 defensive pathway in photo-oxidative stress responses [32]. We too studied the effect of Ectoine mediated antioxidant protein expression in HaCaT cells. Our time curve data indicated that Ectoine mediated expression of all three anti-oxidant proteins (HO-1, NQO-1, γ-GCLC), and Nrf2 were shown to express in a biphasic manner with the increasing time (0.5–12 h) with an observable effect was noted at 4 h time point (Figure 5A). From this, a concentration curve that measures the effect of Ectoine concentration on antioxidant protein expression was also determined at 4 h time point. Figure 5B shows that in comparison to the untreated cells, Ectoine treatment has dose-dependently increased the expression of HO-1, NQO-1, γ-GCLC proteins. We also measured how Ectoine concentration exhibited protective effects in HaCaT cells that were exposed to UVA radiation. Western blot data showed that Ectoine dose-dependently increased the expression of anti-oxidant proteins with a dramatic upregulation in the Nrf2/Keap-1 ratio as well (Figure 5C,D). These results indicated that Ectoine pretreatment (1.5 µM, 4 h) has the potential effect to induce antioxidant protein expression in HaCaT cells that could counteract the deleterious effects posed by UVA exposure.

Later, we determined the signaling pathways that mediated the activation of nuclear translocation of Nrf2 as well as the expression of anti-oxidant proteins. Our pharmacological inhibitor data revealed that p38, PI3/AKT, PKC, and CKII pathways were involved in the Ectoine mediated activation of nuclear NRf2. This data was consistent with the antioxidant expression data as well which showed that pharmacological inhibition of these four pathways down-regulated the expression of anti-oxidant proteins (HO-1, NQO-1, γ-GCLC). Except for the AKT activation (p-AKT), all three pathways (p38, PKC, and CKII) were activated at longer time points (after 30 min). The AKT pathway was demonstrated to be the first pathway activated (within 15 min) after exposure to Ectoine (Figure 6A–C).

Nrf2 knock-down technique has helped us to further demonstrate and confirm the key role played by Nrf2 in Ectoine mediated antioxidant and anti-melanogenic effects in HaCaT cells. Data showed that compared to the control siRNA cells, Nrf2 knockdown cells exposed to 1.5 µM Ectoine exhibited significant downregulation in the expression of HO-1, NQO-1, γ-GCLC antioxidant proteins (Figure 7A). On the other hand, these knockdown cells pre-treated with Ectoine and exposed to the UVA radiation did not affect the α-MSH expression, which confirmed that Nrf2 plays a key role in α-MSH expression in HaCaT cells (Figure 7B). In addition to the α-MSH expression, our DCF fluorescence data also revealed that Nrf2 knockdown is involved in the regulation of intracellular ROS production in UVA irradiated HaCaT cells that were pre-treated with 1.5 µM Ectoine (Figure 7C,D).

5. Conclusions

From the above data, we concluded that low concentrations of Ectoine (0.5–1.5 µM) could downregulate α-MSH and melanin production via the suppression of POMC and tyrosinase pathway in UVA irradiated HaCaT cells, indicating its anti-melanogenesis efficacy. Additionally, Ectoine was also involved in the suppression of intracellular ROS production in HaCaT cells. Unlike HaCaT cells, high concentrations of Ectoine (50–400 µM) were able to show the similar effect in B16F10 melanoma cells that have signified the fact that keratinocytes could play a key role in the Ectoine mediated anti-melanogenesis and skin-whitening effects in skin cells. Most importantly, Ectoine mediated beneficial effects via the activation of the Nrf2 pathway, that induces the expression of antioxidant proteins HO-1, NQO-1, and γ-GCLC. AKT was shown to be the first signaling pathway that initiates the activation of Nrf2 followed by the other pathways (p38, PKC, and CKII). Finally, silencing of Nrf2 directly provided the evidence that Nrf2 plays a key role in the regulation of intracellular ROS as well as the α-MSH production. We concluded that the main whitening mechanism of Ectoine should be reasoned by the inhibition of ROS-p53/POMC-α-MSH pathway in UVA-irradiated HaCaT cells. Therefore, Ectoine or its derivatives could be an active ingredient in the moisturizers and lotions that are used as potential and natural-based skin whitening agents in the cosmetic industry.

Author Contributions: Conceptualization—Y.-C.H. and H.-L.Y.; Methodology—X.-Z.C., Y.V.G., H.-R.Y. and J.-Y.C.; investigation—X.-Z.C., Y.V.G., H.-R.Y. and J.-Y.C.; data curation—X.-Z.C., Y.V.G., H.-R.Y. and J.-Y.C.;

writing—original draft preparation—Y.-C.H. and Y.V.G.; writing—review and editing—Y.-C.H. and Y.V.G.; supervision—Y.-C.H. and H.-L.Y.; funding acquisition—Y.-C.H. and H.-L.Y. All authors have read and agreed to the published version of the manuscript.

Funding: This study was supported by the Ministry of Science and Technology, Asia University, and China Medical University, Taiwan (grants MOST-106-2320-B-039-054-MY3 and MOST-107-2320-B-039-013-MY3, CMU 107-ASIA-15, and CMU106-ASIA-19. This work was financially supported by the "Chinese Medicine Research Center, China Medical University" from The Featured Areas Research Center Program within the framework of the Higher Education Sprout Project by the Ministry of Education (MOE) in Taiwan (CMRC-CHM-8).

Conflicts of Interest: The authors declare no conflict of interest.

References

1. D'Mello, S.A.; Finlay, G.J.; Baguley, B.C.; Askarian-Amiri, M.E. Signaling Pathways in Melanogenesis. *Int. J. Mol. Sci.* **2016**, *17*, 1144. [CrossRef]
2. del Giudice, P.; Yves, P. The widespread use of skin lightening creams in Senegal: A persistent public health problem in West Africa. *Int. J. Dermatol.* **2002**, *41*, 69–72. [CrossRef] [PubMed]
3. Dey, V.K. Misuse of topical corticosteroids: A clinical study of adverse effects. *Indian Dermatol. Online J.* **2014**, *5*, 436–440. [CrossRef] [PubMed]
4. Burnett, C.L.; Bergfeld, W.F.; Belsito, D.V.; Hill, R.A.; Klaassen, C.D.; Liebler, D.C.; Marks, J.G.; Shank, R.C.; Slaga, T.J.; Snyder, P.W.; et al. Final Report of the Safety Assessment of Kojic Acid as Used in Cosmetics. *Int. J. Toxicol.* **2010**, *29*, 244s–273s. [CrossRef]
5. Mata, T.L.; Sanchez, J.P.; Oyanguren, J.D. Allergic contact dermatitis due to Kojic acid. *Dermatitis* **2005**, *16*, 89. [CrossRef]
6. Draelos, Z.D. Skin lightening preparations and the hydroquinone controversy. *Dermatol. Ther.* **2007**, *20*, 308–313. [CrossRef]
7. Lentzen, G.; Schwarz, T. Extremolytes: Natural compounds from extremophiles for versatile applications. *Appl. Microbiol. Biotechnol.* **2006**, *72*, 623–634. [CrossRef]
8. Stepniewska, Z.; Goraj, W.; Kuzniar, A.; Pytlak, A.; Ciepielski, J.; Fraczek, P. Biosynthesis of Ectoine by the Methanotrophic Bacterial Consortium Isolated from Bogdanka Coalmine (Poland). *Appl. Biochem. Microbiol.* **2014**, *50*, 594–600. [CrossRef]
9. Peters, P.; Galinski, E.A.; Truper, H.G. The Biosynthesis of Ectoine. *Fems Microbiol. Lett.* **1990**, *71*, 157–162. [CrossRef]
10. Harishchandra, R.K.; Wulff, S.; Lentzen, G.; Neuhaus, T.; Galla, H.J. The effect of compatible solute ectoines on the structural organization of lipid monolayer and bilayer membranes. *Biophys. Chem.* **2010**, *150*, 37–46. [CrossRef]
11. Meyer, S.; Schroter, M.A.; Hahn, M.B.; Solomun, T.; Sturm, H.; Kunte, H.J. Ectoine can enhance structural changes in DNA in vitro. *Sci. Rep.* **2017**, *7*, 7170. [CrossRef] [PubMed]
12. Sydlik, U.; Peuschel, H.; Paunel-Gorgulu, A.; Keymel, S.; Kramer, U.; Weissenberg, A.; Kroker, M.; Seghrouchni, S.; Heiss, C.; Windolf, J.; et al. Recovery of neutrophil apoptosis by ectoine: A new strategy against lung inflammation. *Eur. Respir. J.* **2013**, *41*, 433–442. [CrossRef] [PubMed]
13. Bünger, J.; Driller, H.J.; Martin, R. Use of Ectoine or Ectoine Derivatives in Cosmetic Formulations. U.S. Patent 6,602,514, 5 August 2003.
14. Buenger, J.; Driller, H. Ectoin: An effective natural substance to prevent UVA-induced premature photoaging. *Skin Pharmacol. Physiol.* **2004**, *17*, 232–237. [CrossRef] [PubMed]
15. Marini, A.; Reinelt, K.; Krutmann, J.; Bilstein, A. Ectoine-containing cream in the treatment of mild to moderate atopic dermatitis: A randomised, comparator-controlled, intra-individual double-blind, multi-center trial. *Skin Pharmacol. Physiol.* **2014**, *27*, 57–65. [CrossRef]
16. Kanapathipillai, M.; Lentzen, G.; Sierks, M.; Park, C.B. Ectoine and hydroxyectoine inhibit aggregation and neurotoxicity of Alzheimer's beta-amyloid. *FEBS Lett.* **2005**, *579*, 4775–4780. [CrossRef]
17. Lapidot, A.; Benasher, E.; Eisenstein, M. Tetrahydropyrimidine Derivatives Inhibit Binding of a Tat-Like, Arginine-Containing Peptide, to Hiv Tar Rna in-Vitro. *FEBS Lett.* **1995**, *367*, 33–38. [CrossRef]

18. Bilstein, A.; Overhagen, S.; Géczi, L.; Baráth, Z.; Mösges, R. Effectiveness, Tolerability, and Safety of Ectoine-Containing Mouthwash Versus Those of a Calcium Phosphate Mouthwash for the Treatment of Chemotherapy-Induced Oral Mucositis: A Prospective, Active-Controlled, Non-interventional Study. *Oncol. Ther.* **2018**, *6*, 59–72.
19. Unfried, K.; Krämer, U.; Sydlik, U.; Autengruber, A.; Bilstein, A.; Stolz, S.; Marini, A.; Schikowski, T.; Keymel, S.; Krutmann, J. Reduction of chronic lung inflammation by inhalation of the compatible solute ectoine: A population-based intervention study with elderly individuals. *Pneumologie* **2017**, *71*, S1–S125. [CrossRef]
20. Yao, C.L.; Lin, Y.M.; Mohamed, M.S.; Chen, J.H. Inhibitory effect of ectoine on melanogenesis in B16-F0 and A2058 melanoma cell lines. *Biochem. Eng. J.* **2013**, *78*, 163–169. [CrossRef]
21. Hseu, Y.C.; Ho, Y.G.; Mathew, D.C.; Yen, H.R.; Chen, X.Z.; Yang, H.L. The in vitro and in vivo depigmenting activity of Coenzyme Q10 through the down-regulation of alpha-MSH signaling pathways and induction of Nrf2/ARE-mediated antioxidant genes in UVA-irradiated skin keratinocytes. *Biochem. Pharmacol.* **2019**, *164*, 299–310. [CrossRef]
22. Yang, H.L.; Lin, S.W.; Lee, C.C.; Lin, K.Y.; Liao, C.H.; Yang, T.Y.; Wang, H.M.; Huang, H.C.; Wu, C.R.; Hseu, Y.C. Induction of Nrf2-mediated genes by Antrodia salmonea inhibits ROS generation and inflammatory effects in lipopolysaccharide-stimulated RAW264.7 macrophages. *Food Funct.* **2015**, *6*, 230–241. [CrossRef] [PubMed]
23. Cawley, N.X.; Li, Z.; Loh, Y.P. 60 YEARS OF POMC: Biosynthesis, trafficking, and secretion of pro-opiomelanocortin-derived peptides. *J. Mol. Endocrinol.* **2016**, *56*, T77–T97. [CrossRef] [PubMed]
24. McGregor, D. Hydroquinone: An evaluation of the human risks from its carcinogenic and mutagenic properties. *Crit. Rev. Toxicol.* **2007**, *37*, 887–914. [CrossRef]
25. Kolbe, L.; Kligman, A.M.; Schreiner, V.; Stoudemayer, T. Corticosteroid-induced atrophy and barrier impairment measured by non-invasive methods in human skin. *Skin Res. Technol.* **2002**, *7*, 73–77. [CrossRef]
26. Desmedt, B.; Courselle, P.; De Beer, J.O.; Rogiers, V.; Grosber, M.; Deconinck, E.; De Paepe, K. Overview of skin whitening agents with an insight into the illegal cosmetic market in Europe. *J. Eur. Acad. Dermatol.* **2016**, *30*, 943–950. [CrossRef] [PubMed]
27. Graf, R.; Anzali, S.; Buenger, J.; Pfluecker, F.; Driller, H. The multifunctional role of ectoine as a natural cell protectant. *Clin. Dermatol.* **2008**, *26*, 326–333. [CrossRef] [PubMed]
28. Henri, P.; Beaumel, S.; Guezennec, A.; Poumes, C.; Stoebner, P.E.; Stasia, M.J.; Guesnet, J.; Martinez, J.; Meunier, L. MC1R expression in HaCaT keratinocytes inhibits UVA-induced ROS production via NADPH oxidase- and cAMP-dependent mechanisms. *J. Cell Physiol.* **2012**, *227*, 2578–2585. [CrossRef] [PubMed]
29. Rousseau, K.; Kauser, S.; Pritchard, L.E.; Warhurst, A.; Oliver, R.L.; Slominski, A.; Wei, E.T.; Thody, A.J.; Tobin, D.J.; White, A. Proopiomelanocortin (POMC), the ACTH/melanocortin precursor, is secreted by human epidermal keratinocytes and melanocytes and stimulates melanogenesis. *FASEB J.* **2007**, *21*, 1844–1856. [CrossRef]
30. Wu, C.Y.; Pang, J.H.; Huang, S.T. Inhibition of melanogenesis in murine B16/F10 melanoma cells by Ligusticum sinensis Oliv. *Am. J. Chin. Med.* **2006**, *34*, 523–533. [CrossRef]
31. Gegotek, A.; Skrzydlewska, E. The role of transcription factor Nrf2 in skin cells metabolism. *Arch. Dermatol. Res.* **2015**, *307*, 385–396. [CrossRef]
32. Marrot, L.; Jones, C.; Perez, P.; Meunier, J.R. The significance of Nrf2 pathway in (photo)-oxidative stress response in melanocytes and keratinocytes of the human epidermis. *Pigment Cell Melanoma Res.* **2008**, *21*, 79–88. [CrossRef] [PubMed]

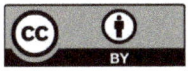

© 2020 by the authors. Licensee MDPI, Basel, Switzerland. This article is an open access article distributed under the terms and conditions of the Creative Commons Attribution (CC BY) license (http://creativecommons.org/licenses/by/4.0/).

MDPI
St. Alban-Anlage 66
4052 Basel
Switzerland
Tel. +41 61 683 77 34
Fax +41 61 302 89 18
www.mdpi.com

Antioxidants Editorial Office
E-mail: antioxidants@mdpi.com
www.mdpi.com/journal/antioxidants

www.ingramcontent.com/pod-product-compliance
Lightning Source LLC
LaVergne TN
LVHW070632100526
838202LV00012B/786